Y0-CAF-499

Men's Health

TOTAL-BODY

HEALTH & FITNESS GUIDE 2014

Men'sHealth®
TOTAL-BODY
HEALTH & FITNESS GUIDE 2014

RODALE.

The information in this book is meant to supplement, not replace, proper exercise training. All forms of exercise pose some inherent risks. The editors and publisher advise readers to take full responsibility for their safety and know their limits. Before practicing the exercises in this book, be sure that your equipment is well maintained, and do not take risks beyond your level of experience, aptitude, training, and fitness. The exercise and dietary programs in this book are not intended as a substitute for any exercise routine or dietary regimen that may have been prescribed by your doctor. As with all exercise and dietary programs, you should get your doctor's approval before beginning. Mention of specific companies, organizations, or authorities in this book does not imply endorsement by the author or publisher, nor does mention of specific companies, organizations, or authorities imply that they endorse this book, its author, or the publisher.

Internet addresses and telephone numbers given in this book were accurate at the time it went to press.

© 2014 by Rodale Inc.

All rights reserved. No part of this publication may be reproduced or transmitted in any form or by any means, electronic or mechanical, including photocopying, recording, or any other information storage and retrieval system, without the written permission of the publisher.

Men's Health is a registered trademark of Rodale Inc.

Rodale books may be purchased for business or promotional use or for special sales. For information, please write to: Special Markets Department, Rodale, Inc., 733 Third Avenue, New York, NY 10017

Printed in the United States of America
Rodale Inc. makes every effort to use acid-free ∞, recycled paper ♲.

Book design by Elizabeth Neal

Library of Congress Cataloging-in-Publication Data is on file with the publisher

ISBN: 978–1–62336–223–2

2 4 6 8 10 9 7 5 3 1 hardcover

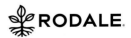

We inspire and enable people to improve their lives and the world around them.
rodalebooks.com

Contents

PART 3: Muscle Up Fast

ESSENTIAL READING

PART 4: Look Better Instantly

ESSENTIAL READING

PART 5: Work Smarter, Grow Wealthier

ESSENTIAL READING

PART 6: Live Longer, Live Better

PART 7: Improve Your Game

Introduction

How would you like to do everything better? That's what you'll learn in this book. With the tips in *Men's Health Total-Body Health & Fitness Guide 2014,* you can take your life to the next level. You'll lose weight, eat better, muscle up, look great, build wealth, stay healthy, and up your game on and off the field.

In Part I, you'll take the first step and Lose Your Gut. Discover how to reprogram your metabolism, determine if you have a food addiction, and learn the truth, for once and for all, about your workout and its effect on your waist.

Life is short; eat better with the strategies and recipes in Part 2. Here you'll find "The Supermarket Survival Guide" and our guide to "Alternative Fuels." Prepare some of *Men's Health*'s best recipes in "Takeout That Delivers" and "Great Bowls of Fire."

Once you've begun to fuel your body properly, you'll be ready to Muscle Up Fast in Part 3. Save yourself the cost of a gym membership with "Power Tools for Your Home Gym." Test out some of the most effective *Men's Health* workouts ever, and transform your body.

You'll Look Better Instantly after reading Part 4. You'll know how to get "The Good Life, Guaranteed." Fake it till you make it with tips from "The Life-Altering Power of Faking It." And use our simple style strategies to master combining timeless essentials with timely trends.

In Part 5, you'll learn from the most savvy financial experts how to Work Smarter, Grow Wealthier. Kick off this section with a financial fresh start, then break free from "The Money Habits That Hold You Back." Finally, get insider advice on how to weather troubled economic times with our "Financial Crisis Survival Plan."

Part 6 will help you to Live Longer, Live Better. Discover how to have your healthiest year ever. Plus you'll learn how you can prevent allergies, cancer—even heart disease.

Last, in Part 7, you can Improve Your Game. Heed these tips to run faster, train harder, and prepare yourself for sidelining injuries. And learn how to do everything better, from mixing a killer Bloody Mary to quashing your opponents at foosball.

We hope that this book will inspire you to change your body—and to change your life. With the simple tips and life-changing strategies in this book, you'll add more years to your life, and more life to your years. Here's to your *better* health!

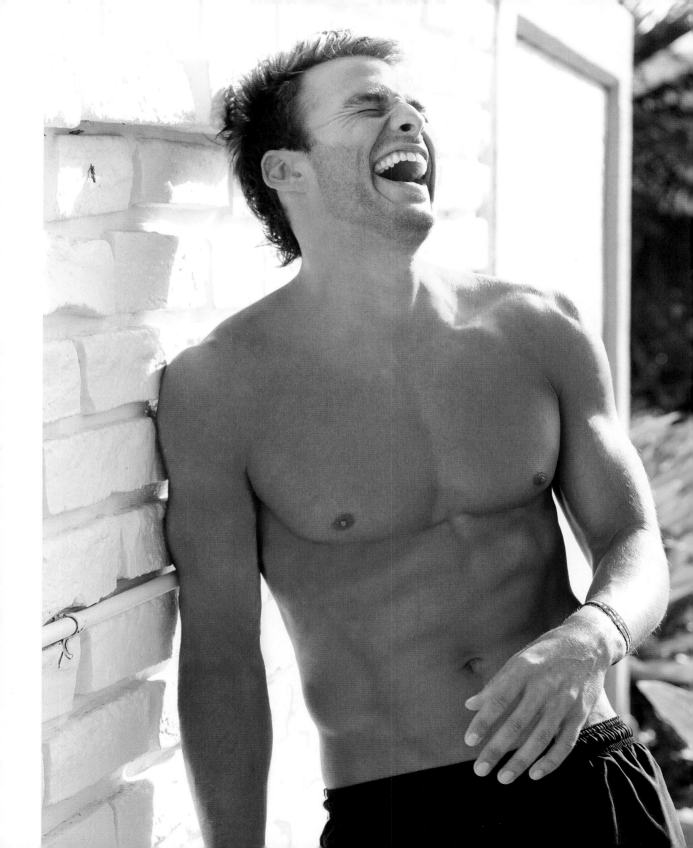

Lose Your Gut

Men'sHealth

Your Metabolism— Reprogrammed

Our modern world conspires to make us fat and keep us fat. Here are the weapons that can help you fight back.

Back in the early 1960s, the average American man in his 30s weighed 170 pounds. Today, a typical guy in his 30s now weighs 196 pounds. A lot of us know from sorry experience that the classic weight-reduction formula—exercise more, eat less—works in the short term, but the fat typically comes back. Sometimes a double chin redoubles, just to show you who's in charge.

The human metabolism is a complex system that evolved to keep our weight stable in times of both abundance and famine. How did it devolve into a coin toss where the choices are "heads, you gain weight" and "tails, you gain even more"?

For many, the problem is a condition called metabolic inflexibility, a bit of complicated science that points the way toward simple diet, exercise, and lifestyle modifications—modifications that can help you become lean and stay lean. But before we dive into the deep end of weight-loss research, let's take a quick detour and look at the reasons the single-generation rise in obesity shouldn't have happened. We'll then see how it did happen, and finally we'll reach the important part: how you can seize your own metabolic destiny and steer it toward lean.

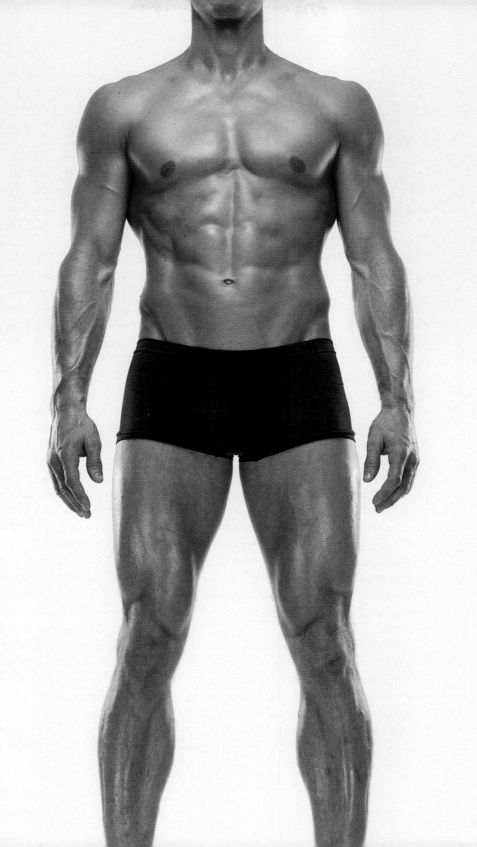

Why We Can't Eat Just One Anymore

From the early 1900s—when obesity was so uncommon that people lined up to gawk at the "fat lady" in circus sideshows—until the 1980s, our per-capita food supply stayed more or less the same.

We could've eaten more food back then. We just didn't crave it as we do now. Consider everything that happens when you eat a normal meal.

The food you eat becomes progressively less appetizing. No matter how good the first few bites of that steak might be, by the end you're just going through the motions.

Your stomach expands, sending chemical messages to your brain, asking it to stop eating.

Your metabolism cranks up as your body works to move the food through your digestive system, burning off 10 percent of the calories you just ate.

Over the following hours and even days, your body monitors your energy balance—the amount of calories coming in and going out. Eat more than you need and you'll compensate with a faster metabolism—or by burning more calories through physical activity, or by producing more hormones like leptin, which lowers your appetite.

These mechanisms also work in reverse. Should you eat less than you need in order to maintain your current weight, your metabolism slows down to preserve energy, and hunger hormones like ghrelin tick up to increase your appetite.

The goal of this complex system is to hit a balance, at which point it's hard to gain or lose weight. Only powerful stimuli can override this system, to literally alter your metabolism so it can't respond the way it should.

Enter your main adversary: the modern food industry, which is to nutrition what lobbying is to Congress—a sure way to twist a good system into one that runs counter to everybody's best interests.

When Lay's potato chips introduced the famous slogan "Bet you can't eat just one" in the early 1960s, the company knew what it was talking about. Its food scientists were in the process of snipping the brake lines on our appetites, and as a society we began running stop signs that had existed for centuries. The food scientists found ways to combine sugar, salt, and fat so that "enough" was never actually enough. If we have a little, we want a lot. Our metabolism wasn't prepared to counteract the hedonic reward of these new foods or the quantities now available. The food manufacturers ramped up food energy production to 3,900 daily calories per person, enough to put most of us at the "who shrunk my seat belt?" end of the body-weight range.

"Food stimulates many parts of the brain, including regions associated with reward," says Stephan Guyenet, Ph.D., a postdoctoral research fellow at the University of Washington and the author of a terrific blog about metabolism and weight control, at wholehealthsource.org. "By stimulating those reward pathways directly, you can have a profound impact on food preference and body fat. Manufacturers are trying to maximize the reward." The upshot, he says: "We're awash in food

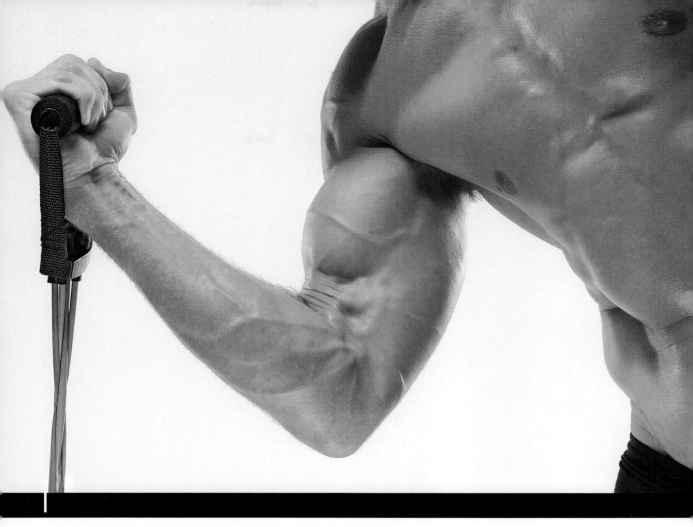

IS YOUR FAT BURNER ON LOW?

The sure way to find out is to measure your respiratory quotient, or RQ—the ratio of carbon dioxide exhaled to oxygen inhaled. That predicts how much fat or carbohydrate you burn at rest or during exercise. Leaner people typically have lower RQs; fatter people almost always have higher RQs.

You can schedule an RQ test, but a basic blood test also provides clues. If your fasting blood sugar is unusually high—100 to 125 milligrams per deciliter of blood—you almost certainly have a problem with insulin. Another sign is a high ratio of triglycerides to HDL cholesterol. One way insulin eliminates excess glucose is by starting a process to transform it into triglycerides. Most of these triglycerides end up in fat cells, but your circulating levels still remain high. A parallel effect is low levels of HDL, the "good" cholesterol. The danger zone is a 3.5-to-1 ratio of triglycer-

ides to HDL, but regardless of the ratio, you should worry about a triglyceride count higher than 150 milligrams per deciliter (mg/dL) or an HDL below 40 mg/dL.

Where you carry the fat also matters. "Belly fat correlates pretty well with insulin resistance," says Stephan Guyenet, Ph.D. If you can rest your hands on your belly while standing, it's too big.

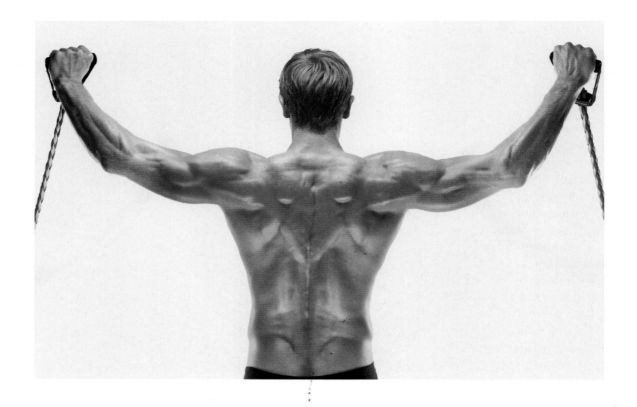

that's easily available, energy dense, highly palatable, and highly rewarding. Commercial food overstimulates those connections in the brain."

So Now Glucose Is Getting Us Down, Too

As we eat massive volumes of overstimulating food—the whole tube of Pringles, washed down with an entire Big Gulp—our digestive processes convert it all into massive amounts of blood sugar. That's where the hormone insulin comes in. It's a kind of bodily butler in charge of showing glucose to safe havens in the body. In our society, and in our bodies, it's one overworked butler.

"Your body is hardwired to survive," says Mike T. Nelson, C.S.C.S., a Ph.D. candidate at the University of Minnesota who has studied this problem for the past 6 years. "If your glucose is too high, it's toxic. Your body will do everything possible to get it out of there." The hormone insulin is your main glucose-disposal tool. The longer it stays elevated, the less effective it becomes; and the less effective it becomes, the longer it stays elevated. Insulin's purpose is to eliminate glucose in the blood by storing it in the body. As a consequence, insulin inhibits our ability to burn fat. Chronically elevated insulin means your body is always using less fat for energy than it otherwise would, so fat gathers where you want it least.

Human bodies are designed to run on a mix of fuels, using fat predominantly at rest or during low-intensity exercise. You gradually shift to a higher dependence on carbohydrates as exercise becomes more difficult. If you're metabolically flexible, you can shift easily from one fuel source to the other, tapping into your body's abundant fat deposits while saving those limited carbohydrates for when they're really needed. Someone with chronically elevated insulin becomes inflexible, burning too many carbs all the time and leaving fat stores untouched. That's a metabolic disaster for a body that has more fat than it could ever use—a body that, under normal circumstances, should be tapping fat like a pool of black gold under the tundra.

"Systems are trying as hard as they can to cooperate with each other," Nelson says. "But they can't."

Why Most Men Can't Jog Their Way to the Promised Land

We all grow hungry when our carbohydrate supplies run down. This is one of our most important survival mechanisms, due to the fact that our brains normally run on pure glucose. We can make glucose from fat, but that's not the easiest way to get it. Our bodies prefer the real thing. So we become ravenously hungry when our glucose supplies suddenly drop. The problem

> Food scientists combine sugar, salt, and fat so that "enough" is never actually enough.

for the metabolically inflexible man is that his supplies are always running low, and his body is always looking for the next food fix. A workout can exacerbate the problem by draining more carbs than the body wants to give up.

So the standard reaction to too much belly—"I have to start jogging"—could actually hurt in two ways. A man who's using the wrong fuel won't get much out of it because of his limited endurance. He could also end up hungrier afterward, as his body panics over depleted glycogen stores.

"You can't burn excess fat without mobilizing it from a fat cell," says Mike Ormsbee, Ph.D., a professor of exercise physiology and sports nutrition at Florida State University. "You have to move it from the fat cells to the blood so you can eventually use it for energy elsewhere."

Strength training offers a workaround for metabolic inflexibility. "Brief, intense activity seems to dump a lot of fat into the bloodstream," says Christopher Scott, Ph.D., who studies strength training and metabolism at the University of Southern Maine. "I think it's to fuel recovery."

When you do a bout of cardio, the goal is to reach one level of intensity that you can maintain for a long time. And there's only one recovery period, during which

Metabolism evolved to keep our weight steady.

you use much less energy than you did while exercising. But when you're recovering from a set of bench presses or squats, you burn more calories: "If you do 12 sets, that's 12 recovery periods," Scott says. That's in addition to the long postworkout recovery period, so your body has a lot of time to be burning fat, as opposed to relatively short periods of using carbohydrates for fuel.

Because strength training is an anaerobic activity—meaning your body burns mostly carbohydrate while you lift—you're burning mostly fat during the recovery period. Moreover, when you leave the weight room, you're burning many more calories than you were before the workout, and you're burning them for hours.

Another argument for strength training—or, really, for any type of exercise in which you alternate hard work with an easier pace—is that you train your body to shift back and forth between fuel sources, making your metabolism more flexible.

We Now Return to Your Regularly Scheduled Metabolism

As important as exercise is—and we'll deal with that later—it runs a distant second to the first change you need to make.

Clean Up Your Diet

"If we came up with a list of 10 things that affect weight loss, 1 through 7 would involve diet and behavior," Scott says. "Then 8, 9, and 10 would cover exercise."

Research shows that just about any mainstream diet regimen can work as long as you stick to it. A diet won't work for you unless it meets two seemingly contradictory standards: It has to be different from what you're doing now, which is to say restricts the stuff you currently eat too much of. And it has to be something you can live with for the foreseeable future, meaning it has to be based on foods you like and to which you have easy access.

That's where behavior becomes the key to success.

"The amount of food you consume is not just the result of conscious processes," Guyenet says. Exposing yourself to highly palatable, superstimulating foods will derail any diet. Nobody has that much willpower.

The following three key actions help you build self-control into your diet.

- Prepare and eat most of your meals at home, with minimal added salt and minimal added sugar.

- Prepare foods so they're as close as possible to their natural state: grilled or baked meat, poultry, and fish; eggs however you like them; raw or steamed vegetables; fruit; beans, nuts, or seeds. For simple recipes to make real food taste better, check out MensHealth.com/guy-gourmet.

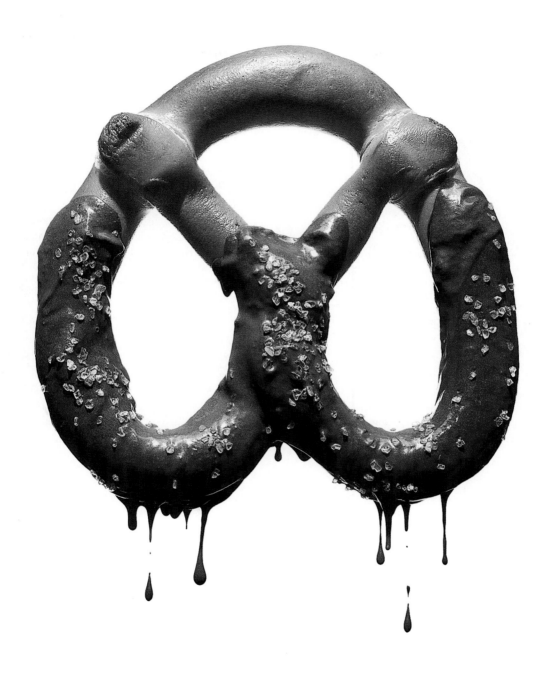

FLEX PLAN

The following workout, based on research from Florida State University, optimizes the way your body uses fuel and burns fat. The goal: more muscular fitness and better glucose storage.

Do 3 sets of each exercise, alternating between the A and B exercise of each pair until you've finished all sets of both exercises. Then move on to the next pair. Choose weights or exercise variations you can do 10 times. Do 8 reps for the first 2 sets, and then do as many reps as you can for the third set. Catch your breath after each set, but stay on your feet the entire workout.

1A: Goblet squat with a bench

Grab a heavy dumbbell or kettlebell and hold it against your chest with both hands. Stand with your back to a bench or a step that's about 18 inches high. Push your hips back and lower your butt to the bench. Touch it lightly and then return to standing.

1B: Standing lat pulldown

Attach a long bar to the high pulley of a cable machine. Grab it with your hands a bit beyond shoulder width, and step back as you face the cable machine, keeping your arms straight and some tension in the cable. This is the starting position. Pull the bar to your lower chest and then return it to the starting position.

2A: Straight-leg deadlift

Grab a barbell overhand, your hands just outside your legs, and hold it at arm's length in front of your thighs. Lower the bar until it's just below your knees, and then pull your shoulders back to return to standing.

2B: Pushup

Choose a pushup variation that's challenging for 10 reps. Do a conventional pushup, or elevate both feet on a bench, or elevate one foot on a bench and keep the other one raised. If you're advanced, you might put your hands on a Swiss ball or on a pair of medicine balls. Keep your body in a straight line from neck to ankles as you lower your chest, and push back up to the starting position.

3A: Reverse lunge and shoulder press

Stand holding a pair of dumbbells at your shoulders. Step back with one leg and lower your body until the top of your front thigh is parallel to the floor and your rear knee comes close to the floor. At the same time, press the dumbbells overhead. Push back to standing as you lower the dumbbells to your shoulders. Repeat with the other leg. That's 1 rep.

3B: Standing EZ-bar curl

Grab an EZ-curl bar or a pair of dumbbells. Stand with the weight in front of your thighs. Tighten your upper-back and core muscles. Curl the weight toward your shoulders without moving your torso forward or back. Lower the weight and repeat.

- Fill half your lunch or dinner plate with lean protein (chicken breast, sirloin steak, scrambled eggs) and half with fiber-rich vegetables. Protein and fiber fill you up fastest and satisfy hunger longest.

It's possible to gain weight from a diet of mostly home-cooked food, especially if it includes a lot of high-calorie, low-fiber starches such as bread, pasta, and potatoes. But you'd have to work at it.

Cut Carbs and Increase Protein

Because a big belly can be a sign of insulin resistance, and insulin resistance manifests functionally as metabolic inflexibility, you will respond best with a lower-carb diet. Even a small decrease in your insulin level will lead to a large increase in fat burning, says Jeff Volek, Ph.D., who studies strength training and nutrition at the University of Connecticut. "Low-carb diets lead to a much greater decrease in fat."

Low-carb doesn't have to mean militantly low-carb. In a yearlong weight-loss study at Stanford, participants assigned to an Atkins-type diet were eating a third of their calories from carbs by the end—more than twice as much as their Atkins-type diet recommended. And they still did better than people assigned to the other diets.

Carbohydrates are less problematic at two times of the day.

First thing in the morning. Whole-grain carbs, such as steel-cut oatmeal, provide an easy-to-access source of glucose for your body and brain.

Even a small decrease in your insulin level will lead to a large increase in fat burning.

Immediately following a workout, when a baked potato helps you refuel and provides a high level of postmeal satiety.

Don't Eat on Thursday, Ever

There's one surefire way to encourage your body to burn stored fat: Stop feeding it. Intermittent fasting—going without a meal for 8, 12, or even 24 hours at a time—is an increasingly popular weight-loss tool.

"Even people who are metabolically inflexible use fat as fuel during a fast," says Nelson. "It ramps up all the processes associated with burning fat."

Entry-level fasters should start with modest expectations. Some find it easy to skip breakfast and extend an overnight fast to 12 or more hours. But it works only if you have the discipline to end the fast with real food rather than by hitting the drive-thru. For others, an early dinner works best, but this plan is easily derailed if you find yourself wide-awake and starving at midnight.

A better strategy: Shoot for a daily 6-hour break between two substantial meals. Work up to 8 hours from time to time. If you feel better—and many fasters say they do—build up to a single 24-hour fast once a week. If you feel worse, stick with a meal/snack schedule built around foods you prepare yourself.

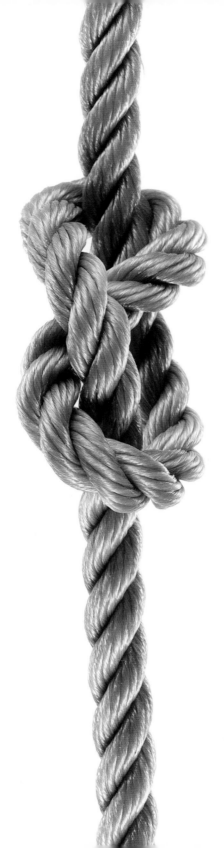

Never Go Jogging

"I don't think low-intensity, steady-state exercise is a very effective stand-alone treatment for existing obesity," Guyenet says. Interval exercise—short periods of hard work followed by longer periods of recovery—pushes your body to shift quickly from carbs to fat and back again while boosting your metabolism for hours afterward.

Here are three ways to light a fire.

Time-specific intervals. You might run hard for 20 seconds and then recover for 40 seconds. An advanced athlete might use a 1-to-1 work-to-rest ratio, so he'd go hard for 30 seconds and recover for 30 seconds. You can also do this with weights or calisthenics. Ten minutes of these intervals—at the beginning or end of a regular workout or as a stand-alone training session—is plenty to start. Fifteen to 20 minutes is the max for anyone.

Volume-specific intervals. Go for a fixed number of repetitions if you're lifting (which is how most of us work out), or a specific distance if you're running or swimming, and then recover for however long it takes. You can train like this for a full workout—30 to 45 minutes of lifting or cardiovascular exercise, plus 5 to 10 minutes of warmups.

Timed volume-specific intervals. You might do 10 pushups, squats, or kettlebell swings every minute. The faster you do the reps, the more time you have to recover. But with subsequent sets, your pace will slow down, which cuts into your recovery time and leaves you with more residual fatigue. That's what you want, because fatigue is what keeps your metabolism elevated long after you leave the gym.

Push Beyond Your Comfort Zone

"We want the quick fix, and we want it to be easy," Scott says. "But what do all successful programs have in common? You're working your butt off. Intense activity, by itself, is going to produce changes."

That doesn't mean kill yourself every time you pick up a dumbbell. But it does mean pushing your body to do more than it currently does.

"Do more" can mean any of the following:

- Higher volume—more sets, reps, or miles.

- Higher intensity—heavier weights, faster rides or runs.

- Higher frequency—the same thing more often.

- Higher difficulty—more challenging lifts, incorporating hills into cardio training.

From time to time, it helps to ask yourself if what you're doing is "hard" or if you're doing something now that you wouldn't or couldn't do last month, or last year. If the answer is no, you probably need to turn it up a notch (or two).

Don't Expect Perfection

"Ninety percent compliance is good enough," Nelson says. "The closer you are to 100 percent compliance, the less you benefit from it. An occasional ice cream or Twinkie, or a couple of Ho Hos shouldn't destroy you."

There's one hard-and-fast rule for indulgence, Nelson adds: "Sit back and enjoy it!" Don't feel guilty, don't try to run a marathon the next day just so you can burn it off, and most of all don't gulp down your treat like a junkie who just escaped from court-ordered rehab. The slower you eat, the more you can savor it and the more quickly you'll feel satiated. Then brush your teeth and recommit to your program.

The science of metabolic restoration might be complicated, but the path to success is refreshingly simple: Do the best you can as often as you can, and blame society for the rest.

Your Food Addiction

Discover the emerging science behind the brain-belly connection and how food companies hook you.

Exercise and watch what you eat.

Simple, right? Or not. What if other forces were at work, trying to put pounds on your frame until you join the 58 percent of the world predicted to be overweight or obese by 2030? Many scientists now believe that it's not your stomach you should worry about; it's your brain. In the past 2 years, scientists have published nearly 40 studies on whether the temptation of food can veer into actual addiction.

Think the addiction concept is an overeater's cop-out? Experts don't. Researchers are currently debating whether food addiction should be included in the *Diag-nostic and Statistical Manual of Mental Disorders*, the go-to reference for members of the American Psychiatric Association.

Scientists speculate that only some people are truly addicted to food. However, a far greater number of us might be vulnerable to the ways food can trick the brain into making us eat more than we want to, says Joe Frascella, Ph.D., of the National Institute on Drug Abuse's division of clinical neuroscience and behavioral research. And with the current profusion of food-themed TV shows and an escalating fast-food arms race, it's becoming more and more difficult for

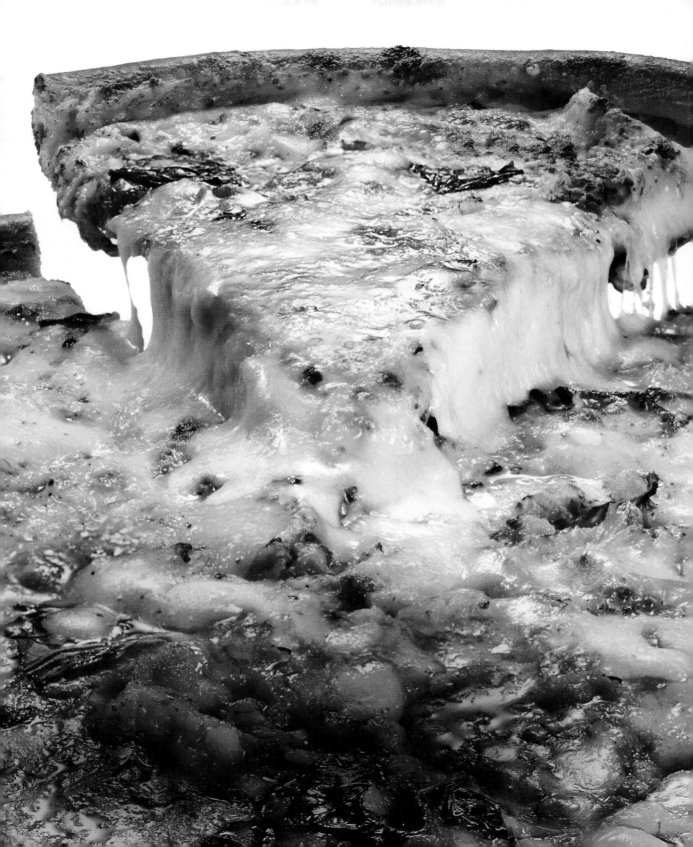

> "Unlike drugs, food keeps us alive. Untangling that association can be difficult."

our brains to resist cues to overeat. So fight back with these tactics, and gain mastery over your meals.

Control Your Survival Instinct

We exist on the planet because of fat and sugar, those valued treasures in the evolutionary struggle. Fat was survival fuel for cavemen, says Nicole M. Avena, Ph.D., a food addiction researcher and assistant professor of psychiatry at the University of Florida. The macronutrient contains more calories per gram (9, in fact) than either protein or carbs. And back in the day, sugar carbohydrates helped keep us alert to potential dangers.

Today we and our deskbound brethren burn far fewer calories, yet we maintain that Cro-Magnon connection to the pleasures that high-fat, high-sugar foods bring to our brains, says Avena. So the food we're wired to desire isn't always the food we need.

A 2010 Scripps Research Institute study found that when rats were presented with a "cafeteria-style" diet of large amounts of high-fat food, they ate almost twice as many calories as rats given only standard laboratory chow. It's another piece of evidence that fatty, sugary foods might be more habit-forming than other foods, Avena says. Yes, humans are more evolved than rats, but who hasn't had a similar experience at an unlimited pizza-and-dessert buffet?

Break the Habit

Make your calories work longer. Because you no longer need to amass large stores of calories until your next mastodon kill, choose foods that have nutrients with staying power.

Aim to eat at least 20 to 40 grams of protein per meal, and about 25 to 35 grams of fiber over the course of the day. These nutrients promote fullness, might dampen the reward response to overeating, and will help you fend off cravings so you eat fewer calories at later meals. Even at that pizza buffet.

Stop Getting High

On food, that is. In a study in the journal *Archives of General Psychiatry*, researchers found that the brains of food-addicted people who consumed a high-calorie milkshake responded the same way the brains of drug addicts respond to a dose of cocaine.

"Food addicts have the same reward signals and signs of dopamine dysfunction as drug addicts have," says Frascella. And like drug addicts, food addicts might relapse when they try to curb their tendencies.

"Unlike drugs, food keeps us alive. Untangling that association can be difficult," Frascella says.

Certain foods might also have the same mood-boosting properties as drugs have. In a 2011 study in the *Journal of Clinical Investigation*, participants who ingested a saturated-fat solution felt happier after listening to sad music than those who ingested a saline solution. It turns out that comfort food might actually comfort us, and that makes it even more challenging to resist.

Break the Habit

You don't need psychotherapy to stop emotional eating. You just need to reverse the reward patterns.

That means hitting the pause button, says Gary Foster, Ph.D., director of Temple University's center for obesity research, who has explored the topic of emotional eating. Recognize triggers for what they are, ride out the emotions, and then praise yourself for doing so, Foster says. "It's difficult at first, but each time you reinforce the positive behavior, you drive emotional eating into extinction," he says.

Avoid Mindless Eating

It's happened to us all: You have a brutal day at work, and the first thing you do after your grueling commute is raid your helpless refrigerator. Feels good, right?

"It's because you've conditioned yourself," says Foster. "People eat for any number of reasons: They're happy, sad, stressed, bored. When the trigger occurs, like Pavlov's dog you start salivating."

The more often you use a fridge raid as a stress buster, the more your brain will come to expect that behavior. Repeating this cycle can reinforce the habit.

Break the Habit

Think of your growing belly, not your growling stomach. Mindless eating is just that: Your brain shuts down as your gullet opens up.

"We've found that most people focus only on the short-term rewards when it comes to foods," says Ashley Gearhardt, a clinical psychology doctoral student at Yale University and author of the high-calorie milkshake study. "But what we've found is that if you can train yourself to focus on the long-term consequences—the weight gain, the sickness—then you'll activate your prefrontal cortex, or the 'brakes' in your brain that may prevent you from overeating."

Escape the Food Traps

It's hard to resist the siren call of the 24-hour meal.

"Our modern eating environment isn't like it was 10,000 years ago. Cheap, high-calorie foods are available on every corner," says Frascella. Fast-food joints pump out aromas to entice you, and "food porn" TV shows are spliced with ads for double-stuffed pizzas and towering burgers. "For people who have a tendency to overeat, these stimulating cues trigger unhealthy food behaviors," says Foster.

Break the Habit

Limit your exposure to triggers. Ask your server for the check before the dessert menu reaches the table. Change the channel if commercials start splashing unhealthy foods across the screen. Think twice about that pizza buffet.

How Fat Attacks

Not all body fat is created equal. Some is fairly harmless. It's the stuff you can't see that can hurt you.

The man on the operating table is under IV sedation, facedown, circles drawn around the flabbiest parts of his body. He's painted with iodine and has two small holes punched through the soft skin of his lower back.

Board-certified New York City plastic surgeon David Shafer, M.D., aligns the tip of a foot-long suction wand, called a cannula, with one of the holes. He carefully places it beneath the skin. It makes a slurping sound like a straw sucking at the bottom of a milkshake. For the next hour, Dr. Shafer will be hoovering adipose fat cells from the man's back, flanks, and stomach.

This is where men tend to collect the most fat, explains Dr. Shafer—above the waist and over the ab muscles. He reaches down to grab a handful of the loose flab on the man's torso.

"This is what we call subcutaneous fat," he says.

It's the soft stuff you feel when you pinch your own belly. Then Dr. Shafer sweeps his hand across the patient's midsection, the soft cavity containing the intestines, kidneys, and liver.

"And see how the gut swells outward? That's the visceral fat pushing from beneath the rectus muscles."

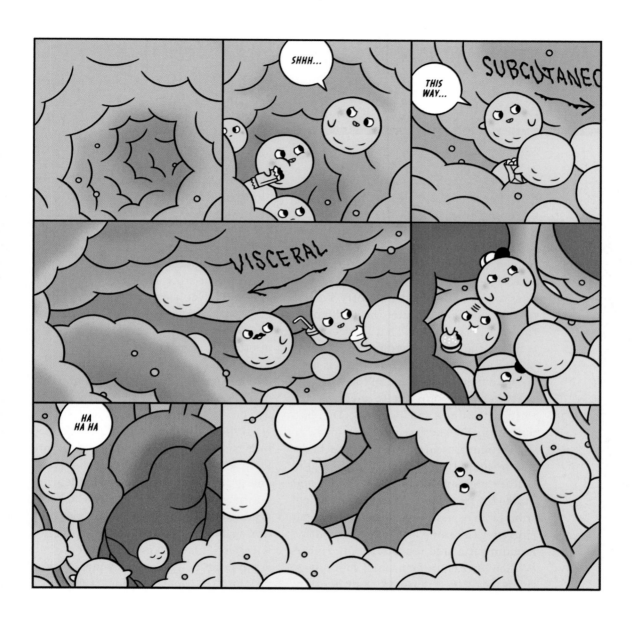

> "Upper-body fat, including visceral fat, is a kind of fight-and-flight depot that both stores and releases energy very easily."

That's the dangerous stuff.

When researchers in St. Louis tracked a group of liposuction patients after surgery, they found zero improvement in blood pressure, triglycerides, glucose tolerance, or HDL or LDL cholesterol profiles. The pale, gloppy fat that a patient pays to have removed isn't pretty, but its absence doesn't guarantee the health profile of a lean, fit person. That's because visceral fat, the kind that wraps around your organs and makes you unhealthy, is also the kind that liposuction can't reach.

"There's no safe way to suck around the heart, kidney, and liver," says Dr. Shafer. "It's just too dangerous."

The more researchers learn about body fat, the more they've come to view it as a multifaceted substance. In a sense, it's not unlike the fat in food. The artery-clogging trans fat in partially hydrogenated margarine isn't the same as the heart-healthy monounsaturated fat in olive oil, right? Well, neither is the fat around your quads the same as the fat around your liver. In terms of its impact on your health, the amount of fat your body carries is less important than where your body stores it.

"It's still not completely understood, but fat behaves very differently on different parts of the body," says Dr. Shafer. The better your grasp of this concept, the better you'll understand the need to target your body's most dangerous fat.

HIDDEN FACT FAT #1
Upper-body fat saved your ancestors.

Say you're a hungry caveman plodding along the tundra, and you spot a 6-ton woolly mammoth wandering on the horizon. You want an energy source that kicks into action immediately so you can chase and kill the beast. That's very likely the reason men store more upper-body fat than women do, says Fredrik Karpe, M.D., Ph.D., a professor of metabolic medicine at the University of Oxford. Men were the hunters.

"Upper-body fat, including visceral fat, is a kind of fight-and-flight depot that both stores and releases energy very easily," he says.

It does this through a process called lipolysis, which breaks clumps of fat into fatty acids that your muscles can use as energy. In visceral fat, lipolysis occurs at an unusually high rate. It's an ongoing process of deconstruction and reconstruction that keeps your bloodstream flooded with fat. This high concentration of fat compounds can bog down your liver and jack up LDL cholesterol and triglyceride levels.

The big problem today is that our bodies still hold on to visceral fat even though we're no longer starving cavemen.

"Those fat depots are no longer useful,"

THE TWO SIDES OF BODY FAT

Your gut might be attacking you from the inside.

OBESE BODY

250 pounds

40 percent body fat

Fat infestation: Visceral fat wraps around your liver, kidneys, and pancreas, releasing compounds that promote inflammation. This is also the fat that pushes out your gut, giving you a Buddha belly.

Bumpy bulges: Subcutaneous fat (just under the skin) creates bulges on your body. The effect is primarily cosmetic, though.

HEALTHY BODY

150 pounds

18 percent body fat

Flatter gut: When you lose visceral fat, your abdominal cavity contracts, giving you a narrower waistline and flatter belly. This has a positive domino effect that can result in lower LDL cholesterol and triglycerides, and improved insulin sensitivity.

Low-fat flesh: Exercise can't eliminate all of the fat on your frame, nor would you want it to. "Even elite athletes rarely dip below 6 percent body fat," says *Men's Health* nutrition advisor Alan Aragon, M.S. "We need at least that much to protect our organs and regulate body temperature and hormones."

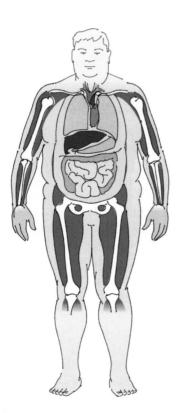

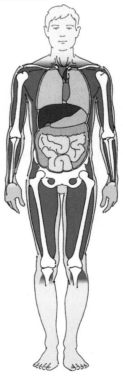

says Dr. Karpe. "It comes at a price to have such easily mobilized fat."

But regular exercise can help neutralize those cardiovascular risks, says Dr. Karpe. When you put your muscles to work, they release enzymes that pluck circulating triglycerides from the blood and burn them off as fuel, which can help clear danger from your arteries.

HIDDEN FAT FACT #2
Body fat below the waist is not as dangerous.

Visceral fat is a threat for another reason: It's highly susceptible to inflammation.

"As the amount of stored fat increases, it triggers a cellular response designed to recruit immune cells," says Michael Schwartz, M.D., director of the diabetes and obesity center of excellence at the University of Washington. This leads to inflammation and can result in insulin resistance and a host of diseases associated with metabolic syndrome.

Fat below the waist behaves differently than visceral fat.

"From an evolutionary standpoint, we believe that lower-body fat is intended as long-term storage. It's packed away, so it doesn't harm the rest of the body, and we use it as a last reserve," says Dr. Karpe.

According to a 2010 review conducted by Dr. Karpe, below-the-belt fat produces fewer inflammatory compounds, which means less cardiovascular damage. This gives women a health advantage because they tend to store more fat in their lower bodies than men do. The fat women tend to carry on their hips? "That's one of the reasons we think women are more resistant to heart disease," Dr. Karpe says.

HIDDEN FAT FACT #3
Body fat is far more than a calorie storage tank.

Five or 10 years ago, researchers and physicians viewed fat merely as a storage system for energy—a soft balloon filled with calories. But they've since come to recognize it as an instrument that plays a critical role in your body's metabolic function.

"Fat is the largest endocrine organ in the body," says David Piston, Ph.D., a professor of molecular physiology and biophysics at Vanderbilt University.

Even a 160-pound man with 13 percent body fat (that's a lean guy) has more than 20 pounds of fat. And that fat—or more specifically, the adipose cells that store fatty triglycerides and keep them out of the blood—is extremely important to his body's hormone regulation.

Consider leptin. This hormone is produced inside fat tissue, and without it you could theoretically eat until your stomach burst. Leptin regulates how responsive your body is to the "I'm full" signals coming from your stomach. The more fat cells you have, the more leptin you have circulating in your blood, so you'll feel full on less food. But while this important signal registers well in lean people, it seems to be ineffective in overweight people.

And that's just one of about 300 compounds coming from fat, says Dr. Karpe.

YOUR 4-POINT VISCERAL-FAT ACTION PLAN

The fat is hidden, but the solutions are easy to see.

Worried that you're harboring dangerous belly fat? Your waist circumference tends to be related to the amount of visceral fat you have, a study in the *American Journal of Epidemiology* found.

The American Heart Association recommends keeping your waist below 40 inches. To check, wrap a tailor's measuring tape snugly around your bare abdomen, just above your hip bones. Relax, exhale, and measure. If your number comes up a little elevated, here's what you need to do to target visceral fat.

QUIT THE FRUCTOSE.

A diet packed with fructose can make your belly bulge. In fact, adolescents in a Georgia Health Sciences University study who consumed the most fructose had about 20 percent more visceral fat than those who ate the least.

Your move: Avoid fruit juice or foods that have added sugar or high-fructose corn syrup. Don't worry about whole fruit, though. It accounts for less than 20 percent of the fructose in the typical American's diet, say Emory University researchers.

SWEAT THE CARDIO.

Resistance training is great for adding lean body mass, but cardio is better for burning visceral fat. In a Duke University study, people who trained on treadmills, elliptical trainers, and stationary bikes for 8 months (at the cardio equivalent of jogging 12 miles a week) lost about 8 percent of their visceral fat. Those who performed equally intense resistance workouts saw no change in visceral fat.

EAT WHOLE GRAINS.

Foods such as barley and quinoa do more than just help fill you up. In a 2010 study in the *American Journal of Clinical Nutrition*, people who ate three or more daily servings of whole grains had 10 percent less visceral fat than those who ate hardly any or no whole grains, even when the researchers adjusted for other lifestyle and diet factors.

One benefit, they speculate, might come from prebiotic compounds that feed beneficial bacteria in your gut.

SLEEP SMART.

The right amount of shut-eye is key. A study in the journal *Sleep* showed that people who logged 6 to 7 hours a night had the lowest levels of visceral fat. Above or below that range was associated with more visceral fat, with the worst numbers going to those who slept less than 5 hours. Over a 5-year span, these sleepers put on visceral fat about five times faster than the healthy sleepers did.

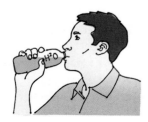 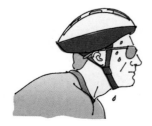 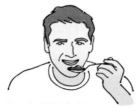 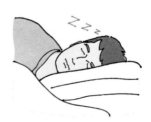

Alas, not all of them are as benign as leptin.

"When tissue is inflamed and overfilled with fat, it can pump out a lot of nasty stuff," he says.

That "stuff" can hijack your appetite, reprogram your fat-storage mechanisms, contribute to conditions such as arthritis, and drive your triglyceride levels to deadly heights.

The best way to cut inflammation? Yep, pack some physical activity into each day. Researchers at Appalachian State University recently determined that highly fit people who reported frequently engaging in moderate exercise such as cycling, swimming, or jogging had nearly 50 percent less C-reactive protein, a marker for inflammation, in their blood than people who were unfit and rarely exercised.

HIDDEN FACT FAT #4
Visceral fat undermines your manhood.

There's a concrete connection between testosterone and visceral fat, and it works in two ways, says Farid Saad, Ph.D., head of scientific affairs for Men's Healthcare at Bayer Pharma in Berlin, Germany.

First, inadequate testosterone levels direct muscle cells to turn into (or "differentiate" into) fat, and second, visceral fat produces substances that suppress testosterone production. So as the visceral bulge grows in your belly, testosterone drops, and your body is less likely to grow muscle. If the spiral goes unchecked, you can end up overweight with no motivation to

change. It may take no more than a couple of ounces of some types of body fat to threaten your life.

"Men with testosterone deficiency are also quite low on energy," says Saad. "You can tell them a thousand times to exercise, and they won't do it."

According to Saad, short-term testosterone supplements might be a viable solution. A 2012 study published in the *Journal of the American Medical Association*, for instance, found that men who received 20 weeks of testosterone supplementation gained fat-free, lean mass.

"For men with deficiencies, 1 or 2 years of supplementation might completely break the cycle," says Saad.

HIDDEN FAT FACT #5
Skinny people are not immune.

Low body fat is a pretty good indicator of health, but a dangerous clump of fat can still hide behind a flat belly. In a study published in the journal *Nature Genetics*, researchers discovered a gene that causes those with it to carry less body fat than those without it. Surprisingly, though, people with that gene (especially men) had a higher ratio of visceral fat to subcutaneous fat. They also had higher triglycerides and lower HDL cholesterol, which is a risky combo that can contribute to heart disease.

What's more, it might take no more than a couple of ounces of some types of body fat to threaten your life. Researchers at the University of Cincinnati have recently begun looking into a type of fat called perivascular fat, which clumps around the arteries leading into your heart.

"For so long the dogma has been that all of the disease was coming from within the artery and traveling outward," says David Manka, Ph.D., lead researcher. "What we're showing is that the fat growing around these arteries is causing the disease on the inside. This perivascular fat tends to be loaded with inflammatory cells in a way that even visceral fat isn't."

You can't tell how much perivascular fat a man has by looking at him, so it's not easy to diagnose. And even though it might seem related to overall body fat, Manka's collaborators found plenty of perivascular fat on otherwise lean organ donors when they harvested samples. His team recently

Low body fat is a pretty good indicator of health, but a dangerous clump of fat can hide behind a flat belly.

received government funding for further research into this heart flab, but in the meantime, eating smart and exercising are always good ideas even if you're at your ideal weight.

"Perivascular fat seems very sensitive to changes in the nutritional state," he says. "Keep an eye on your overall fitness level. That's going to have a big impact."

The Truth about Exercise

Is exercise fattening? We've uncovered the truth about how your workout affects your metabolism, appetite, weight, and overall health.

While you were toiling away on the treadmill, a slow-burning debate among fitness experts was catching fire: Is exercise an effective strategy for losing weight? Or is the effort ultimately a wash, triggering hunger pangs that make you replace everything you burned and then some?

A decade ago no one thought to ask this. Too much food makes you fat. Exercise burns calories. Ergo, exercise makes you less fat. Then research began to find that not everyone who exercises loses weight. Impossible as it may seem, some people actually gain a pound or two.

Here's the problem: The range of individual responses to exercise is huge, says veteran weight-loss researcher Timothy Church, M.D., Ph.D., a professor of preventive medicine at Pennington Biomedical Research Center in Baton Rouge, Louisiana. "We don't understand all of it," he says. Fortunately, however, we understand enough to throw cold water on four of today's most insidious weight-loss myths.

MYTH #1
Exercise won't help you lose weight.

That would be news to all the people who've lost double-digit poundage by pounding the pavement. But it would seem

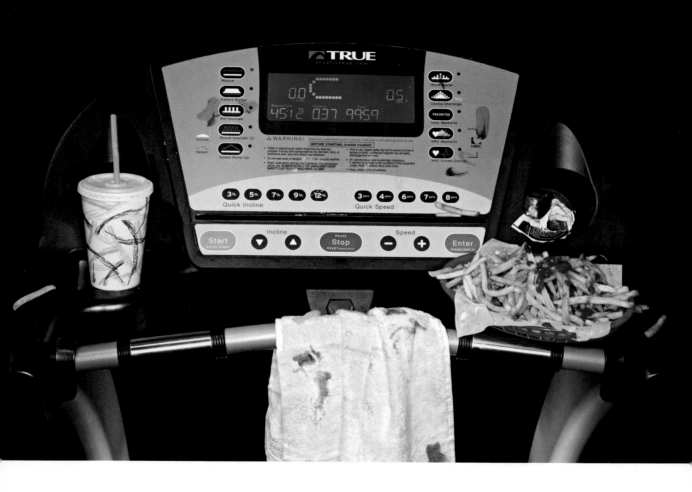

to validate the experience of your buddy who trained for a marathon and finished 2 pounds heavier.

Dr. Church explains: "The degree to which you respond is probably dependent on genetics. Researchers have found 20 specific genes related to this, and how you score across those genes impacts your responsiveness."

Your diet and the kind of exercise you engage in may play a role, too. For most of us, the response is in the middle. Exercise, in fact, helps out in three specific belly-off zones.

Limiting Weight Gain

"A ton of data shows that leading a physically active life is critical for not putting

> Exercise can help rewire your brain so you're less likely to seek out indulgent foods.

on weight," says Dr. Church.

Beyond the obvious calorie-burning rewards, regular exercisers become more attuned to their body's needs, reap mental benefits, and have a better quality of life, research shows. Regular workouts also help you maintain better body composition (more muscle, less fat), which means a lower risk of chronic diseases in your future.

Losing Weight

A recent Cochrane Collaboration review of 43 exercise and weight-loss studies determined that exercise helped people lose some weight—about 2 pounds. Crank up the intensity to "high" and you can lose 3 pounds—without dietary intervention.

Preventing the Pounds from Coming Back

Losing weight isn't easy, but keeping it off is even harder, Dr. Church says. Your metabolism downshifts, and hormonal processes kick in to encourage your body to regain those pounds.

The latest data from the National Weight Control Registry shows that people who successfully keep pounds off exercise for 45 to 60 minutes a day. And as long as you're not taking in more calories than you burn, daily exercise might remodel your metabolism, so your body burns more fat.

Fat Blaster

Intensity trumps all. You burn more calories while you're working out, and you also help your metabolism stay in a higher gear for hours afterward, thanks to a mechanism called EPOC, or excess postexercise oxygen consumption.

In a recent study in the journal *Medicine & Science in Sports & Exercise*, men who cycled hard for 45 minutes burned an average of 519 calories during the workout and another 193 calories in the next 14 hours. The tipping-point intensity level seems to be about 75 percent to 80 percent of your maximum heart rate (which is roughly 220 minus your age).

MYTH #2
Exercise just makes you hungrier.

Doesn't happen, at least in the short term, says David Stensel, Ph.D., who studies exercise metabolism at Loughborough University in England. In Stensel's 2010 study, people who exercised for 90 minutes ate just as many calories on the days they worked out as on the days they didn't.

Numerous other studies have shown that vigorous exercise briefly down-regulates the appetite-stimulating hormone ghrelin. And while the blood levels of ghrelin rebound quickly after exercise,

Stensel says they don't rise beyond where they were before the activity.

Over the long term, however, your body reacts to a serious fitness program as it would to any sustained reduction of its available fuel stores. No matter how much you want that 32-inch waist, your body wants homeostasis more. The degree to which appetite amps up varies among individuals and depends on a combination of genetic, behavioral, and contextual factors, says Barry Braun, Ph.D., an associate professor of kinesiology at the University of Massachusetts at Amherst.

"It's complex, because in most studies we see a poor correspondence between appetite hormones and changes in perceived hunger," he says.

And there's no clear link between appetite and what people actually eat.

Fat Blaster

Increasing your incidental activity—calories you burn when you're not working out—always pays dividends, says *Men's Health* nutrition advisor Alan Aragon, M.S.

For instance, a study from the University of Missouri found that active nonexercisers burned more calories than people who ran 35 miles each week but were otherwise sedentary. And one of Braun's recent studies shows that standing instead of sitting can burn an extra 750 calories each day without triggering an appetite increase.

But don't leave it up to chance: Get an activity recorder, such as Actiheart or Fitbit, and try to boost your numbers in whatever way you can.

MYTH #3
You can "reward" yourself for working out.

Okay, you can, but you shouldn't—at least not with food. The reason is simple: A few seconds of indulgence can undo an hour's worth of exercise. Let's say you run for 40 minutes at a 9-minute-mile pace. That's a good workout, burning about 550 calories. Now suppose you grab a Starbucks Venti Mocha Frappuccino on the way to work. That's 500 calories—almost what you just sweated off.

Dr. Church is now studying dieters who exercise and either gain weight or don't lose as many pounds as they'd expected to. Why? Because they tend to treat themselves with high-calorie foods after workouts.

"The problem is, the reward is disproportionate to the activity," he says.

In a 2010 University of Ottawa study, 16 normal-weight people walked on treadmills until they had burned 300 calories. Then they had to estimate how much energy they'd expended. Some guessed 896—almost triple the actual burn. An hour later, they were told to eat a meal that, in their estimation, would replace the calories they'd burned. This group selected 607 calories—double the energy they'd used.

But there's some good news: Emerging evidence suggests that exercise can help rewire your brain in a way that makes you less likely to seek out indulgent foods. In a study published in 2012, researchers at California Polytechnic State University in

San Luis Obispo asked two groups to either sit quietly or pedal hard on a stationary bike for an hour. When the time was up, the scientists wired them up to measure brain activity and showed them pictures of either high-calorie foods or healthy fare. The people who had exercised showed no preference for any particular category of food. But when the non-exercisers saw images of cookies and sundaes, the reward regions of their brains lit up.

"Being fit can have psychological effects," says Todd Hagobian, Ph.D., the study's author and an assistant professor of kinesiology at Cal Poly. "Regular exercise may increase your desire to consume a better diet—and shed pounds."

Fat Blaster

First, find an exercise you enjoy; that way doing it becomes the reward. Second, keep a closer eye on the calories you burn exercising. (For most activities, it's under 400 for every 45 minutes; you can check at myfitnesspal.com.) Finally, track your portion sizes. You could be in for a shock.

Another key strategy is learning how to fill up on less. Weight loss requires an energy deficit (burning more than you take in), and any time you're managing a deficit, your body will notice. You can't count on self-discipline alone. To win the hunger game, you need to eat foods that fill you up with the fewest calories, says Aragon.

Those tend to be foods packed with protein and/or fiber. He advises consuming 30 to 40 grams of protein at every meal (and snack) and hitting your daily fiber quota of 35 grams by eating plenty of beans, oatmeal, fruits, and cruciferous vegetables. A recent study published in the *New England Journal of Medicine* associated three foods—yogurt, nuts, and fruit—with successful weight loss. Yogurt and nuts offer protein; fruit satisfies your sweet tooth while providing fiber and water. Most fruits have a lot of water, which lowers their energy density—the number of calories per unit of mass. Low-calorie soups have the same effect; the extra fluid helps you feel full with less total food. You can also create the effect by drinking a glass of water before every meal and snack and sipping another one while you're nibbling.

MYTH #4

As a society, we're exercising more but still growing fatter.

This is a phony correlation on two levels. First, it suggests that people who exercise consistently are also gaining weight. There's no evidence of that happening. Then it assumes that more people are actually working out. Research flat-out refutes this idea. The peak years of the obesity epidemic—when the average weight of Americans rose by double digits—were roughly 1980 to 2000. In 1980, about 8 percent of men exercised five times a week, according to University of Minnesota research. In 2000, that increased to 9 percent.

But there was one important change: The number of people who said they sat for

MANAGE YOUR DEFICIT

Weight loss is the opposite of accounting. Your goal: Accumulate red ink, spending more calories than you bring in. We asked *Men's Health* nutrition advisor Alan Aragon, M.S., and Mike Roussell, Ph.D., author of *The Six Pillars of Nutrition,* to give us a budget-busting plan.

PART 1: METABOLIC MATH

How many calories are you eating?

Track everything you eat and drink for 3 days and tally your daily total at fitday.com or with an app like Lose It!

How many calories do you actually need to maintain your weight?

Use Aragon's formula. These are sample calculations for a 185-pound man.

Zero workouts: Multiply your weight by 10. (At 185 pounds, that's 1,850 calories a day.)

One or two workouts a week: Your weight x 12 (2,220 calories)

Two to four workouts a week: Your weight x 14 (2,590 calories)

Five or more workouts a week: Your weight x 16 (2,960 calories)

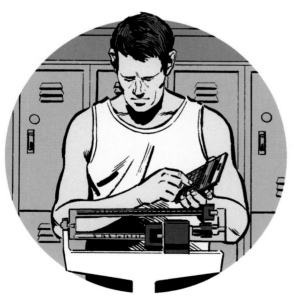

PART 2: BURNING MAN

Aragon recommends a maximum daily deficit of 500 calories when you're trying to shed some pounds. Our 185-pound man is working out 2 to 4 days a week, so 2,590 calories a day maintains his weight. Here's how his body allocates those calories and ways he can create some extra burn.

RESTING METABOLISM: 60 percent to 75 percent: This is the cost of not being dead, including energy used by everything from your organs to individual cells.

70 percent = 1,813 calories

Bonus burn: High-intensity exercise can elevate your metabolism for 14 to 36 hours after exercise. 100 to 240 calories

THERMIC EFFECT OF FOOD: 10 percent: These are the calories burned by digestion.

10 percent = 259 calories

Bonus burn: You use 25 percent of protein calories for digestion—far more than with fat or carbs. By eating your target weight in grams of protein daily, you can burn more sans effort. 100 calories

PHYSICAL ACTIVITY: 15 percent to 30 percent: These are the calories you expend through exercise and movement.

20 percent = 518 calories

Bonus burn: You don't have to sweat through two-a-days to get the benefit of moving more. Minimize your sitting time, take the stairs, fidget—it all adds up. 200 to 600 calories

more than half the day increased by 14 percent. To explore this, Dr. Church and his colleagues at Pennington examined how much physical activity people engaged in at their jobs in the 1960s and in 2008. They found a 58 percent decline in work-related physical activity, with men burning 140 fewer calories a day.

"Background physical activity has plummeted," Dr. Church says. "You have to make up for that somewhere. If you don't, you're going to gain weight."

Fat Blaster

All movement matters. Even a simple evening walk can make up for the calories we no longer burn at work.

When we focus on what exercise doesn't do, we miss a bigger story that goes beyond appetite and even weight control. Exercise pays off in ways that can't be measured on a scale or seen in a mirror. A 2011 study published in the journal *Circulation* found that the fitter you are, the lower your chance of having a heart attack or of premature death from any cause, regardless of your girth.

Other research reveals that even when dieters regain lost weight, they still come out ahead by maintaining their workout routines. A 2010 study from the University of Missouri shows that the still-exercising dieters were healthier than a matched group of people who'd regained weight but stopped working out. The exercising group had higher levels of HDL (good) cholesterol, greater insulin sensitivity, and lower blood pressure.

It's also worth noting that your own workout routine isn't part of a controlled scientific experiment. What you take out of it has a high correlation with what you're willing to put into it and how consistently you adhere to it. And that's no myth.

FOOD, ON THE BRAIN

Emerging science shows that the minds of overeaters might look like those of drug addicts.

The proof is in the neuroimaging scans at right, from Gene-Jack Wang, M.D., of the Brookhaven National Laboratory. When Dr. Wang's team scanned the brains of obese overeaters and meth addicts, they found that the people in both groups had fewer dopamine receptors available in their brains than healthy individuals (dopamine receptor availability is shown in red).

What's the big deal? Just as meth users need more and more of the drug to get high, obese overeaters might need more and more food to produce the same intensity of dopamine "high," which is a cycle that can reinforce addictive behavior, according to Dr. Wang.

Control   Methamphetamine user

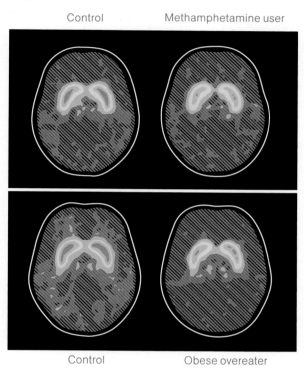

Control   Obese overeater

Six Six-Pack Solutions

Here are six fast ways to lose your gut and sculpt the ripped body of your dreams.

One fitness target is universally understood by all guys: abs.

A ripped core signals good health, a fit body, and sex appeal. But when it comes to sculpting one, we make excuses: genetics, work, a regular Sunday menu of football, wings, and beer.

Truth? Excuses are bull. Arm yourself with these six simple steps—and exercises—from *The Men's Health Big Book: Getting Abs* to finally reveal your six-pack, and enjoy a flatter belly for life.

Sleep More

Here's a truth you'll appreciate: One of the best things you can do for your body is spend more time in bed. Harvard University researchers who studied more than 68,000 people found that those who slept less than 5 hours a night were 5.4 pounds heavier and more likely to become obese than those who slept more than 7 hours.

One reason: Just a single night of inadequate sleep might increase activity in your brain's reward center, particularly

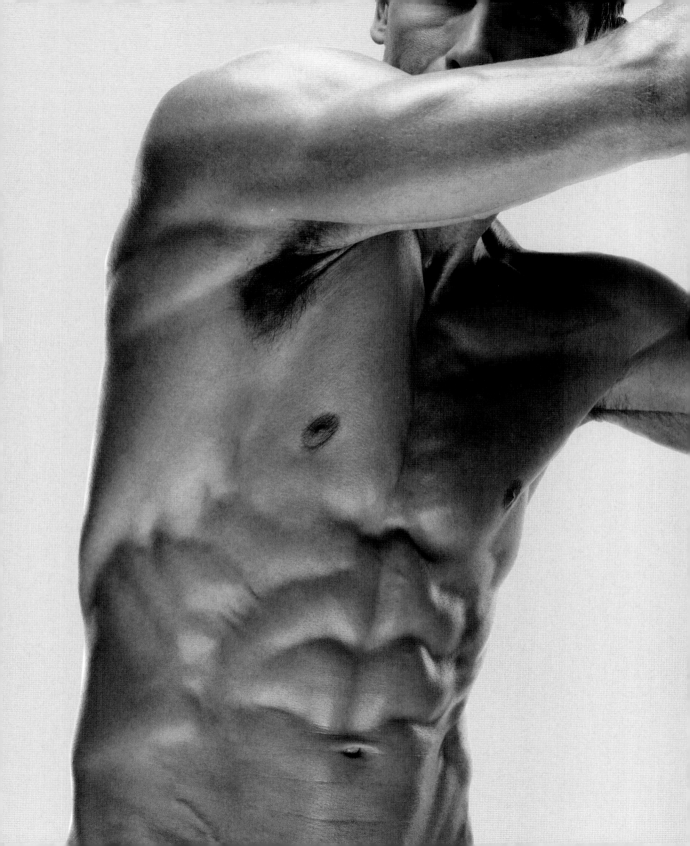

regarding food. To point: A University of Chicago study found that "short sleepers" took in an average of 220 more calories a day than those who logged adequate z's.

Quick Fix

Unplug the bedroom TV and try for 8 hours of sleep a night—and never settle for less than 7. Here's a scary fact for some added inspiration: If you are a habitual short sleeper, your chance of an early death rises by as much as 12 percent, Italian researchers say.

Lift More Often

Your treadmill's calorie tracker might make cardio seem like a fat-loss genie, but don't be fooled. The more miles you log, the more efficient at running you become and the fewer calories you may burn. Plus, running long distances can take a physical toll that can dampen your enthusiasm. All that pain and boredom causes many people to burn out and give up.

Quick Fix

Weave "The Best Abs Workout Ever" (see page 38) into your fitness plan. Just 3 days of resistance training a week can offer the metabolic boost you need to slash fat and finally fit into slimmer, more flattering clothes.

Lift Heavier Weights

Now that you've made it to the gym (or dusted off your weights at home), reach for the larger dumbbells. Lifting heavy weights burns more calories during your workout, and it might also increase your sleeping metabolism by about 8 percent, according to researchers at Washington University school of medicine in St. Louis.

Yep: You'll burn more calories as you lie on your back and dream of Scarlett Johansson. That 8 percent might not sound like much, but it can add up to about 5 pounds a year.

Quick Fix

Push your limits. As you feel yourself becoming stronger and more comfortable during a workout, don't be afraid to go bigger.

Eat When You Want

You've heard that you need five or six meals a day for fat loss. The simple rationale is this: Digestion requires energy, so spreading your calories over many small meals throughout the day keeps your metabolism humming and your hunger at bay.

The problem? It's not how frequently you eat but rather what you eat that affects how many calories you burn at mealtime. So if you take in 2,000 a day, it doesn't matter how many meals you've eaten; your calorie burn from digestion remains the same.

Quick Fix

Take a week and write down when you feel most hungry. Then adjust your eating

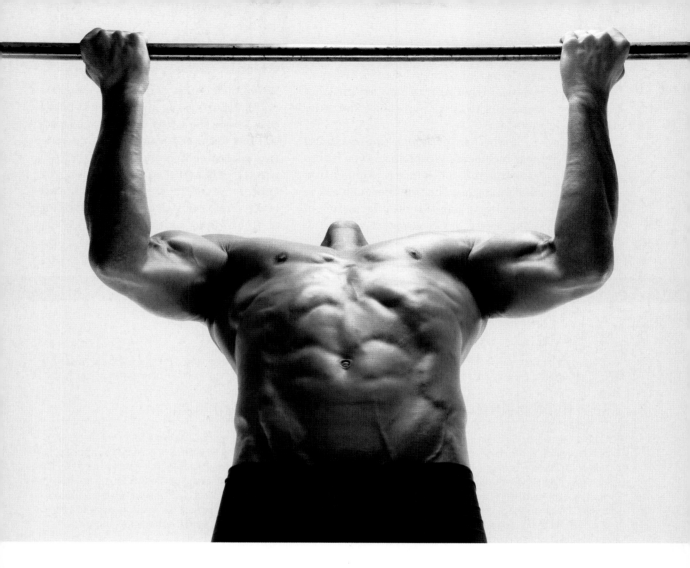

patterns accordingly. The key is to pack each meal with foods that provide the greatest metabolic boost.

Load Up on Protein

Every time you eat a meal that doesn't include protein, you're telling your body you don't want to burn more calories. Here's why: Protein helps control your blood sugar, keeps you fuller, reduces hunger, and burns more calories during digestion. So you can stay lean and still enjoy your favorite foods. Also, the protein stops muscle breakdown and provides the raw materials for laying down new muscle.

Quick Fix

Despite what you might have heard: Carbohydrates are not evil. But when you eat them alone, they set off a series of events—including a rise of insulin—that cause you to crave more food and store more fat.

So whether you're snacking or eating a meal, include some protein and you'll drop fat. For meals, a 6-ounce portion of fish, chicken, or lean beef is reasonable. For snacks, try a handful of nuts, a stick of string cheese, or Greek yogurt.

Snack Smarter

While the number of meals you consume doesn't matter, the size of your snacks does. Since the 1970s, the average snack size has increased from 360 to 580 calories, according to research from the University of North Carolina. When you consider that the average man snacks twice during a workday, you're looking at almost 500 additional calories every

THE BEST ABS WORKOUT EVER

This no-crunches core workout is designed to make you stronger with each visit to the gym and will force you to bring your A-game with each rep, says Nashville-based strength coach J.C. Deen, founder of jcdfitness.com.

Trap Bar Deadlift

Load a trap bar and stand between its handles with your feet hip-width apart. Bend down and grab the handles; this is the starting position. Keeping your lower back naturally arched, drive your heels into the floor and push your hips forward, lifting the bar until it's in front of your thighs. Return to the starting position. Do 5 sets of 3 to 5 reps. For the first set, use 85 to 90 percent of your 1-rep max. For each subsequent set, reduce the load by 5 percent. Rest 2 minutes between sets.

Medicine Ball Slam

Grab a medicine ball and set your feet shoulder-width apart. Hold the medicine ball in both hands above your head with your arms slightly bent. Reach back as far as you can and then slam the ball to the floor in front of you as hard as you can. Catch the ball on the rebound and repeat for 45 seconds. Do 3 sets, resting 30 seconds between them. For an added challenge, do this on one leg.

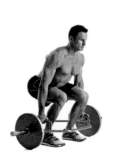
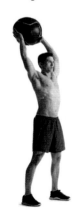
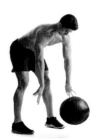

24 hours because of the increased snack size. Over the course of a week, that can contribute to an extra pound of fat.

Quick Fix

Use one hand to defeat your cravings. (Mind out of the gutter, fellas.) If a portion does not fit into your hand—whether it's almonds, a chicken breast, cheese, or fruit—then the portion is probably too large. If it's packaged, read the label. You want 200 to 300 calories in each serving, with 15 to 20 grams of protein and about the same amount of carbs—what you might find in a cup of Greek yogurt and some dried cherries.

For more simple six-pack solutions, pick up your copy of *The Men's Health Big Book: Getting Abs* at mhbigbookofabs.com/mh.

Barbell Row

Hold a barbell at arm's length and lower your torso until it's almost parallel to the floor. Your knees should be bent and your lower back arched. Squeeze your shoulder blades and pull the bar to your upper abs. Pause; lower the bar. Your goal: 30 reps total. Pick a weight that will allow you to do 10 to 12 reps on your first set, but stop 1 or 2 reps short of failure. Rest 20 seconds; perform as many reps as you can, stopping 1 rep short of failure. Continue this pattern until you complete 30 reps.

Cable Core Press

Attach a handle to a cable machine at chest height. Hold the handle against your chest with both hands, your right side toward the weight stack. Spread your feet shoulder-width apart. Step away from the stack until the cable is taut. Slowly press your arms in front of you until they're straight. Hold for 2 seconds and then bring them back to your chest. Do 6 to 8 reps, turn around (left side toward the stack), and repeat. That's 1 set. Do 3 sets with 60 seconds of rest between them.

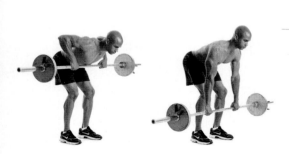
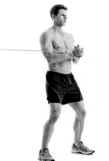
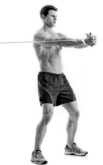

WIN THE HUNGER GAME

An empty stomach might cloud your thinking and turn you into an eating machine. New research from Yale University confirms that the hungrier you are, the harder you might find it to resist high-calorie foods. In the study, when people's blood-sugar levels dropped, they expressed more desire for belly busters such as burgers, pizza, brownies, and ice cream than they did when those levels were normal.

When your blood sugar drops, all your body cares about is feeding itself to boost those levels, say the scientists. Your strategy: Keep hunger at bay with smart snacks (including protein) every few hours.

STOP THE POP

Soda layers on the worst kind of lard. In fact, soft drinks might lead to dangerous belly blubber. A study from Denmark found that heavy people who drank 1 liter

THE HARD TRUTH
81

The number of calories men eat per minute at lunch, according to the Obesity Society 2011 annual scientific meeting.

THE HARD TRUTH
52

The number of calories women eat per minute at lunch, according to the Obesity Society 2011 annual scientific meeting.

of the sweet stuff daily for 6 months had a 23 percent boost in visceral fat and a 139 percent increase in liver fat compared with diet-soda drinkers.

Try a little fruit juice. At least it contains nutrients.

GRAB SOME BUDS

Need a good excuse for a guys' night out? Research in the *Journal of Applied Social Psychology* found that men choose food with more calories when they're around women. In the study, men who ate with only male buddies downed about 952 calories—but when a woman joined them, that number shot up to 1,162. Guys might try to eat more food to demonstrate manliness, the scientists say.

PIN HIM DOWN

Are doctors too polite? More than half of primary care physicians say that they sometimes skip giving specific weight-loss advice to their patients, even when those patients have weight-related health issues,

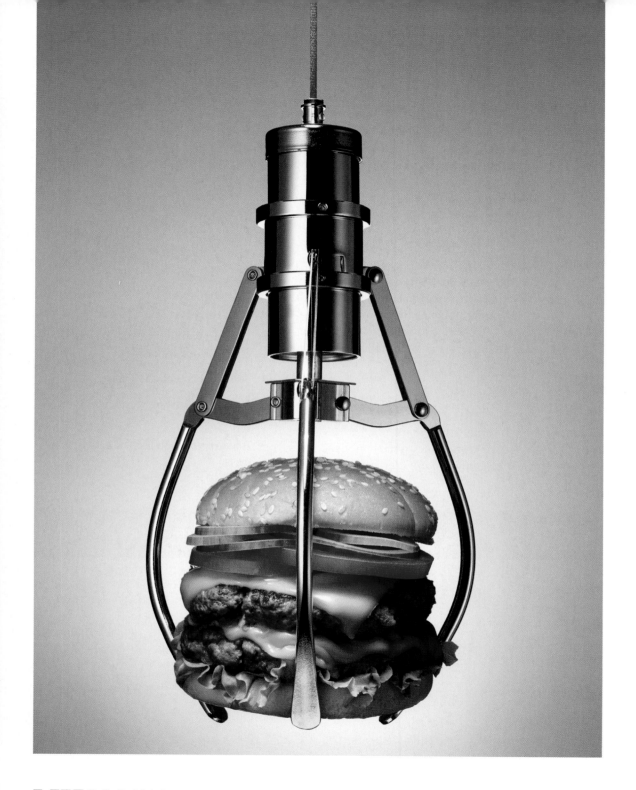

a new study finds. The researchers are exploring whether doctors' practices are understaffed or if the doctors' own diet behaviors may play a part.

Is your doctor holding back on you? Researchers at Virginia Commonwealth University discovered that physicians failed to recommend nearly half of the preventive services their patients were due to receive at yearly checkups. People were even less likely to receive screenings if they took time during their visits to mention health concerns. See how often doctors missed key tests in the chart below—and when you should push for them, according to the U.S. Preventive Services Task Force and Ted Epperly, M.D., *Men's Health* family-medicine advisor.

SET BETTER GOALS

Fads don't work. A new study published in the *American Journal of Preventive Medicine*

pinpointed many elements of successful weight-loss and weight-maintenance programs.

Weight Loss

- Do exercises you enjoy.

- Limit sugar. Limit sweets to no more than 10 percent of your daily calories.

- Think about how much better you feel when you're thinner.

Weight Maintenance

- Remind yourself why you need to control your weight.

- Track motivation in a journal.

- Carve out time for a consistent exercise routine.

- Reward yourself for sticking to your diet.

TEST	PERCENTAGE OF VISITS DURING WHICH THE TEST WAS MISSED	WHEN TO TEST
Diabetes	63 percent	If your blood pressure exceeds 135/80, if you have a diabetic parent or sibling, or if you've noticed extra thirst and urination
Cholesterol	45 percent	If you're 35 or older, or if you're 20 or older and are obese or have high BP, diabetes, or heart disease or a family history of it
Hypertension	8 percent	At every visit or at least every 2 years

Both Weight Loss and Maintenance

- Make grocery lists.

- Weigh yourself often.

- Eat fruits and vegetables. People were more than twice as likely to lose weight when they ate fruits and vegetables often.

Another study, this one at New York University, found that revealing weight-loss goals can make you less likely to follow through. People who shared their resolutions with others were less likely to enact them. One reason: Calling attention to your good intentions can create a premature sense of attainment, the researchers say.

HAIL TO THE CHEESE

Don't be afraid to grab some cheese if you're trying to build muscle—or lose weight. The latest news: A Danish study reports that a daily dose won't raise your total or LDL cholesterol levels.

Go ahead, enjoy this muscle-building, hunger-killing snack.

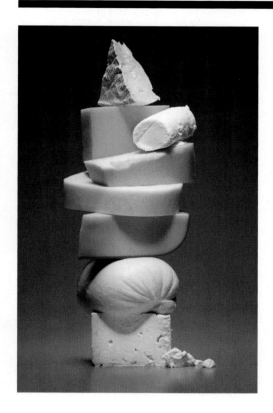

CHEESE (1-OUNCE SERVING)	PROTEIN	CALORIES
Brie	6 grams	95
Cheddar	7 grams	114
Goat (semisoft)	6 grams	103
Gruyère	8 grams	117
Provolone	7 grams	100
Gouda	7 grams	101
Mozzarella	6 grams	85
Feta	4 grams	75

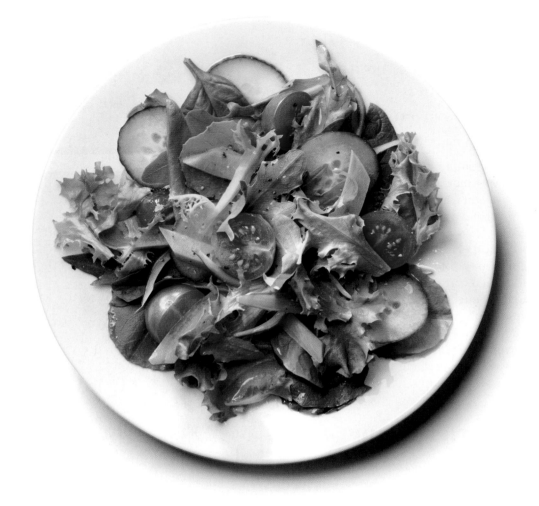

"Even though full-fat cheese has more calories than diet versions, it keeps you satiated for a much longer time," says Alan Aragon, M.S., a *Men's Health* nutrition advisor. "Plus, it tastes a million times better."

More good news: Eating cheese won't raise your cholesterol. When people consumed 13 percent of their daily calories from cheese, they saw no rise in their total or LDL (bad) cholesterol levels, a study in the *American Journal of Clinical Nutrition* found. The fermentation process in cow's milk cheese might be responsible for negating cholesterol-raising effects. So go ahead and have three deli slices of cheese a day. It's a great way to boost your protein and calcium intake.

Just be careful not to overindulge, because the calories can add up. Limit your cheese snacking to once in any given day—and know the stats. (See the chart on page 43.)

EAT GREEN; GET LEAN

Use that salad fork. Adding food to your meal can actually save you calories, according to Penn State University researchers. In the study, people who added a salad to their entree consumed 11 percent fewer calories than when they ate no greens with their meal. The reason: Eating a salad increases your satiety levels without packing on calories, say the scientists.

BE PRO PROTEIN

Beware: Failing to eat enough protein might cause you to gain weight, say researchers from Australia. In the study, people who consumed 10 percent of their diet as protein took in 1,000 more calories over the course of 4 days than those who consumed 15 percent from protein.

The lower-protein group probably wasn't as satiated, the scientists say. Eat 1 gram of protein for every pound of your target body weight.

KEEP IT OFF

Know your limit. To stay slim, set an upper weight limit and use it as a cue to take action. British researchers found that successful dieters typically have an "allowable" weight range (with a fluctuation leeway of 2 to 7 pounds). Your limit is a signal to change your diet, the scientists say.

CLIMB OUT OF THE GENE POOL

Don't worry if fatness runs in your family. A new multinational study reveals that being active lowers a person's genetic risk of obesity. Carriers of the FTO gene (which is associated with obesity) who exercised were 30 percent less likely than their sedentary counterparts to be obese. The scientists speculate that a healthy lifestyle could influence the FTO gene.

Q My dad is very overweight, and I need to lose about 20 pounds. Could "fat" be in my genes?

A: We'd like to say "fat chance," but odds are good that your double helix can predispose you to a double chin. Research in the *International Journal of Obesity* estimates that about 79 percent of your BMI is determined by DNA, with environmental factors making up the difference.

But don't panic—your genes aren't the final word on your weight, says Jeanne McCaffery, Ph.D., an associate professor of psychiatry and human behavior at the Miriam Hospital and the Warren Alpert School of Medicine at Brown University. "A healthy diet and exercise plan can turn down the effect these genes have on your weight."

Start with your diet: If you make sure that at least 25 percent of your calories come from protein, you might lessen the effects of certain obesity-related genes, according to Harvard University research. Then turn up the exercise dial: In a study from the Lawrence Berkeley National Laboratory, men who ran 1.9 to 3.7 miles a day reduced the influence of genetics on their BMI by 29 percent.

Q How should I talk to my 12-year-old son about his ballooning weight?

A: Keep the focus off his fat. Start by mentioning that you've noticed the whole family needs to adopt healthier habits, says Ellen Rome, M.D., M.P.H., head of the Center for Adolescent Medicine at Cleveland Clinic Children's Hospital.

"Kids who feel teased or berated by their parents about their weight don't cope with it well," she says. "What you say and do matters."

So here's your script: Outline the changes that you'll all try to make together, such as eating more vegetables and taking walks after dinner. Next, identify soft spots in your son's routine. Does he eat breakfast? A study in the *International Journal of Obesity* found that kids who skipped breakfast had greater increases in BMI than morning eaters did. If he's pressed for time in the morning, stock up on portable foods, such as bananas and small nut packages, that he can eat on his way out the door.

Another red flag: He parks it in front of the TV every day. According to research from the Netherlands, children who watch 90 minutes or more of TV a day are 70 percent more likely to be overweight than those who view less. Bottom line: Set limits on everyone's TV time. If you notice your son sliding from husky into truly heavy territory, ask your pediatrician to help you devise a customized diet and exercise plan, or look for a dietitian who specializes in pediatric nutrition (eatright.org/iframe/findrd.aspx).

Q Is it true that we can never really get rid of fat cells?

A: Hear that sucking sound? It's from all the liposuction procedures being performed around the world. Although lipo is the only way to eliminate fat cells, you can shrink them by losing weight. Think of your fat cells as plastic grocery bags filled with sticks of butter. You can discard the butter and shrink the bag by (you guessed it) watching what you eat and how you exercise.

Sleep is also critical: Scientists in Canada recently found that dieters lost an extra 1.6 pounds of fat, on average, for each additional hour they slept at night.

Q How can I control cravings?

A: One word: Abstraction.

This mind trick can help you resist temptation. To do it, mentally distance yourself from the present and look into the future—by considering the consequences one action could have on your ultimate goal, says Kentaro Fujita, Ph.D., an assistant professor of psychology at Ohio State University.

"The key is to think beyond the moment when you feel like grabbing a doughnut or some chips." Ask yourself: Does indulging suggest that I am mentally weak? How many squats will I have to do tomorrow to burn off these calories?

Q What is carb cycling?

A: It's a strategy for bulking up while keeping your body fat down.

"Most men who are trying to build muscle tend to gain some fat, too," says Mike Roussell, Ph.D., a nutrition consultant in State College, Pennsylvania. That's like taking one step forward and one step back.

Carb cycling, by contrast, "is like taking two steps forward and one step back." See, when you eat more carbohydrates than you need for fueling your metabolism, your body turns the carbs into glucose and shuttles it off to your fat and muscle cells. This causes your belly to grow along with your biceps. That's where carb cycling kicks in: You boost your carb intake on days you exercise and cut back on days you don't. With this strategy, your body must draw on its stored energy reserves for power, which means you'll be burning fat.

To give carb cycling a spin, use this menu: On workout days, eat a balanced carb-fat-protein diet, emphasizing high-fiber carbs like beans, whole grains, and fruit. On rest days, go with leafy greens and fibrous vegetables, and keep your carb intake under 100 grams.

CRUNCHY PB: WOODSTOCK FOODS ORGANIC CLASSIC

Crunchy yet easy to spread, it has a hint of sugar that sweetens without cranking the calorie count. Use it as a dip with celery and carrot sticks or apple and banana slices.

190 calories, 7 grams protein, 2 grams fiber, 55 milligrams sodium

SMOOTH PB: CREAM-NUT NATURAL

A three-time winner in our 125 Best Foods for Men, Cream-Nut impressed tasters with its fresh-roasted flavor. The velvety consistency makes it easy to blend into smoothies. Just stir before using.

190 calories, 8 grams protein, 2 grams fiber, 35 milligrams sodium

ON-THE-GO PB: POCKETFUEL

Protein makes PB an ideal post-workout snack, but in a jar? Toss squeeze packs in your bag instead.

263 calories, 10 grams protein, 5 grams fiber, 60 milligrams sodium (per 50 gram pack)

NUT ALTERNATIVE: SUNBUTTER ORGANIC UNSWEETENED

This spread, made with roasted sunflower seeds in a nut-free facility, is ideal for anyone with a nut allergy. Note: Some tasters found it slightly bitter, so pair it with something sweet, such as honey.

220 calories, 6 grams protein, 2 grams fiber, 30 milligrams sodium

ALMOND BUTTER: JUSTIN'S CLASSIC

Almonds have more fiber than peanuts, making this a filling alternative to traditional PB. Justin's stands out for its smoothness and subtly sweet flavor.

180 calories, 4 grams protein, 3 grams fiber, 65 milligrams sodium

Nutrition figures are based on a 2-tablespoon serving unless otherwise noted.

Can I really lose weight by eating more peanut butter?

A: Remember how Elvis looked toward the end? All those PB-and-banana sandwiches didn't help him fit into a slimmer jumpsuit. So no, peanut butter will not magically melt your middle.

What it might do, however, is help you avoid a king-size gut in the first place. Researchers in Spain found that men who ate about 3½ tablespoons of nut butter twice a week were 40 percent less likely to be overweight or obese than those who didn't dig in.

"Peanut butter is a good source of healthy unsaturated fats and protein," says Cyril Kendall, Ph.D., a researcher of nutritional science at the University of Toronto. "These nutrients are highly satisfying and help regulate your blood sugar so you don't have cravings."

Before you spread PB on your bread, check out our picks for the best-tasting peanut butters with less than 100 milligrams of sodium in a 2-tablespoon serving, and no hydrogenated oils (a source of trans fats). You might have to stir them, but you can keep the oils mixed by storing the jars upside down. Oh, and guys? Go easy on the jelly.

What's the best body-weight move to build muscle and burn fat?

A: Step onto the mat: Greco-Roman wrestlers swear by this sequence, called the Gut Wrench, says Zach Even-Esh, a trainer at Underground Strength Gym in Edison, New Jersey.

"Grapplers explosively push, pull, twist, and squat hundreds of pounds, all at a fast pace," he says. "This series trains them to do just that, which is one reason wrestlers have among the best strength-to-weight ratios in sports."

Do the moves on pages 50 and 51 as a sequence. Start a stopwatch, do 1 repetition, and rest for the remainder of 1 minute. In minute 2, do 2 reps and rest for the balance of that minute. In the third minute, do 3 reps and rest for the remainder. Continue adding reps until you can't complete the allotted number of reps in 1 minute. That's 1 set. As a full workout, do enough sets to fill 15 minutes. Or as a fat-burning finisher to a regular workout, do 2 sets.

Sit-through

Assume a bear-crawl position, with your hands and toes on the floor and your knees bent and held slightly off the floor under your hips (A). Lift your right foot and bring your right knee toward your chest as you lift your left hand and rotate your body up to the left. Straighten your right leg (B). Return to the starting position and repeat to your other side, lifting your left foot and right hand (C).

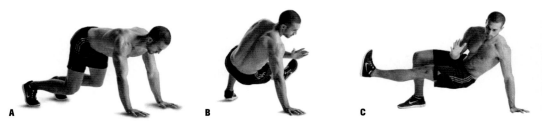

Burpee

Return to the bear-crawl position, straighten your legs (D), and do a pushup (E). Pull your feet toward your hands (F).

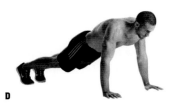 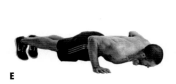 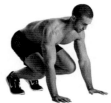

Pullup

Jump up (G) and grab a pullup bar using an overhand grip. Squeeze your shoulder blades together and pull your chest to the bar (H). Pause, and lower your body back to a dead hang.

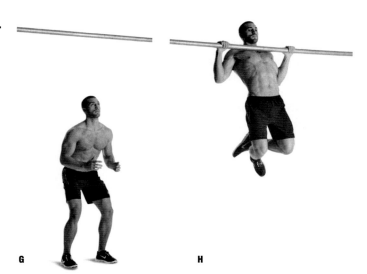

Squat

Drop to the floor and squat (I). Keeping your lower back naturally arched, push your hips back, bend your knees, and lower your body as deeply as you can into a squat, placing your hands on the floor in front of you (J). Kick your legs back into a bear-crawl position (A). That's 1 rep.

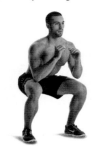

I

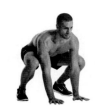

J

Q **Is that moneymaker muscle pure genetics, or is there an exercise that can shape my abs that way?**
A: No chromosome comes with the assigned function "create inguinal crease."

As for an exercise, well, Mike Boyle, C.S.C.S., of Mike Boyle Strength and Conditioning in Woburn, Massachusetts, does have a move in mind: "The table pushaway—you know, push away from the table and focus on eating less."

That's because the only way to reveal your moneymaker is to reduce your body fat to less than 10 percent. And no, it's not going to be easy. Boyle recommends eating more lean protein and high-fiber foods, and staving off cravings by drinking green tea or water.

While you're melting off the top layer, strengthen the muscles underneath. Boyle likes the Swiss ball rollout because it activates both the lower and upper portions of your six-pack, and it targets your transversus abdominis, which lies beneath it.

Swiss Ball Rollout

Kneel directly in front of a Swiss ball and place your forearms and fists on top of it (A). Slowly roll the ball forward, straightening your arms and extending your body as far as you can without letting your lower back collapse (B). Flex your core muscles to pull the ball back to your knees. (Keep your core braced, and don't let your hips sag.) That's 1 rep. Do 3 sets of 10 reps at the end of every workout.

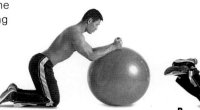

A

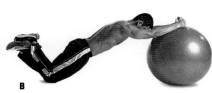

B

Q I drop pounds but always end up back at my starting weight. Why?

A: The reason you keep rebounding is something called set-point weight: This is the weight that your hormones and metabolism try to maintain—typically plus or minus about 10 pounds—in order to regulate fat stores.

Starvation or dieting, which often look the same to your body, conserves fat, says Mike Roussell, Ph.D., author of *The Six Pillars of Nutrition*. "When you cut your calorie intake, your metabolism slows to compensate and your body releases more appetite-boosting hormones, such as ghrelin."

Luckily, Roussell says, there's a single way to combat both reactions: intense exercise. A British study found that resistance training can suppress ghrelin levels for 2 hours. Other research suggests that resistance training and interval training can raise your metabolism for up to 24 hours after you stop exercising.

To successfully keep weight off, exercise 7 hours a week (or about 3,300 calories' worth of activity), combining strength training and intervals, says Roussell. Along with a diet low in refined carbs, this approach can also improve your insulin sensitivity, so your body stores less fat, effectively lowering your set-point weight.

Q Zumba is helping my girlfriend tone up. Should I try it?

A: You're wondering whether you should check out a fad workout for women that your gym buddies wouldn't be caught dead doing? Absolutely. Zumba's fast-paced Latin dance steps could help you burn as much as 550 calories in an hour while tacking on a mental challenge you just won't find on a treadmill.

What's more, because Zumba sessions mash up dance moves with exercises like squats and lunges, "it's a fun, fat-burning, fitness-improving, flexibility-enhancing workout," says BJ Gaddour, C.S.C.S., CEO of StreamFit. His only caution: While that cha-cha slide can crush calories, it won't stress your muscles enough to spark growth. That's why Gaddour advises strength training twice or three times a week and then doing Zumba on your off days.

Q **I know fruits and vegetables such as broccoli can help with weight loss. I'd eat more broccoli if it tasted better. How can I do that?**

A: Mustard is a must. Mix this yellow with that green, and the result is a more bearable broccoli. It'll also be more nutritious, says Elizabeth Jeffery, Ph.D., a professor of nutritional sciences at the University of Illinois.

"Mustard triggers the release of sulforaphane and indoles, compounds in broccoli that help your liver destroy carcinogens and other toxins." In fact, eating three to five servings of cruciferous vegetables a week can decrease your risk of prostate cancer by about 40 percent, says Jeffery.

You can also try these other flavor-masking tricks.

- Toss the florets in olive oil and 1 teaspoon of sugar and roast for 10 minutes at 450°F—the broccoli will caramelize, becoming less bitter.

- Chop up a head of broccoli and add it to chicken broth; simmer for 5 minutes and puree in a blender to make soup.

- Use broccoli sprouts instead of lettuce in a sandwich.

- You can also add horseradish or mix some broccoli into coleslaw or another cabbage dish; horseradish and cabbage work in synergy with broccoli, just as mustard does.

Whatever strategies you use, remember to keep some mustard on hand to add to your florets.

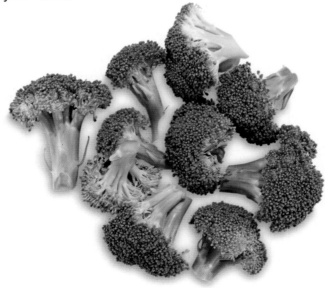

Eat Better

Men'sHealth

The Supermarket Survival Guide

The first step to eating better?
Navigating the aisles of the grocery store.

A hundred years ago, food was simple. People didn't worry about trans fats in their cheese crackers or artificial colors in their fruit snacks. They didn't have to: They were eating real cheese and real fruit. And food companies used to focus more on making food than on enticing people to buy it. That's why supermarkets are so daunting today: It's easy to make a false move, even when you're trying to eat healthy.

In the first half of 2010, supermarket ad spending increased by 19 percent over the first half of 2009.

"The influence of marketing on what Americans eat has been gigantic," says Frederick J. Zimmerman, Ph.D., chairman of the health services department at UCLA's school of public health. "We tend to eat 'typical' meals, but marketers are the ones who define what that is." It's time to follow our own rules.

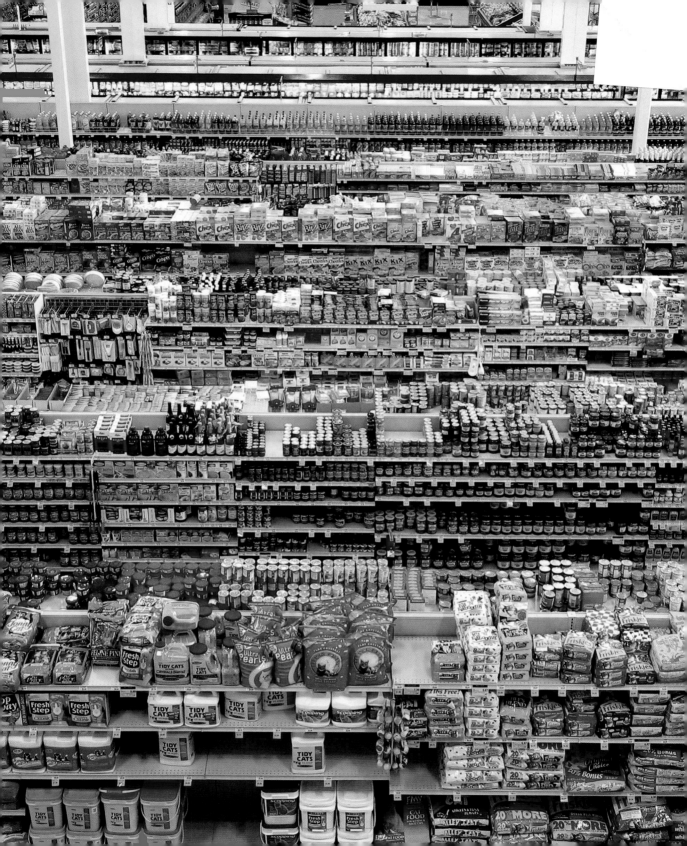

Ignore the packaging billboards.

Time for a turnaround. "The front of a food package is real estate owned by the manufacturer, whose goal is to sell you something," says *Men's Health* weight-loss advisor David Katz, M.D., M.P.H. Flip the package over to find the information you need on the one part that's well regulated by the FDA: the Nutrition Facts label.

Calories: A University of Minnesota study showed that 91 percent of shoppers often bypass the calorie count before buying an item. That's bad: If each meal exceeds your energy needs by just 170 calories, you can gain a pound a week.

Fat: Plenty of men still assume that if a food is low in fat, it's good for them and vice versa. Far from it, says Dr. Katz. A better approach: Seek out healthier omega-3 and monounsaturated fats to reap heart-health benefits.

Sodium: Some studies suggest that healthy men don't need to watch their sodium, but the more sodium a food has, the more processed it's likely to be. Rule of thumb: Don't buy foods with higher sodium counts than calories.

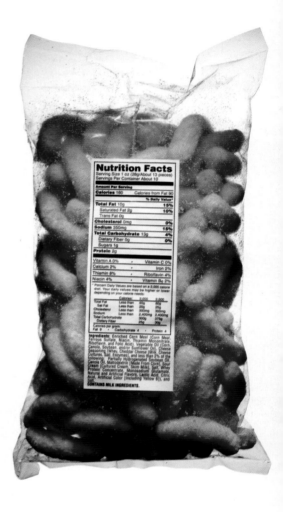

SKIMMER IN AISLE 9

Speed-reading can be unhealthy. In a simulated online shopping trip, most people read only the first five items on the Nutrition Facts panel, a study in the *Journal of the American Dietetic Association* found. That means they tended to skip critical data about carbohydrates, fiber, sugar, and sodium. Read on and you'll form a fuller picture of your food's nutrition.

Protein: An average active guy should take in at least 115 grams of protein a day, says *Men's Health* nutrition advisor Alan Aragon, M.S. Plus, protein-rich foods keep you full longer, so they might help prevent overeating.

Serving size: "Don't assume the amount listed is an accurate serving size for you," says Chris D'Adamo, Ph.D., a nutritional epidemiologist at the University of Maryland school of medicine. Assess how much you'll actually eat, and judge the impact accordingly, D'Adamo says.

Fiber: The USDA recommends 38 grams a day for men. To reach that, be sure to eat grain products that contain at least 2 grams of fiber per 100 calories.

Sugar: We consume about 10 percent more caloric sweeteners today than we did 30 years ago, the USDA reports. In that same period, adult obesity has doubled. Coincidence? Keep the sugars below 10 percent of total calories: That's 2½ grams of sugar per 100 calories, says Dr. Katz.

RULE #2
Challenge the cashier.

Every industry employs tools that make routine tasks easier. For register jockeys, it's the UPC bar code. UPCs let the cashier become a brainless automaton that dutifully drags cans and boxes over a static scanner. Fruits and vegetables are the cashier's enemy—no bar codes.

"I tell clients all the time to move from bar codes to bags," says nutrition consultant Mike Roussell, Ph.D.

In other words, the harder your cashier works, the healthier your purchase tends to be. You'll reap the rewards when you step on the scale: A 2009 *Journal of Nutrition* study of nearly half a million people found that men with diets high in

HOW AN ACTOR SHOPS

British actor Adewale Akinnuoye-Agbaje, best known for steely roles in *Oz* and *Lost*, is a busy man, starring in three feature films in a single year. After he gained weight for his role, in *Best Laid Plans*, he enlisted a nutritionist to help him drop 25 pounds. Here's how he thrives (and shops) now.

Focus on fish. Akinnuoye-Agbaje eats fish every day for lunch and dinner, so he looks for substantial cuts that will keep him satisfied. "My favorite is ahi tuna, because it's a thick, meaty fish," he says. It's also important to buy it fresh. Just look at the corners and be wary if it's changing color, he says.

Pass the carb aisles. Nowadays, Akinnuoye-Agbaje limits his carbohydrates, so for most supermarket trips, he avoids the cereal, grain, and bread aisles entirely.

Spice things up. "I tend to eat a lot less when I add chile peppers to my food," Akinnuoye-Agbaje says. "The spice helps me feel full." A Purdue University study supports the link between spiciness and satiety. He also deploys spice between meals, stifling hunger pangs by drinking water spiked with cayenne and lemon juice.

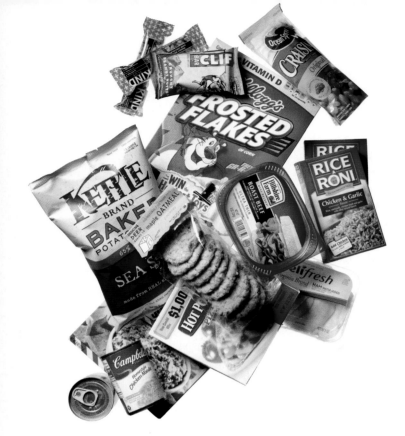

vegetables, seafood, legumes, fruits, nuts, and cereal grains—all foods typically purchased in bulk and without bar codes—had smaller waist circumferences.

Consider the recipe.

Twinkies, Pop-Tarts, French's Classic Yellow Mustard—they all have their recipes printed right on the package. It's near the Nutrition Facts label, buddy, under the word "ingredients."

"If the contents cannot be placed in any part of the universe you're familiar with—animal, vegetable, or mineral—then step away from the box and nobody will get hurt," says Dr. Katz. Here are three companies that have come clean and eliminated certain mystery additives.

HOW A DOCTOR SHOPS

Travis Stork, M.D., host of *The Doctors* and a *Men's Health* contributor is in his 40s. "When I was in my 20s it was all about muscle-building protein. But now when I shop, I pay more attention to foods that improve heart health," he says. "It's amazing how 'heart-healthy' translates to overall health. More energy, better sex—it's all related." So how does Dr. Stork navigate his cart? With this three-point approach.

Start in produce. "This guarantees that I'll put some fruits and vegetables in my cart," says Dr. Stork. "That's always a tough thing for guys." Two foods he routinely picks up are avocados and berries. One provides healthy fats that unclog arteries, and the other offers heart-healthy antioxidants that bring big flavor to oatmeal and whole-grain cereal.

Work the periphery. Once the bottom of his cart is sufficiently layered with produce, Dr. Stork takes a full lap around the edges of the store. That's where he finds the minimally processed foods—eggs, chicken, fish, cheese, Greek yogurt, and low-fat milk.

Balance your meals. With lean protein, dairy, and produce accounted for, Dr. Stork examines his cart and decides which packaged foods he needs for complete, balanced meals. "If I have chicken, then I might grab whole-wheat pasta and marinara. For my avocado, I'll probably pick up low-sodium black beans and whole-grain tortillas.

Eden Foods

What it eliminates: Bisphenol A

U.K. scientists have linked BPA, a chemical used to line metal cans, with heart disease and diabetes. Worse, a CDC study detected it in the urine of 95 percent of Americans tested. Recently, Eden Foods became the first U.S. producer of BPA-free canned goods.

Hormel Natural Choice

What it eliminates: Added nitrates and nitrites

In 2010 a Harvard University meta-analysis linked processed meats (not red meat itself) to coronary heart disease and listed nitrates and their by-products as some of the likely culprits. Hormel's Natural Choice line uses a high-pressure processing method instead.

Oh Boy! Oberto

What it eliminates: Hydrolyzed protein

Oberto's new all-natural jerky line skips this additive, which is chemically similar to MSG. That's good news: A study in the journal *Obesity* found that people who consumed the most MSG were almost three times as likely to be overweight as MSG avoiders were.

RULE #4
Call your rep in Congress.

The average U.S. household kicks in about $1,500 in annual subsidies, and the foods we subsidize most are among the least healthy, says Thomas Kostigen, author of *The Big Handout*. Check out the following foods (and nonfoods) your tax dollars support (U.S. subsidies from 1995

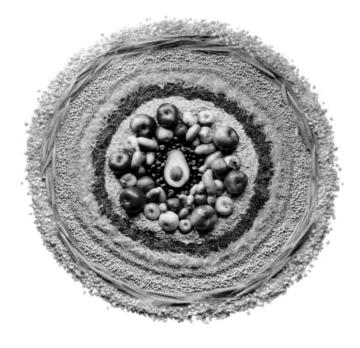

to 2010, according to the Environmental Working Group).

- Corn: $77.1 billion
- Wheat: $32.4 billion
- Soybeans: $24.3 billion
- Sorghum: $6.1 billion
- Dairy: $4.9 billion
- Tobacco: $1.1 billion
- Oats: $267 million
- Apples: $262 million
- Potatoes: $665,698
- Blueberries: $207,659
- Avocados: $6,984
- Tomatoes, broccoli, lettuce: $ 0

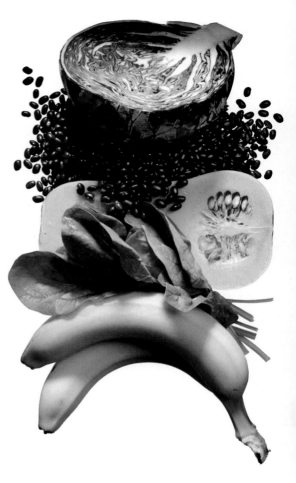

RULE #5
Master your impulses.

Easy-grab items at the market tend to be built from bottom-of-the-barrel ingredients—sugar, starch, and cheap fats. Use the following strategies to resist their siren song.

Grab a cart. A study in the *Journal of Marketing Research* shows that shopping with a basket instead of a cart makes you nearly seven times more likely to purchase vice foods like candy and chocolate. The researchers say that curling your arm inward to carry a basket increases your desire to embrace instant rewards—like sweet foods. With a cart, you tend to extend your arm—a motion associated with avoiding negative outcomes. That makes you more likely to shop smart.

Avoid lines. The longer you're exposed to tempting snacks at the checkout, the more likely you are to succumb to them, say University of Arizona researchers. Avoid the wait by shopping during off-peak hours, such as the middle of the week or late at night.

Leave the kids at home. "Children shouldn't have a vote in supermarket decisions," says Greg Critser, author of *Fat Land: How Americans Became the Fattest People in the World.* About 80 percent of parents report they'll probably buy snacks or frozen desserts if their kids ask for them at the grocery store, according to a 2011 Mintel report.

RULE #6
Shop the rainbow, cheaply.

To build a recession-ready cart, we compared prices of foods that scored 90 or higher on the NuVal scale, a sophisticated system used to rank their overall nutritional values. Then we chose the cheapest common items per serving from five spots on the color wheel. (All prices are per serving.)

Purple: Red cabbage, 15¢

A dose of vitamin A, fiber, and glucosinolates, which might help prevent some types of cancer

Black: Dry black beans, 12¢

Loaded with fiber and plenty of brain-boosting anthocyanins

Orange: Butternut squash, 19¢

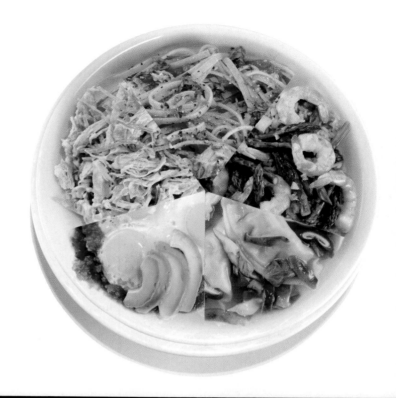

HOW A CHEF SHOPS

Seamus Mullen grew up on an organic farm in Vermont. Needless to say, Funyuns were never a big part of his diet. But when the chef-owner of Manhattan's Tertulia (and former *Next Iron Chef* contestant) was diagnosed with rheumatoid arthritis 5 years ago, his interest in food took a new turn. He's the author of *Seamus Mullen's Hero Food*. Now, he shares the "hero foods" that keep him healthy and satisfied.

Go in with a plan. "One of the biggest challenges in going to the supermarket is arriving there and not being sure what to buy," he says. "So I always shop with a plan for the next three meals I want to cook, plus any pantry items I need so I can throw something together."

Shell out for meat. The idea of an animal sitting in a feedlot with antibiotics and hormones coursing through its veins doesn't sit well with Mullen. "A rib steak from a grass-fed cow is going to have more omega-3 fats than one from a cow that's never seen pasture," he says. And when he's craving a hot dog, he heads to the butcher or looks for organic brands such as Applegate Farms.

Stock up on umami. Mullen always makes sure his kitchen is stocked with flavorful, savory foods such as cured meat, mushrooms, and blue cheese so he can add a hit of umami to platefuls of vegetables and whole grains.

Lots of beta-carotene, and less than half the calories of a sweet potato

Green: Spinach, 38¢

Packed with folate, a B vitamin shown to bolster cognitive performance

Yellow: Bananas, 13¢

Potassium-rich, with prebiotic fiber that promotes good gut bacteria

RULE #7
Shop for shortcuts.

Not all boxed, bagged, and jarred food is terrible, says J. Lynne Brown, Ph.D., R.D. Shortcut products with honest ingredient lists can save you time—and make a home-cooked dinner on a weeknight a viable option.

Start with the following meals; they all take less than 5 minutes and use five ingredients, max.

- Cook whole-wheat pasta. Simmer tomato sauce with crumbled tuna for 5 minutes. Toss together; top with chopped parsley.

- Stir-fry shrimp and asparagus in olive oil; add minced garlic at the last minute if you like. Top with a squeeze of lemon and serve over rice.

- Cook dumplings in simmering broth; add sliced shiitake mushrooms for the last 3 minutes and stir in spinach right before serving.

- In a small pan, heat salsa to simmering. Crack in eggs, cover, and cook until the whites are set. Serve with avocado and Wasa bread.

- Skin and shred rotisserie chicken; toss with bagged coleslaw mix. Add sriracha to yogurt and toss with the chicken slaw.

HOW AN ATHLETE SHOPS

A couple of years ago, Raul Ibanez, clutch-hitting left fielder for the Philadelphia Phillies, was constantly sore and short of breath. He ended up in a nutritionist's office, where Robert Pastore, Ph.D., told him he had delayed food allergies to gluten and casein, a dairy protein. He cut them out and started buying better foods, and his cholesterol dropped 40 points. Here's his game plan.

Pick your organics. All organics are not created equal. "If I'm going to eat the peel, I'll buy organic," he says. "Otherwise, I don't see the point." An Environmental Working Group study confirms the theory; it found that fruits eaten unpeeled tend to have higher pesticide levels.

Embrace healthy fat. Ibanez always puts nuts, avocados, olive oil, and coconut oil in his cart. "Your body needs the fat," he says. "I just like mine to be from natural sources."

Think 80 percent. "A friend says, 'If you can't pick it, pull it, hunt it, or fish it, don't eat it.' I follow that 80 percent of the time," Ibanez says.

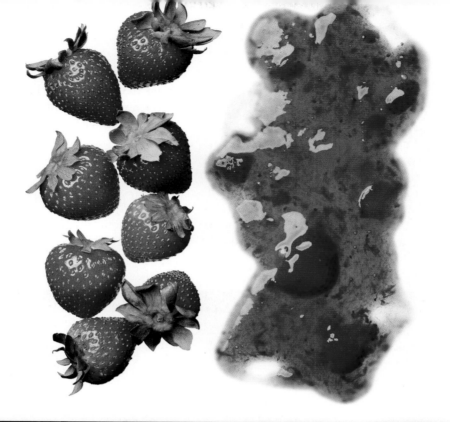

EAT $1 OF . . .	INSTEAD OF $1 OF . . .	YOU EARN
Sweet potatoes 1 lb	Ore-Ida Sweet Potato Fries 5.3 oz	More than quadruple the fiber, nearly five times the bone-building calcium, and more than 19 times the vitamin A
Broccoli 0.6 lb	Campbell's Cream of Broccoli Condensed Soup 7.75 oz, unprepared	Almost four times the fiber, twice the muscle-building protein, and an extra dose of vitamin K
Blueberries 2.9 oz	Kellogg's Blueberry Pop-Tarts (unfrosted) 3½ tarts	A dose of vitamins C and K, plus plenty of disease-fighting phytonutrients
Tomatoes 0.4 lb	Heinz Ketchup half of a 20 oz bottle	Twice the fiber—and less of a post-eating blood-sugar spike
Oats 3 cups (uncooked)	Nature Valley Oats 'N Honey Crunchy Granola Bar 4 bars	Four times the protein, six times the fiber, and nearly six times as much iron
Strawberries 4 oz	Smucker's Strawberry Topping 7½ Tbsp	Your RDA of vitamin C and get a dose of plant protein and fiber in the bargain

RULE #8
Invest in nutrients, not calories.

Conventional wisdom says that healthy food costs more than junk food. "The notion of food value that everyone embraces is calories per dollar," says Dr. Katz. The problem is, we're no longer starving Paleolithic hunters. We live in an age of pandemic obesity, and processed foods have made calories abundant and nutrients scarce. Shop for nutrients, not calories, and see where the real value lies.

RULE #9
Fill your cart with dark.

When it comes to whole foods, more pigment often means more nutrient power.

UPGRADE FROM . . .	TO . . .	THE PAYOFF
Light beer	Dark beer	More iron and cancer-fighting polyphenols
Honeydew melon	Cantaloupe	Double the vitamin C, plus nearly 70 times the vitamin A and beta-carotene
White wine	Red wine	A dose of sleep-regulating hormone melatonin and the heart-healthy antioxidant resveratrol
Chicken breast	Dark-meat chicken	Nearly triple the iron, 245 percent more zinc, and extra vitamin B12
Iceberg lettuce	Spinach	Triple the protein, a higher concentration of powerful antioxidants like beta-carotene, and 19 times the vitamin A
White rice	Brown rice	Thirty percent more of the antioxidant selenium and 4½ times the fiber
Table sugar	Maple syrup	100 times the heart-healthy potassium
Apple juice	Pomegranate juice	Vitamin K, cell-building folate, and abundant antioxidants
Potato	Sweet potato	More than a day's worth of vitamin A, 2½ times the calcium, and 50 percent more fiber
Milk chocolate	Dark chocolate	Three and a half times the iron, plus extra antioxidants
White mushrooms	Baby bellas	Six times the calcium, 40 percent more potassium, and almost triple the selenium

RULE #10
Beware the natural food store.

Fancy food shops can still wreck your waistline.

Don't assume it's healthy. In a study in the *Journal of Consumer Research,* people estimated familiar foods to have up to 35 percent fewer calories when they came from a "healthy" place. But be warned: Trader Joe's, Whole Foods Market, and Fresh Market all stock plenty of stuff that can make you fat. One cup of Trader Joe's Pecan Praline Granola has as many calories as two twin-wrapped packages of Reese's Peanut Butter Cups.

Watch out for the free samples. Stanford researchers discovered that a tasty sample can make you more likely to engage in reward-seeking behavior, such as buying foods you normally wouldn't go for.

Don't fall for fads. Just because that scone is vegan, lactose-free, and made with positively charged ions doesn't mean it isn't still loaded with calories. Whole Foods' Gluten Free Vanilla Cupcake has 480 calories, but you wouldn't know that, because foods prepared in-house don't have to carry nutrition labels.

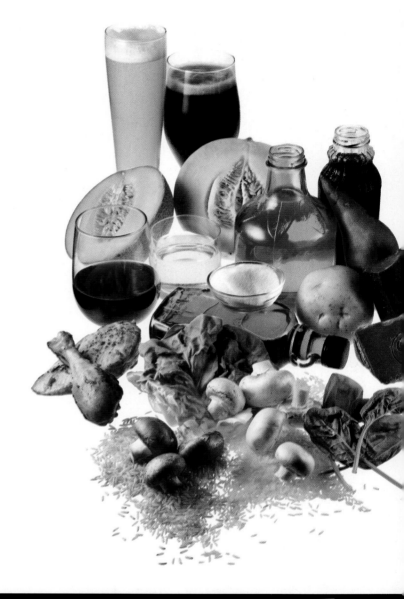

READ THIS!

Make your next trip to the supermarket a healthier one: Pick up a copy of the new updated edition of *Eat This, Not That! All New Supermarket Survival Guide,* by former *Men's Health* Editor-in-Chief David Zinczenko and Matt Goulding, in stores and online at eatthisnotthatbook.com/sm.

Alternative Fuels

We've debunked taurine and guarana for years. But energy drink makers have found new ways to entice you. Don't be fooled.

America is in the midst of an energy crisis. We're guzzling energy drinks and shots at record rates but feeling more lethargic than ever. Sales of these products have more than doubled in the past 5 years, with 35 percent of men ages 18 to 24 drinking them regularly, a new Mintel survey reveals.

"Guys create an up-and-down trap with energy drinks and with whatever they take at night to help slow down," says Matthew Edlund, M.D., author of *The*

Power of Rest. "They never feel completely rested."

Or, even scarier, they end up on a gurney in the E.R. Hospital visits related to energy drinks have surged more than tenfold since 2005, reports the U.S. Center for Behavioral Health Statistics and Quality. And most of those amped-up patients are men.

"Energy drinks emphasize vigor, power, all the things that appeal to men," says Cecile Marczinski, Ph.D., an assistant

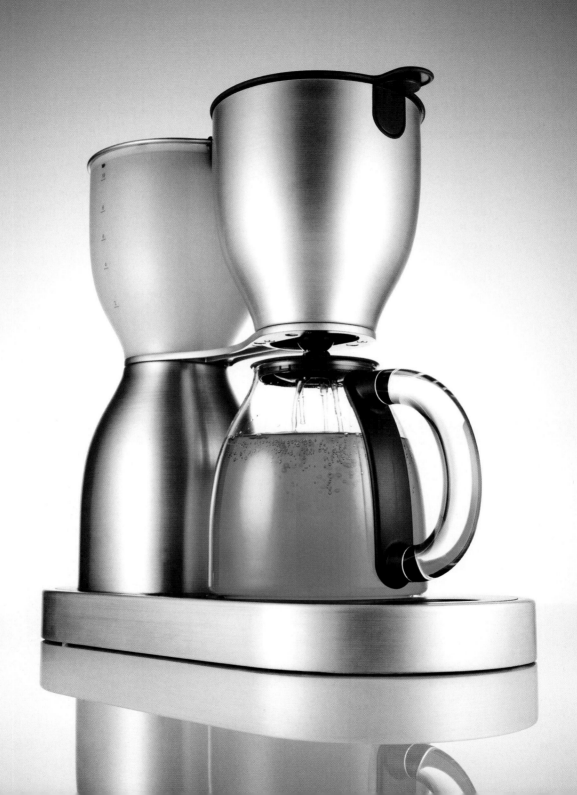

It's no wonder we walk around like zombies—and treat these drinks like liquid life support.

professor of psychology at Northern Kentucky University. Guys willingly swallow the bottled boosters' claims, when they should really be asking, "Why am I so damn tired?"

"We don't use our bodies the way they're built to be used," says Dr. Edlund. "We guzzle energy drinks and then can't sleep at night. We sit all day and then read e-mails at 3 a.m." It's no wonder we walk around like zombies—and treat these drinks like liquid life support. As sales and heart rates spike, it's a good time to question the trends and find healthier ways to power up.

ENERGY SPIKE #1
Decaf Energy Drinks

Marketers of energy drinks are clever. They remove a well-known, often worrisome compound and then tout the resulting drink as a "healthier" version of the original. The first vilified ingredient was sugar. Now it's caffeine. Hydrive and 5-Hour Energy have both unveiled decaf options. Makes sense: Some 38 percent of men who buy energy drinks now look for low caffeine content, the Mintel survey found.

So what's the alleged alternate energy source? Most often, B vitamins. A decaf 5-Hour Energy shot, for example, packs several thousand times your daily recommended B_{12} and B_6, plus 100 percent of

RELAXATION IN A BOTTLE?

Don't rely on these drinks to wind down. The science is too foggy.

If energy drinks are the bad boys of the cold case, relaxation drinks are the stoners. Currently, an estimated 400 "anti-energy" drinks are sold in the United States, and they share one common promise: "Drink this, and you'll chill." So what's their alleged soothing secret? A blend of ingredients such as melatonin, valerian, GABA, and 5-HTP, all of which are purported to induce sleep, relieve anxiety, or both. The effect might be very different from what is advertised because only the individual ingredients, not the combinations, might have been studied.

Or there may be no effect at all: "Many of these ingredients degrade in water," says Joe Vinson, Ph.D., a professor of chemistry at the University of Scranton.

Your alternative: a noncaffeinated herbal tea. In a 2012 Australian study, drinking caffeine-free beverages was linked to increased relaxation and work-stress recovery.

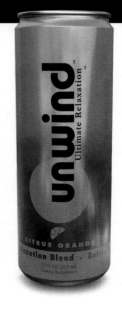

your folic acid. But here's the thing: You won't feel a B-induced boost, because the energy provided by B vitamins isn't stimulating like caffeine.

"They simply help extract energy from your food, and you need only a little bit," says Tod Cooperman, M.D., president of ConsumerLab.com, an independent tester of health and nutritional products. "The science is misused to lead people to believe that a megadose of B vitamins will somehow energize them. It won't."

Plus, if you eat fortified foods or take a multivitamin, energy shots could send you over the folic-acid edge—which in the long term, he warns, could raise your cancer risk.

Your Move

For a caffeine-free boost, sip on FRS Healthy Energy drinks. They're free of folic acid and contain reasonable levels of the other B vitamins. What makes FRS effective is quercetin, an antioxidant that can help you fight fatigue during exercise, a 2010 University of South Carolina study found. Like caffeine, quercetin also blocks brain receptors for adenosine—a chemical that makes you sleepy—to make you feel energized, says study author Mark Davis, PhD.

"Over time, it can also increase the number of mitochondria in your cells," he says, "which provide energy for your muscles."

ENERGY SPIKE #2
Coffee Energy Drinks

Herbal ingredients might trigger a guy's skepticism, but coffee appeals to the average Joe.

"Coffee is a commonly consumed, relatively safe product," says Marczinski. "So people may assume coffee energy drinks are safe, too."

But even if the label says "coffee," you might still be downing an alphabet soup of ingredients. Java Monster, for example, which claims to contain "premium coffee and cream," is actually a blend of coffee extract, milk, taurine, panax ginseng, caffeine, and guarana.

"Panax ginseng has been linked to pretty significant side effects, including abdominal pain and headaches," says University of Massachusetts toxicologist Richard Church, M.D. And guarana is just an herbal guise for an extra shot of caffeine. Its seeds pack about four times the caffeine of coffee beans.

Your Move

Fire up the coffeepot instead.

"In addition to the caffeine boost, coffee can lower your risk of depression, diabetes, and Parkinson's disease," says Dr. Edlund. "Plus, it has a healthy social element. You're often with others when you drink coffee."

If you're brewing at home, opt for light-roast blends, such as the new Starbucks Blonde Roast. These offer significantly more antioxidants than dark roasts, a 2011 Portuguese study found.

ENERGY SPIKE #3
Energy Shots

Red Bull recently introduced giant cans, but the bigger trend is toward shrinking drinks.

The lure of energy shots—
the promise of instant
crash-free energy—is
exactly what makes them
dangerous.

According to a Mintel estimate, Americans dropped about $1.3 billion on energy shots in 2011—more than 17 times the $73 million they spent in 2006. What's the lure? The promise of crash-free energy in just a couple of sips—in other words, the very effect that makes these drinks dangerous.

"Shots contain all the stimulants of large energy drinks," says Marczinski. "But because they're only a couple of sips, people often drink more than one. They're using energy shots to stay up all night."

Your Move

There's a better way to fuel up before a night out.

"Drink a lukewarm cup of coffee really quickly, and then close your eyes for 15 to 20 minutes," says Michael Breus, Ph.D., a sleep specialist in Virginia Beach. "You'll get enough rest to decrease your sleep drive. Then after you start moving again, the caffeine will kick in to keep you awake."

Before you head out, grab a protein-rich snack, too, such as a handful of almonds. "Protein helps increase insulin production, and insulin can have an alerting effect," he says.

ENERGY SPIKE #4
Juice and Tea Drinks

About half of energy drink consumers are interested in juice- or tea-based alternatives, according to Mintel. That's a bright spot: Juices contain many of the same vitamins added to energy drinks, but in their natural form.

"Food is not one substance or vitamin," Dr. Edlund says. Whole foods provide a matrix of nutrients, some of which might enhance others' effects in your body, he says. So isolating a single nutrient could rob you of the whole food's full benefits. And while Red Bull might amp you up more effectively than tea, the liquid in that silver can lacks tea's disease-fighting antioxidants.

Your Move

Check the label: Juice and tea should replace, rather than accompany, energy drink ingredients such as guarana and B vitamins. We like the new V8 Berry Blast Energy Shot—each 50-calorie serving offers a blend of 10 juices and green tea extract, and it's refreshingly devoid of unpronounceable additives.

Or just grab a bottle of tea. According to a 2008 study in the journal *Psychopharmacology*, the combination of caffeine and theanine, an amino acid in tea, might boost alertness without raising blood pressure as much as caffeine does alone. Try Honest Tea Community Green Tea; it's lower in sugar than most bottled brews.

Nonliquid Energy

Energy boosts no longer require a bottle. Rockstar and Amp now come in gum form, with 40 milligrams of caffeine in a single piece; products like LiveWire and High Octane energy chews claim to pack as much caffeine as a cup of coffee.

The danger: "People think a stick of gum is a stick of gum. Before they know it, they've crammed five pieces into their mouths," says Dr. Church. That's like drinking a pot of coffee—but with a side of artificial sweeteners or, in the case of the chews, corn syrup and evaporated cane juice.

What's brewing in those energy drink bottles? The answer just might be an eye-opener.

Your Move

Close your eyes and focus on a specific place of tension on your head or neck, Dr. Edlund says. "Removing one spot of tension can help your entire body relax. Focus and energy are closely related."

The Butcher Is Back

There's a new class of chefs picking up their cleavers to reclaim and revive the art of butchery. With some basic skills—and the right recipes—you can, too.

Think about the best burger you've ever had. Was it the tomato slice that made it so memorable? The lettuce leaf? The bun? In all likelihood, you're thinking, hell no, it was the savory, tender, juicy beef patty that gave that burger its identity.

The customers in line at the 4505 Meats stand know this in their bones. The Saturday sun is just beginning to bathe San Francisco's Ferry Plaza Farmers Market, but even at this early hour, hungry patrons are waiting for a taste of a freshly ground 4505 burger. This one needs little more than a soft but sturdy bun, a swipe of coriander aioli, and some sliced scallions. Bite in, and the elemental meatiness will likely unseat whichever burger currently holds your top spot.

So who's the genius chef behind this burger of burgers? Actually, the man is more than just a chef. He's also a butcher. And what he and others like him can teach you about meat will help you unlock the true potential in your protein.

The State of the American Butcher

We've never eaten more meat than we're eating today. The average American consumed 66 more pounds of the stuff in 2009 than in 1950. The irony is that most men pick up their proteins at the supermarket; they know little about where the

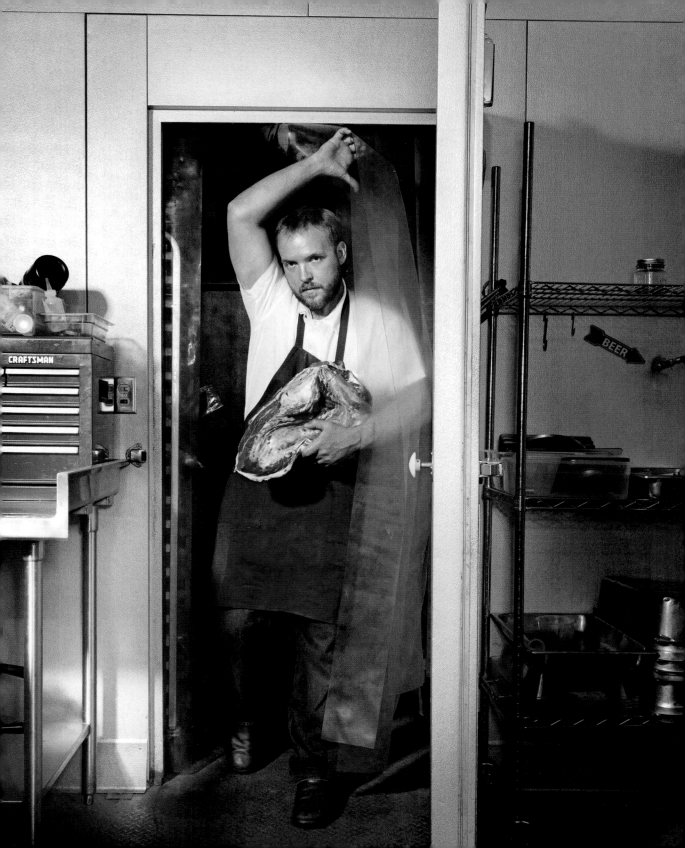

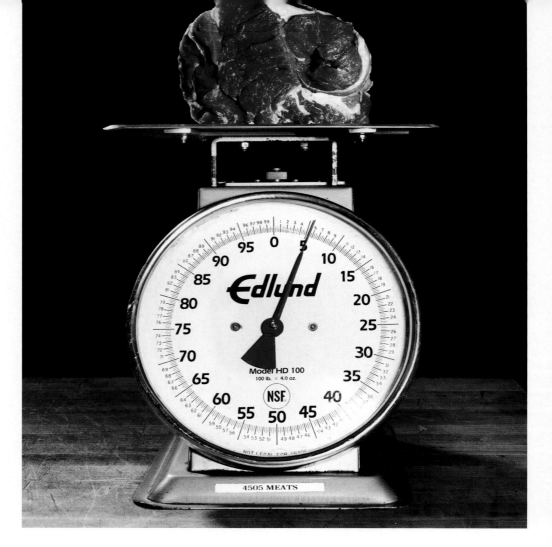

TIP #1

"Ask your butcher where the meat comes from and how the animal was raised. The less distance it travels, the better it ends up tasting."

—RYAN FARR

animals came from or how they were raised, or whether tastier cuts might be available elsewhere. And despite our ever-increasing appetite for meat, butchers are in danger of extinction. Well, real butchers, anyway.

Nowadays it's more common to find meat wrapped in plastic than in butcher paper. The Bureau of Labor Statistics projects only a 1 percent increase in jobs for butchers from 2008 to 2018, but an average 5 percent growth for slaughterers,

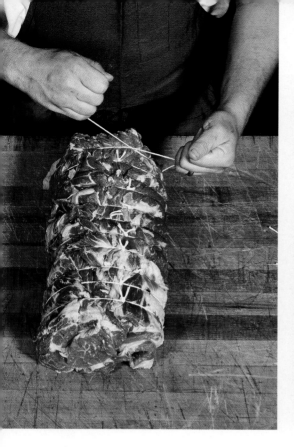

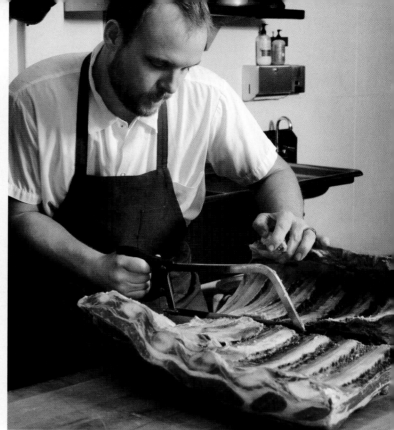

meatpackers, and "cutters and trimmers." Increasingly, these lower-paid, generally less skilled workers are the ones slinging your meat at the supermarket.

So what, right? As long as your shrink-wrapped protein is in the meat case, who cares who sold it to you?

"Well, first of all, people are missing out on flavor," says Brady Lowe, founder of Cochon 555, a nationwide competition that showcases pig butchering. "We fell asleep one night and woke up to flavorless meat products packaged on an industrial scale, and commodity cuts wearing meat diapers in the grocery store because they've been pumped with water and other untasty things.

"Butcher shops have to carry flavorful,

natural meat because if they didn't, they'd lose customers," Lowe adds. "Supermarkets don't have to do that. They assume their customers have few other options."

But butchers are more than just good sources of quality meat. They're resources themselves. It's like the difference between taking your car to a Jiffy Lube and entrusting it to the master mechanic you've known for years.

"The butcher shop used to be a place you'd visit once a week," says Jessica Applestone, co-owner of Fleisher's Grass-fed and Organic Meats in Kingston, New York. "Your butcher could put in special orders, tell you about the farm the meat came from, make suggestions based on your tastes, give you recipes, and make

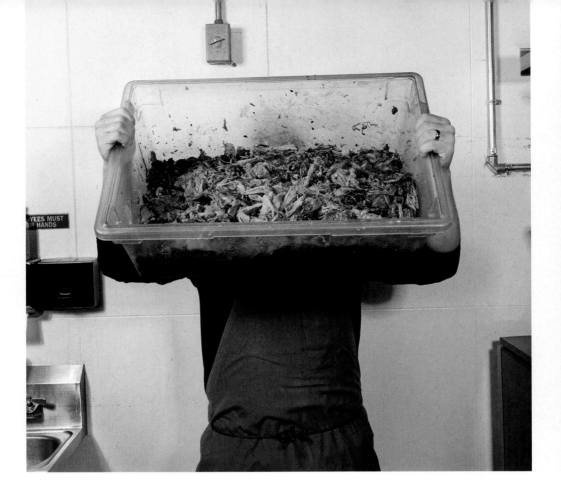

cuts to your specifications. Today we've lost that connection and the wealth of knowledge that goes with it."

It's no surprise, then, that a butcher created that perfect patty at 4505 Meats. If he could elevate a burger to best-ever status, what else can butchers teach us?

Welcome to Meat School

Ryan Farr, the 30-something owner and head butcher of 4505 Meats, doesn't run your typical butcher shop operation. It's more of a studio, really, with no storefront or dining tables—like a butchery garage, he says.

The Friday before market day, while the patty machine clanks to a beat—cha-CHUNK, cha-CHUNK—Farr's team members prepare turduckens (a kind of poultry nesting doll) for 4505's mail-order business. They also churn out his trademark bacon-studded hot dogs and handmade *chicharrones* (fried pork rinds).

Farr's burger process starts with cutting grass-fed, dry-aged beef from the Magruder Ranch in Potter Valley, Califor-

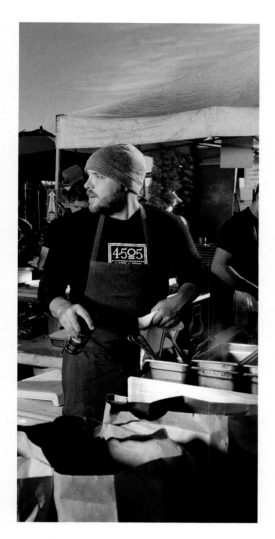

TIP #2

"Always quiz butchers about their favorite cuts of meat and how they like them prepared. Go for offbeat choices. Mix it up."

—EVAN LOBEL

nia, into 1-inch chunks. Then he sidles up to a meat grinder and passes the meat through a large die for a rustic, coarse texture.

Next, Farr turns to a whole forequarter of a cow that he has lugged from his storage fridge. He breaks it down into skirt steak, rib sections, and chuck that he'll pack up to sell at the market. It's more than simple knife work: The toughest part is pushing a hacksaw through a bone the diameter of a beer can. He uses his free hand to splay the massive cut of meat, drawing the saw back in strong, swift pulls.

But his work doesn't always involve movements as brutal as sawing bone. Farr spends much more time wielding a slim, curved butcher's scimitar, dancing its tip

THE RED SCARE

Do you feel pangs of guilt when you sink your teeth into a steak? It's probably because you've heard that red meat is bad for you. This claim arose in the 1950s, when researchers began to link saturated fat with heart disease. But the latest science is debunking that belief: A 2010 Harvard review found no higher risk of heart disease from eating red meat. Previous research has found that replacing carbs with saturated fat raises HDL (good) and LDL (bad) cholesterol but doesn't adversely affect their ratio—and that's what's important. Focus on quality, and there's no need to fear the steer.

around tendons and gracefully pulling excess fat away from marbled meat.

Farr is accustomed to guiding novices in the art of butchery. He offers classes (dubbed "Tasty Education" and described at 4505meats.com) that routinely draw sellout crowds of people looking to make sausage, break down sides of meat, master cut-specific recipes, store protein properly, and, of course, take home plenty of high-quality cuts.

"Part of my job as a butcher is to make people care about the meat as much as I do. And if what most people know about meat is from the supermarket, sometimes we're starting at a very basic level," Farr says.

TIP #3

"The key to preparing a tougher cut like tri-tip or hanger steak is searing it first, and then finishing it in a 350°F oven. The gentle cooking is necessary to break down the meat for maximum tenderness and flavor."

—TOM MYLAN

The New Breed of Butcher

Luckily for your belly, Farr isn't the only butcher practicing the trade in an innovative way. A new guard of meat maestros armed with vast knowledge are picking up knife, cleaver, and bone saw. They're also sustaining a growing number of old-school cattlemen and pig farmers, who in turn are coddling new generations of heritage breeds that are far superior to the feedlot zombies we've become accustomed to eating. These kitchen-savvy butcher-cooks are allowing eaters to take home the sustainable, acorn-fed, local bacon, and they're also frying it up in a pan.

They're guys like Adam Sappington, who put in 20 years as a butcher before he opened the Country Cat, a restaurant in Portland, Oregon, known for its house beef jerky and bacon. Or Tom Mylan, who trained at Fleisher's before opening the Meat Hook, home to a staggering sausage menu in Brooklyn. Or the Lobel family, a Manhattan cleaver dynasty whose members are converting acolytes with their cookbook *Lobel's Meat Bible*.

Sure, the tricks of the trade that these butchers use will work with meat from the supermarket, and you'll eat better than ever. That will suffice . . . until the day you reach the protein promised land: a butcher shop you can call your own.

Recipes

Divide, conquer, and feast upon these five meals from the boldest butchers in the land.

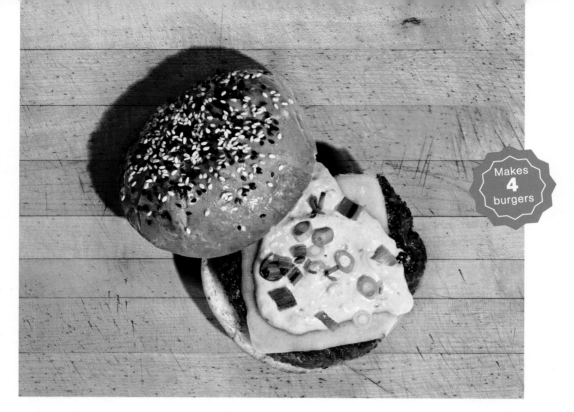

Makes
4
burgers

Ryan Farr's Fresh Lamb Burger with Harissa and Scallions

1 pound lamb sirloin, ground (see Skill 1 on page 87)

½ teaspoon ground coriander

½ teaspoon freshly ground pepper

1 teaspoon salt, divided

1½ tablespoons mayonnaise

1½ tablespoons sour cream

1 tablespoon milk

1 tablespoon harissa paste (find it in the international section of the supermarket)

4 slices Gruyère cheese (1 ounce slices)

4 potato buns, toasted

⅓ cup chopped scallions

1. Sprinkle the lamb with the coriander, pepper, and 1 teaspoon of the salt; fold until blended, about 1 minute. Divide the meat into quarters and form into ½-inch-thick patties. Refrigerate for 15 minutes.

2. In a bowl, combine the mayo, sour cream, milk, harissa, and remaining ½ teaspoon salt. Set aside.

3. On a hot, well-oiled grill or cast-iron pan set on medium high, cook the patties until seared, 1 to 1½ minutes. Flip them and top each with Gruyère. Cook until medium rare, 1 minute more.

4. Place the burgers on the bottom part of the buns. Slather the cut sides of the top buns with the sauce and sprinkle with the scallions. Close the buns.

Per serving: 561 calories, 33 g protein, 31 g carbohydrates, 35 g fat, 17 g saturated fat, 1 g fiber, 1,045 mg sodium

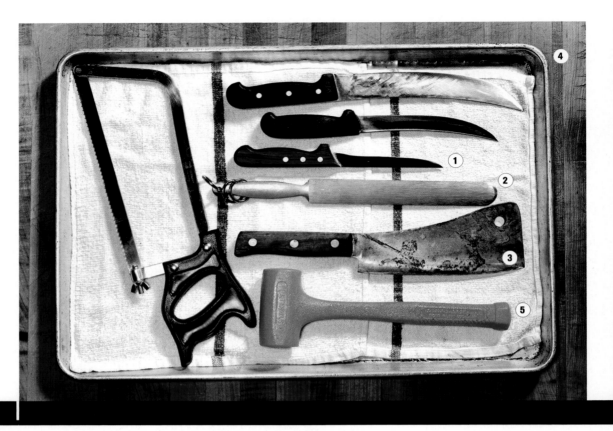

OWN THE TOOLS OF THE TRADE

Ryan Farr wields a wide array of weapons in his shop, but meat-eating home cooks don't need the whole set. Here's a butchery starter kit.

1. BONING KNIFE: Use this medium-length, thin-bladed knife to deftly debone a leg of lamb, trim fat, or french a roast. Try the sturdy Wüsthof Classic 5-inch Boning Knife ($100, metrokitchen.com).

2. STEEL: A dull knife adds to your workload; you end up sawing, not slicing. The result? Uneven, sloppy cuts. Try the Friedr. Dick 14-inch round regular-cut sharpening steel ($40, twinsupply.com).

3. CLEAVER: Butchers depend on this wide, heavy knife far less than they do their scimitar. It's best for tasks like snapping smaller or softer bones, pounding meat into flatter portions, or dividing ribs into chops. Pick up the TWIN Four Star II Meat Cleaver ($140, zwillingonline.com).

4. CUTTING BOARD: You want an "end grain" chopping block. It's durable, and the perpendicular grain actually helps keep your knife sharp. We like the Catskill Craftsmen End Grain Chopping Block ($89, catskillcraftsmen.com).

5. MEAT MALLET: Use the flat face to flatten cutlets without tearing the flesh. We like Oxo's Meat Tenderizer ($15, oxo.com).

6. POULTRY SHEARS: If you take a pair of scissors to the spine of a chicken, you'll shred the bird to bits. You need a tougher tool, like Wüsthof's Classic Poultry Shears ($80, williams-sonoma.com), which have two pincerlike blades with teeth that snip and tear through skin and fowl flesh, no sweat.

Eat Better **MH**

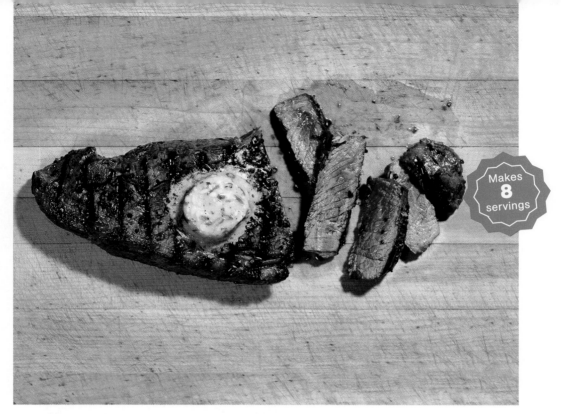

Makes **8** servings

Tom Mylan's Thick-Cut Sirloin Steaks with Bacon-Blue Cheese Butter

1   stick salted butter at room temperature

2   tablespoons bacon fat (save from your next batch of bacon)

2   tablespoons crumbled blue cheese

2   tablespoons thinly sliced scallions

    Salt

    Freshly ground pepper

1   top-sirloin roast (6 to 7 pounds), cut into 8 steaks (see Skill 2 on page 87)

1. Preheat the oven to 375°F. In a bowl, combine the butter, bacon fat, cheese, and scallions. Season with a pinch of salt and pepper. On a piece of plastic wrap, roll the mixture into a log. Put it in the freezer.

2. Season the steaks with salt and pepper. Heat two heavy ovenproof pans on high. (Open the windows and turn on your stove's fan.) When they're blazing hot, add one or two steaks to each pan; sear until a crust develops, 2 to 3 minutes on each side.

3. Transfer the pans to the oven and cook to medium rare, 5 to 7 minutes. Slice the butter into ½-inch-thick rounds, place them on the steaks, and let the meat rest 5 minutes before serving.

Per serving: 542 calories, 71 g protein, 0 g carbohydrates, 29 g fat, 13 g saturated fat, 0 g fiber, 330 mg sodium

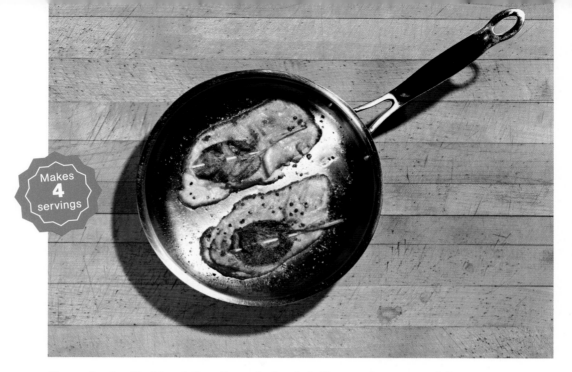

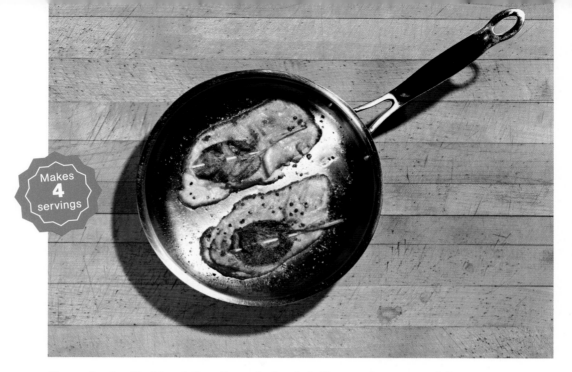

Makes **4** servings

Evan Lobel's Veal Scaloppini with Prosciutto and Sage

6–8 thin slices prosciutto

6–8 large fresh sage leaves

6–8 thin veal cutlets (1 pound total), pounded (see Skill 3 on page 87)

Kosher salt

Freshly ground pepper

3 tablespoons extra-virgin olive oil, plus more as needed

All-purpose flour for dredging

½ cup dry white wine

⅔ cup chicken broth

1. Trim each prosciutto slice to about the same dimensions as a cutlet. Place a slice and a sage leaf atop each cutlet. Working lengthwise, weave a toothpick in and out of the cutlet to secure them, keeping the veal flat. Season lightly with salt and pepper.

2. In a large skillet, heat the oil on medium high. Meanwhile, dredge the cutlets in flour, shaking off any excess.

3. When the oil starts to smoke, add half of the cutlets to the pan, prosciutto side down. Cook them until the prosciutto crisps, about 1 minute. Flip and cook until golden brown, 1 minute more. Transfer to a serving platter; repeat with the second batch of veal, adding oil to the pan if necessary.

4. Add the wine to the pan and cook, scraping the pan, until it's reduced to a couple of spoonfuls. Add the broth and reduce to ⅓ cup. Serve the veal with the pan sauce.

Per serving: 458 calories, 30 g protein, 7 g carbohydrates, 31 g fat, 9 g saturated fat, 0 g fiber, 814 mg sodium

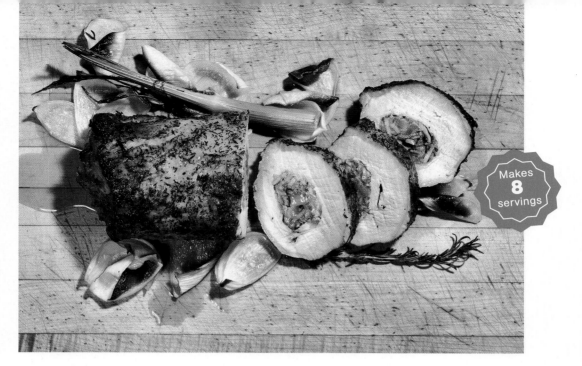

Adam Sappington's Ham-and-Pear-Stuffed Pork Loin

1 boneless center-cut pork loin (4 pounds)

2 tablespoons thyme salt (equal amounts of dried thyme and kosher salt mixed together)

3 tablespoons unsalted butter

5 ounce ham, roughly chopped

3 shallots, peeled and thinly sliced

2 Bosc pears, peeled and diced

1 cup apple cider

1 bunch fresh thyme, stemmed and chopped

3 fresh rosemary sprigs

3 fennel fronds

3 onions, peeled and cut into quarters with onion layers separated

1. Thoroughly massage the pork with the thyme salt. Place it on a baking rack and refrigerate it overnight.

2. An hour before cooking the pork, take it out of the fridge. Preheat the oven to 375°F.

3. In a large sauté pan, melt the butter on medium. Add the ham and cook until caramelized, 15 to 20 minutes. Add the shallots and cook until golden, 5 minutes. Add the pears and cook until softened, 15 minutes. Add the cider, turn the heat to high, and cook until the stuffing is chunky. Chill it on a baking sheet for 15 minutes.

4. Stuff the pork loin with the ham mixture (see Skill 4 on page 87). On a foil-lined baking sheet, place the thyme, rosemary, fennel, and onions and top with the pork. Roast until an instant-read thermometer inserted into the center reads 140°F. Transfer the pork to a cutting board and let it rest for 5 minutes before slicing.

Per serving: 474 calories, 56 g protein, 14 g carbohydrates, 21 g fat, 8 g saturated fat, 1 g fiber, 1,306 mg sodium

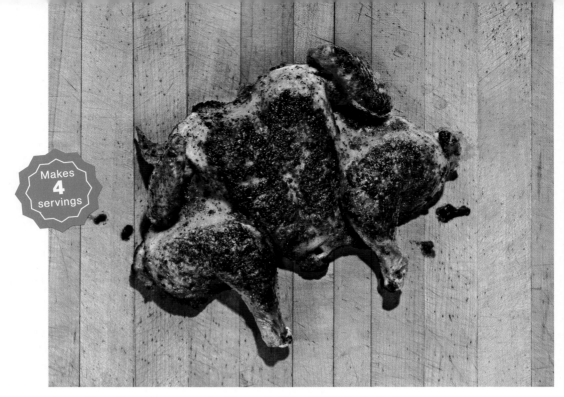

Makes **4** servings

Jessica Applestone's Butterflied BBQ Chicken

¼ cup kosher salt

¼ cup (packed) dark-brown sugar

¼ cup paprika

3 tablespoons freshly ground pepper

1 tablespoon garlic powder

1 tablespoon onion powder

1 teaspoon cayenne pepper

1 teaspoon mustard powder

½ teaspoon celery seed

1 whole chicken (3½ to 4 pounds), giblets removed, butterflied (see Skill 5 on page 87)

Olive oil

1. Preheat the oven to 350°F. In a medium bowl, combine the salt, brown sugar, and spices. Brush the chicken with olive oil and season it with 2 tablespoons of the rub.

2. Heat a cast-iron skillet on medium high. Add the chicken (breast side down) and sear it until golden brown, about 3 minutes. Then turn it over, place another heavy ovenproof pan directly on the bird, and cook that side until golden, 3 to 5 minutes more.

3. Transfer the pans and chicken to the oven; roast about 15 minutes. Remove the pan you used to weigh down the chicken, flip the chicken (so it's breast side down), and roast until the internal temp reads 160°F. Let rest 5 minutes before carving.

Per serving: 589 calories, 49 g protein, 6 g carbohydrates, 40 g fat, 11 g saturated fat, 1 g fiber, 1,626 mg sodium

FIVE ESSENTIAL BUTCHER SKILLS

Even if you can't find a butcher shop in your neighborhood, you can steal the following tips from the masters of meat to make your meals more flavorful. Study up, and then see the recipes beginning on page 81 you can use to test your new skills.

SKILL 1:
GRIND BURGERS

Here's why: Freshly ground meat makes mind-blowing burgers. No grinder? Try our food processor method.

HERE'S HOW:

1. Cut the meat into 1½-inch cubes and place them, along with the blade and bucket of a food processor, onto a baking sheet. Pop everything into the freezer until the cubes are slightly frozen around the edges.

2. Put the cold meat into the cold food processor. Pulse until it's chopped but still slightly chunky. Place it into a bowl and refrigerate until you're ready to use it.

SKILL 2:
CUT THICK STEAKS

Here's why: Supermarket steaks cook up dry because they're too thin. It's time to cut your own.

HERE'S HOW:

1. Place a roast on a cutting board and examine it for its striations—the "grain." Position it so the grain runs perpendicular to your knife. (If you cut parallel to the grain, your meal will turn out tough.)

2. Holding the roast in place, use a chef's knife to slice it into steaks 1½ to 2 inches thick; use long, even strokes, drawing the knife toward you. (Resist the urge to saw with the knife.)

SKILL 3:
POUND MEAT FLAT

Here's why: for the thinnest, most tender scallopine, you need to flatten cutlets without crushing them.

HERE'S HOW:

1. Place a veal cutlet between two pieces of waxed paper.

2. Using a mallet, the flat side of a cleaver, or the bottom of a heavy skillet, deliver firm, solid whacks to the meat, starting from 6 to 8 inches away. If the veal isn't flattening enough, then start pounding from about a foot away. Don't overdo it; if you pound too hard, the meat will break into mushy pieces. You're ready to go when the cutlet is about ⅛ inch thick.

SKILL 4:
STUFF A ROAST

Here's why: A roast feeds a crowd with ease, but you need to infuse flavor from the inside out.

HERE'S HOW:

1. Insert a long, thin slicing knife into the middle of one end of the roast as far as you can. Repeat on the other end to form a tunnel.

2. Move the knife back and forth to enlarge the hole.

3. With the stuffing in a resealable plastic bag, cut a 1½-inch hole in one corner. Insert the tip into one end of the loin, grip the open end of the bag, and squeeze the filling into the loin. Turn the loin and stuff it from the other end.

SKILL 5:
BUTTERFLY A BIRD

Here's why: Removing the backbone and flattening the flesh helps it cook quickly and carve easily.

HERE'S HOW:

1. Place the chicken on a cutting board so its wing tips point down and the drumsticks are closest to you. Feel out the spine and use kitchen shears to cut along each side of it, starting at the tail. Snip off the spine at the neck.

2. Flip the chicken over so its wing tips face up. Now use the heel of your hand to press down on the center of the breastbone hard enough to break it and flatten the flesh.

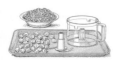 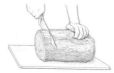 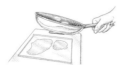 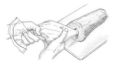 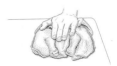

Takeout That Delivers

Hungry for Asian? Make fast, fresh DIY versions of delivery classics.

Odds are, your food delivery guy is bringing trouble to your doorstep. Inside that innocuous bag, he carries unhealthy versions of virtuous, protein-packed Asian dishes like salmon teriyaki and shrimp pad thai. Loaded with gloppy, neon-colored sauces, limp vegetables, MSG, and excess oil, the food may blunt your hunger, but it won't optimally fuel your body. And that #2 combo isn't doing your waistline any favors, either: A 2011 study in the *Journal of the American Dietetic Association* reports that people who eat takeout just once a week may significantly increase their body fat as well as other risk factors for heart disease and diabetes.

Time to reclaim takeout. Where to start? From scratch. In less time than it takes the delivery dude to reach your doorstep, you can create vibrant home-made versions of your go-to Asian orders. Just deploy lean protein, produce for fiber and disease-fighting phytonutrients, and fresh aromatics like garlic and ginger. Stock up on a few Asian pantry staples, and prep can be even easier. The only thing that'll make your meals better? A strategic dose of spicy sriracha.

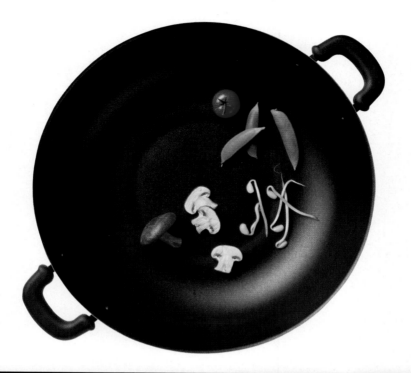

TOOLS OF THE TRADE

Keep a few basic weapons in your arsenal to ensure stir-fry success. Grace Young, author of *Stir-Frying to the Sky's Edge*, recommends these three key items.

14-inch carbon steel flat-bottom wok: Inexpensive carbon steel helps meats and vegetables sear superbly.

Slotted metal spatula: A wide, flexible metal spatula (also called a fish turner) can follow the sides of a wok and easily slips under foods that have a tendency to stick. Try Oxo's version ($13, oxo.com).

Peanut oil: A high smoke point makes peanut oil popular in Asian kitchens. Grapeseed oil and canola oil are other options that can take the heat. We like the oils from spectrumorganics.com.

  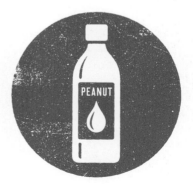

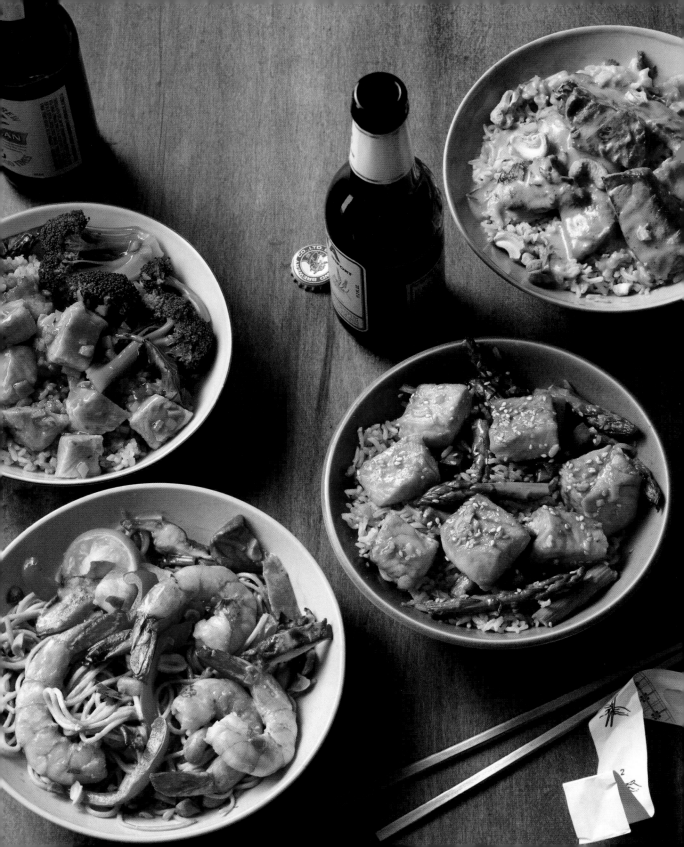

Thai Red Curry with Beef

UPGRADE: *Swapping in sweet potatoes for the classic white variety gives this curry a beta-carotene boost. Serve this over rice, garnished with unsalted, roasted cashews and cilantro.*

- 2 tablespoons vegetable oil (preferably peanut), divided
- 1 pound steak (round, loin, or flank), cut into ½-inch-wide strips
- 1 large shallot, chopped
- 1 tablespoon minced fresh ginger
- 1 tablespoon Thai red curry paste
- 1 can (13.5 ounces) light coconut milk
- 1 teaspoon grated lime zest
- 1 tablespoon fish sauce
- 1 medium sweet potato, peeled and diced
- Juice of ½ lime

1. Heat a wok or skillet on medium high. When it's hot, add 1 tablespoon of the oil and swirl to coat the pan. Add the beef and sear it until browned, tossing occasionally, 2 to 3 minutes. Transfer the beef and its juices to a plate.

2. Return the wok to medium heat and swirl in the remaining 1 tablespoon oil. Add the shallot and ginger; stir-fry for 3 minutes. Stir in the curry paste and heat for 30 seconds. Stir in the coconut milk, lime zest, and fish sauce; heat for 2 minutes.

3. Add the sweet potatoes to the wok and bring the mixture to a boil. Reduce it to a simmer, cover, and cook until the potatoes are tender, about 15 minutes. Stir in the lime juice and beef and heat through.

Per serving: 350 calories, 27 g protein, 12 g carbohydrates, 21 g fat, 8 g saturated fat, 1 g fiber, 611 mg sodium

Makes **4** servings

Soba Shrimp Pad Thai

UPGRADE: *Pad thai typically uses nutritionally void rice noodles. Use Japanese soba noodles instead for a bonus dose of fiber and nutty flavor.*

- 2 garlic cloves, chopped
- 2 tablespoons natural peanut butter
- 1 tablespoon honey
- 2 teaspoons roasted sesame oil
- 1 tablespoon reduced-sodium soy sauce
- 1 tablespoon sriracha chili sauce
- 1 tablespoon fish sauce
- ¼ cup water
- 2 tablespoons vegetable oil (preferably peanut), divided
- 1 pound peeled large raw shrimp (thawed and drained if frozen)
- 2 red bell peppers, thinly sliced
- 1 cup sliced shiitake mushrooms
- 6 ounces soba (buckwheat) noodles, cooked, rinsed, and drained
- 3 scallions, sliced
- ¼ cup roasted peanuts, coarsely chopped
- 2 limes, quartered, for serving

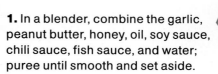

Makes **4** servings

1. In a blender, combine the garlic, peanut butter, honey, oil, soy sauce, chili sauce, fish sauce, and water; puree until smooth and set aside.

2. Heat a wok or large skillet on medium high. When it's hot, add 1 tablespoon of the oil and swirl to coat the pan. Then add the shrimp and cook until opaque, about 2 minutes. Transfer them to a plate.

3. Add the remaining 1 tablespoon oil to the wok and swirl. Add the peppers and mushrooms; stir-fry for 2 minutes. Return the shrimp to the pan along with the peanut sauce, cooked soba, and scallions; stir-fry for 1 minute.

4. Serve with the peanuts and limes.

Per serving: 490 calories, 29 g protein, 54 g carbohydrates, 20 g fat, 39 g saturated fat, 5 g fiber, 1550 mg sodium

Salmon Teriyaki with Asparagus

UPGRADE: *A helping of in-season asparagus adds potassium and folate to this Japanese stir-fry. Serve this over brown rice and garnish with sesame seeds.*

2 tablespoons reduced-sodium soy sauce

2 tablespoons mirin (Japanese rice wine)

1 tablespoon honey

1 tablespoon sriracha chili sauce

1 teaspoon cornstarch

1 teaspoon Asian sesame oil

1 tablespoon minced fresh ginger

2 garlic cloves, finely chopped

1 tablespoon vegetable oil (preferably peanut)

1 pound skinless salmon (preferably wild), cut into 1-inch cubes

1 bunch asparagus, trimmed and cut into thirds

1. In a small bowl, whisk together the soy sauce, mirin, honey, sriracha, cornstarch, sesame oil, ginger, and garlic. Set the mixture aside.

2. Heat a wok or large skillet on medium high. When it's hot, add the vegetable oil and swirl to coat the pan. Add the salmon pieces and cook, stirring occasionally, until they just begin to turn opaque, about 2 minutes. Transfer them to a plate.

3. Add the asparagus to the wok and stir-fry until crisp-tender, about 2 minutes. Return the salmon to the wok and stir in the soy sauce mixture. Heat, stirring, for 1 minute. If the sauce seems too thick, add a couple of tablespoons of water.

Per serving: 271 calories, 28 g protein, 12 g carbohydrates, 11 g fat, 2 g saturated fat, 3 g fiber, 344 mg sodium

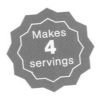

Makes
4
servings

General Tso's Chicken with Broccoli

UPGRADE: *Why weigh down chicken chunks with bland, oil-logged batter? Bake them instead to cut calories without sacrificing taste. Then pile on the fresh vegetables. Serve it over brown rice.*

1 pound boneless, skinless chicken breasts, cut into 1-inch cubes

2 tablespoons + 2 teaspoons cornstarch

2 teaspoons vegetable oil (preferably peanut)

2 garlic cloves, minced

1 tablespoon minced fresh ginger

¼ cup reduced-sodium chicken broth

1 tablespoon reduced-sodium soy sauce

1 tablespoon hoisin sauce

1 tablespoon rice-wine vinegar

1 tablespoon honey

1 tablespoon sriracha chili sauce

2 tablespoons water

4 cups steamed broccoli florets

1. Preheat the oven to 375°F.

2. On a foil-lined baking sheet, toss the chicken with 2 tablespoons of the cornstarch. Spread out the cubes and bake until cooked through, about 12 minutes.

3. Meanwhile, in a medium saucepan, heat the oil, garlic, and ginger on medium for 2 minutes, stirring often. Add the broth, soy sauce, hoisin, vinegar, honey, and sriracha; simmer for 3 minutes.

4. In a small bowl, whisk the remaining 2 teaspoons cornstarch into the water; add that to the saucepan and cook until the mixture thickens, about 30 seconds.

5. Add the cooked chicken to the pan with the sauce and toss together. Serve alongside the broccoli.

Per serving: 222 calories, 27 g protein, 16 g carbohydrates, 6 g fat, 1 g saturated fat, 2 g fiber, 396 mg sodium

Makes
4
servings

Great Bowls of Fire

Remember that campfire feast in *Blazing Saddles?* That's healthy eating at its best. Indulge!

You never know with those bowl games. It's 50-50 whether the college kids will produce fourth-quarter heroics or second-quarter blowouts. Not so with the traditional halftime meal, the Chili Bowl. It reliably unites heat, spice, protein, and fiber, with spectacular results. (Cue the flatulence effects.) And if you follow our simple rules, it's also a health-boosting meal. You don't have to tell your football-mad guests that, though. What they don't know just might help them. A lot.

STRATEGY #1
Amp up the Scoville units.

Leverage a range of hot peppers for your next batch of chili. According to a study in the *British Journal of Nutrition*, eating foods with capsaicin (the compound that gives chiles their burn) can rev your metabolism. Spicy foods like this incendiary chili can also keep you satisfied for longer.

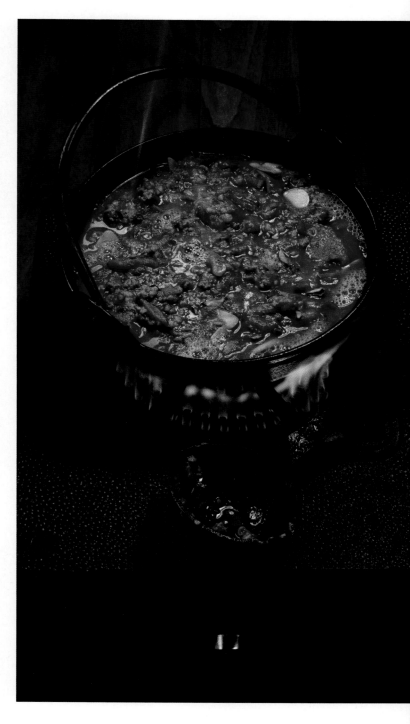

STRATEGY #2
Boost the fiber factor.

Chili purists might argue the virtues of a beanless bowl, but the fiber in beans keeps you feeling satisfied and might also help regulate blood pressure and boost heart health. To ramp up the fiber even more, add bulgur, a type of cracked wheat that's a ground-beef look-alike and adds even more meaty texture.

STRATEGY #3
Go for a leaner cut that packs flavor.

Like some NFL playoff teams, lean meats are overrated. Zero-fat ground turkey breast has zero taste. If you want to cut calories while still creating a championship bowl of Texas red, stick to relatively lean cubed dark-meat chicken or beef sirloin. They both turn tender and flavorful when slow-simmered.

STRATEGY #4
Double up on vegetables.

On paper, vegetarian chili sounds like a smart idea—the hidden-ball trick for your daily servings. The problem: All-veg varieties taste like . . . vegetables! The solution: Choose produce that actually works with Mexican flavors, and don't stint on fresh toppings such as tomato, avocado, and pickled jalapeños.

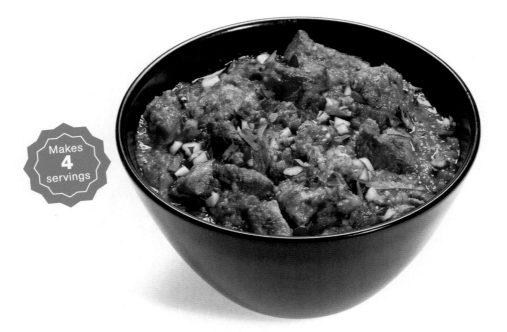

Makes **4** servings

Four-Alarm Green Chili with Pork

1 pound fresh tomatillos, husks removed

2 poblano chile peppers, stemmed and halved

2 serrano chile peppers, stemmed and halved

1 pickled jalapeño chile pepper, stemmed and halved

1 small onion, cut into chunks

3 garlic cloves, smashed and peeled

½ cup fresh cilantro leaves

1 teaspoon dried oregano

1 teaspoon ground cumin

½ teaspoon ground coriander

½ teaspoon chipotle chili powder

¼ teaspoon ground allspice

¼ cup water

2 tablespoons olive oil

1½ pounds boneless pork shoulder, cut into 1-inch chunks

1½ teaspoons coarse salt, divided

1 tablespoon fresh lime juice

1. In a medium pot of boiling water, cook the tomatillos until softened, about 5 minutes. Drain and transfer to a blender along with the peppers, onion, garlic, cilantro, and spices. Add the water and puree until smooth.

2. Meanwhile, in a 5-quart pot, heat the oil on medium high. Season the pork with ½ teaspoon of the salt and, working in two batches, sear it until browned, about 7 minutes per batch. Transfer the pork to a bowl.

3. Add the tomatillo puree to the pot and cook for 3 minutes. Add the seared pork, lime juice, and remaining 1 teaspoon salt; bring to a boil. Reduce to a simmer, cover, and cook, stirring occasionally, until the pork is tender, about 1¼ hours.

Per serving: 407 calories, 29 g protein, 13 g carbohydrates, 27 g fat, 8 g saturated fat, 4 g fiber, 839 mg sodium

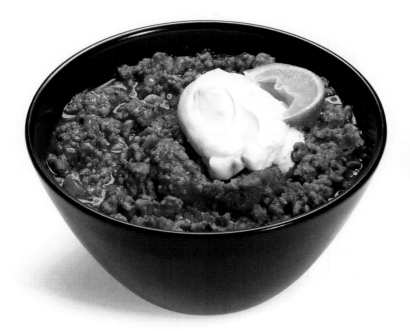

Makes **4** servings

Ancho, Beef, and Bulgur Chili

1 tablespoon + 1 teaspoon olive oil

1 large onion, coarsely chopped

1 green bell pepper, diced

1–2 serrano chile peppers, stemmed, halved, seeded, and chopped

3 garlic cloves, thinly sliced

1½ teaspoons ground cumin

1 teaspoon ancho chili powder

¾ teaspoon dried oregano

½ teaspoon ground cinnamon

⅓ cup bulgur wheat

1 pound 90%-lean ground sirloin

1 can (15 ounces) plum tomatoes in puree

1 can (15 ounces) black beans, rinsed and drained

½ cup water

1 teaspoon coarse salt

Lime wedges (optional)

1. In a 5-quart pot, heat the oil on medium. Add the onion, peppers, and garlic; cook, stirring occasionally, until the onion is golden brown and the peppers are tender, about 10 minutes.

2. Add the cumin, chili powder, oregano, and cinnamon and cook, stirring, for 1 minute to lightly toast them. Stir in the bulgur. Add the beef and cook, breaking it up with a spoon, until it's no longer pink, about 3 minutes.

3. Stir in the tomatoes with puree, beans, water, and salt; bring to a simmer. Cover and cook until the flavors are blended and the meat and bulgur are tender, about 30 minutes. Serve with lime wedges if desired.

Per serving: 386 calories, 30 g protein, 31 g carbohydrates, 17 g fat, 5 g saturated fat, 9 g fiber, 1047 mg sodium

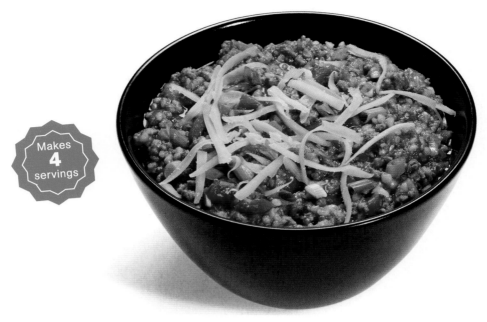

Makes **4** servings

Chunky Tex-Mex Chili

4 teaspoons olive oil, divided

1 small fresh chorizo sausage (3 ounces) removed from its casing (optional)

1¼ pounds boneless beef sirloin (choose the most marbled) or boneless, skinless chicken thighs, cut into ½-inch chunks

1 medium onion, coarsely chopped

3 garlic cloves, thinly sliced

¼ cup ancho chili powder

2 teaspoons dried oregano

¼ cup tomato paste

1 tablespoon red-wine vinegar

1¼ cups water

1 teaspoon coarse salt

2 tablespoons cornmeal

1. In a 5-quart pot, heat 2 teaspoons of the oil on medium. Add the chorizo (if using) and cook until it has rendered its fat, about 5 minutes. With a slotted spoon, remove the chorizo to a bowl.

2. Working in two batches, add the beef or chicken to the pot and cook until browned, about 5 minutes per batch. With a slotted spoon, transfer to the bowl with the chorizo.

3. Add the onion, garlic, and remaining 2 teaspoons oil and cook, stirring frequently, until the onion is tender, about 7 minutes. Stir in the chili powder and oregano, and cook for 1 minute. Stir in the tomato paste and vinegar.

4. Return the meat and chorizo to the pot. Add the water and salt and bring to a boil. Reduce to a simmer, cover, and cook, stirring occasionally, until the meat is tender, about 1 hour. Stir in the cornmeal and simmer until slightly thickened, about 5 minutes.

Per serving: 298 calories, 34 g protein, 14 g carbohydrates, 12 g fat, 3 g saturated fat, 5 g fiber, 829 mg sodium

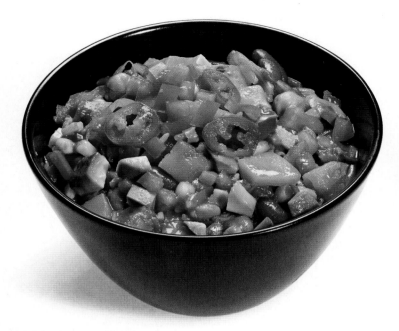

Makes
4
servings

Winter-Vegetable Chili

2 tablespoons olive oil

1 large onion, coarsely chopped

3 garlic cloves, thinly sliced

1 red bell pepper, diced

2 cups finely chopped cabbage (you can use preshredded coleslaw mix)

1 tablespoon unsweetened cocoa powder

1 teaspoon chipotle chili powder

1 pound butternut squash, peeled and cut into 1-inch chunks (3 cups)

¼ cup tomato paste

2 cups vegetable broth

1 can (15 ounces) red kidney beans, rinsed and drained

1 can (15 ounces) chickpeas, rinsed and drained

1½ teaspoons coarse salt

1½ cups frozen corn kernels, thawed

Chopped avocado, tomato, and pickled jalapeños for topping

1. In a 5-quart pot, heat the oil on medium. Add the onion, garlic, and bell pepper and cook, stirring frequently, until the onion is golden brown and tender, about 10 minutes.

2. Stir in the cabbage and cook, stirring frequently, until wilted, about 5 minutes. Add the cocoa powder and chili powder; cook for 1 minute. Add the squash and tomato paste and cook for 1 minute.

3. Add the broth, beans, chickpeas, and salt and bring to a boil. Reduce to a simmer, cover, and cook until the squash is tender, about 30 minutes. Stir in the corn and heat through, about 3 minutes. Serve topped with avocado, tomato, and jalapeños.

Per serving: 349 calories, 13 g protein, 60 g carbohydrates, 10 g fat, 1 g saturated fat, 14 g fiber, 1480 mg sodium

HAVE THAT CAFFEINE FIX

Here's a perk for coffee lovers: In a new study published in the *American Journal of Clinical Nutrition,* people who drank at least 4 cups of coffee a day were 23 percent less likely to have type 2 diabetes later in life. According to the authors, who used data from 42,659 participants, the polyphenols in coffee might reduce oxidative stress linked to the development of chronic diseases. Even better, a 2011 study from Japan found that men who drank a cup or two of coffee a day had a 16 percent lower risk of cardiovascular disease.

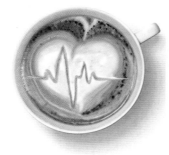

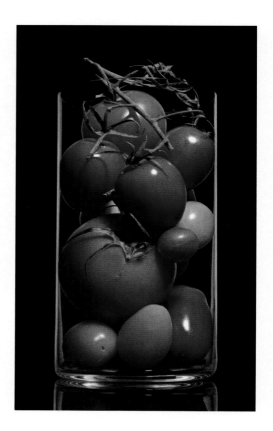

TEA UP

Buy some cup protection: Black tea might improve your blood pressure, say Australian scientists. People who drank 3 cups of black tea every day for 6 months saw a 2-point drop in both diastolic and systolic blood pressure. Tea flavonoids might reduce concentrations of endothelin-1, a protein that constricts blood vessels, the researchers report. Less than 3 cups a day may work, too.

POWER UP YOUR JUICE

You say tomato, we say tomato juice. Researchers have known for years that processing tomatoes increases the power of their lycopene, which is an antioxidant that might help prevent prostate cancer. But for an even more potent pour, go with a glass of organic tomato juice instead: A 2011 Spanish study found that organic tomato juice has up to 23 percent more disease-fighting polyphenols than the regular red stuff.

The researchers say that tomatoes grown with pesticides might lose their natural defense mechanisms, of which polyphenols are a key component.

CRACK THAT HABIT

Eating more nuts might protect you from the harmful effects of diabetes. In a study published in the journal *Diabetes Care*, people with type 2 diabetes who ate a handful of nuts daily had more-stable blood sugar than other people who ate whole-wheat muffins instead.

By replacing some carbs with the

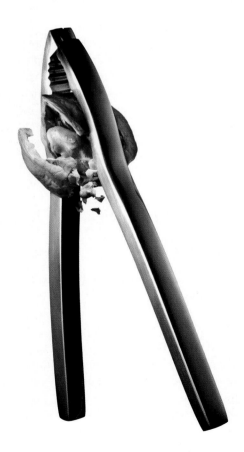

healthy fats of nuts, you might regulate your blood sugar, and you might even stave off diabetes, says lead study author Cyril Kendall, Ph.D. You could eat walnuts as a snack, mix them into a salad, or crush them and use them to top roasted green beans as a side.

BE BERRY GOOD

Pick some protection: Find a berry farm. According to new research in the journal *Neurology*, eating berries regularly might help shield you from Parkinson's disease. In the study, men who ate the most strawberries and blueberries (two or more weekly servings) were 23 percent less likely to develop Parkinson's disease later in life than other men who ate the least servings of berries.

Why? One theory is that berries are rich in anthocyanins, which are flavonoids that might trigger the production of protective brain enzymes, the researchers say.

BE A GRAIN MAN

Pour some cereal as a snack. People who regularly ate at least seven servings a week of whole-grain cereal had a 19 percent lower risk of hypertension later in life than people who ate none, according to a study in the journal *Clinical Nutrition*. Whole-grain cereals might lessen inflammation and improve insulin sensitivity, the study noted. We like Health Valley Organic Fiber 7, with 7 grams of fiber in every cup.

FIGHT CANCER— WITH FOOD!

Colorectal cancer is the second leading cause of cancer death in the United States. Protect your plumbing with this Asian dinner, from the journal *Nutrition and Cancer*.

1 fillet cooked salmon: It's packed with vitamin D, which might help fight colon cancer. Top with scallions, sesame seeds, and hot sauce.

1 cup sautéed spinach: Study participants who ate at least a daily serving of cooked greens were 24 percent less likely to have rectal or colon polyps.

1 cup brown rice mixed with ½ cup peas: Eat a serving of brown rice every week and you might reduce your risk of rectal or colon polyps later in life by 40 percent.

½ cup dried fruit: Dried fruit's high fiber content may reduce the effect of potential carcinogens.

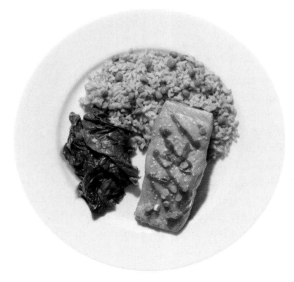

KNOW YOUR PROTEIN

Look for a change in your grocery's meat case, thanks to a new USDA rule: Major cuts of meat and poultry will now be labeled with nutrition facts that include calories, total fat, and saturated fat. Remember: You need fat. It helps you absorb nutrients. But it's also high in calories, so watch how much you eat.

BEAT YOUR GENES!

Scientists have already linked heart disease to variations in a certain chromosome region. Now a study published in the journal *PLoS Medicine* reveals that people who eat several servings of raw fruit or vegetables a day are less likely to suffer from heart disease linked to that chromosome region than people who eat little produce. More research is needed to determine exactly what mechanism is at work.

GET SOME STEALTH HEALTH

Here are some surprisingly good for you super foods.

Anchovies
These small, salty fish fillets are intensely savory and contain loads of beneficial nutrients.

Why they're healthy: Five canned anchovies have 6 grams of protein and only 42 calories. Plus, they're a good source of niacin (which helps your body metabolize fat) and selenium, an essential mineral.

How to eat them: They're delicious draped over a slice of pizza, minced and mixed into olive tapenade, or chopped finely and simmered into a spicy tomato-caper sauce for pasta.

Artichoke Hearts

They're the greenish yellow centers of the artichoke plant's flower buds. These hearts are tender, with a mild, vegetal flavor.

Why they are healthy: Artichoke hearts are a good source of iron and dietary fiber.

How to them: They're great in salads, or paired with roasted red pepper and pesto on a sandwich, or as a topping for homemade pizza.

Arugula

It's a peppery salad green. Younger leaves have less of a bite than mature ones do.

Why it's healthy: Arugula has vitamin A (for vision), vitamin C (for immune function), and vitamin K (for clotting). Plus, it contains heart-protecting compounds known as flavonols.

How to eat it: Toss arugula into cooked rigatoni; add a drizzle of olive oil along with some roasted cherry tomatoes and shaved Parmesan. Or use it instead of lettuce on a burger or sandwich.

Guava

It's a fruit with sweet white, yellow, pink, or red flesh inside its yellow-green rind.

Why it's good for you: Guava delivers fiber and vitamin C. Plus, its antioxidants are more active than those in apples, bananas, mangoes, or papayas, a 2010 study from India revealed.

How to eat it: Bite into it like an apple, or slice it in half and scoop out the pulp. You can also blend some of the flesh into a yogurt smoothie for a hint of tropical sweetness.

Horseradish

When cut or grated, this root releases a biting aroma and sharp taste that can ratchet up the kick in a range of foods.

Why it's healthy: Low-calorie, high-flavor horseradish has glucosinolates, which might help fight cancer cells, according to a 2009 review by Indian researchers.

How to eat it: First, peel and finely grate it. Then, for an instant sauce for grilled fish or beef tenderloin, mix it into half a cup of sour cream. It's also great in a Bloody Mary.

Mussels

These mollusks cook up plump and have a faintly briny yet sweet flavor.

Why they're healthy: Mussels are quite low in fat and pack a big protein punch—40 grams in a 6-ounce, 292-calorie serving. They're also a good source of vitamin B12 and omega-3 fatty acids.

How to eat them: Scrub under cold water, removing the attached "beards." Then steam them in a covered pot over medium heat with white wine, garlic, and herbs until they open, 5 to 10 minutes.

Q Should I pay attention to supermarket food-rating systems?

A: The theory behind these scorecards is that people are more likely to buy healthy foods if they can identify them at a glance rather than, say, freezing their fingers comparing the Nutrition Facts on three different brands of frozen pizza.

About 1,600 supermarkets feature NuVal, a system that ranks a food's nutritional value from 1 (poor) to 100 (excellent), while about the same number of stores use Guiding Stars to rank foods from zero stars (poor) to three stars (excellent). Both use algorithms to crunch nutrition data down to a simple score.

The two systems haven't been compared head-to-head, but research suggests that each has its benefits. A 2011 Harvard study linked the consumption of foods with higher NuVal ratings to a 9 to 12 percent lower risk of developing a chronic disease. As for Guiding Stars, a 2010 study published in the *American Journal of Clinical Nutrition* found that people using these rankings purchased a significantly higher percentage of healthy food.

"Summary ratings can help you quickly figure out what's in packaged foods, which are often covered in marketing phrases like 'low in fat' or 'all natural,'" says James C. Hersey, Ph.D., a nutrition researcher at RTI International, a nonprofit institute.

Q What's the difference between "organic" and "natural" on food labels?

A: Both words sell a greener eating experience, but only organic delivers the full grocery cart of nutritional goods. For a food to bear the USDA Organic logo, it must meet strict criteria, including no synthetic ingredients, no petroleum-based fertilizers, no synthetic pesticides, and no genetic modification. In the case of meat, poultry, and eggs, animals should have been fed 100 percent organic feed.

The bar is a lot lower for the word "natural"; the FDA requires only that these foods contain no added color, artificial flavors, or synthetic substances.

"'Natural' is a marketing gimmick," says Marion Nestle, Ph.D., M.P.H., a nutrition professor at New York University and the author of *Food Politics*. "Food companies have always used 'natural' to market products, but its use increased after the USDA passed its organic standards in 2002. The word 'natural' should serve as a warning for you to scan the ingredient label."

Be especially wary of ice cream, cereals, and fruit snacks, which often contain chemically processed ingredients, such as corn syrup, alkalized cocoa, partially hydrogenated soybean oil, vanillin, and maltodextrin. What's more, foods labeled "natural" are allowed to have genetically modified ingredients and to be grown using pesticides; and meat, fish, and poultry bearing that label can be raised with growth hormones and antibiotics.

Which lunch meats are the healthiest?

A: The devil is in the deli case: Gaze through the glass and you'll see three types of lunch meat: whole (slabs, such as roast beef), formed (chunks of meat cooked together, like some types of ham), and processed (meat stuffed in a casing, like salami).

"Whole cuts generally have the most nutrients and fewest additives," says Valerie Berkowitz, M.S., R.D., director of nutrition at the Center for Balanced Health in New York City. Meat additives, particularly nitrates and nitrites, might be harmful.

A new British review suggests that your colon cancer risk rises 24 percent for every 1.7-ounce increase in your daily intake of processed meat. Colleen Doyle, M.S., R.D., the American Cancer Society's director of nutrition and physical activity, advises eating no more than two servings a week. To be extra safe, we found the following tasty meats without heavy processing or added nitrates or nitrites.

PROSCIUTTO

LA QUERCIA PROSCIUTTO GREEN LABEL

Health facts: 140 calories, 18 grams (g) protein, 1,140 milligrams (mg) sodium

Flavor: This organic, dry-cured leg of ham has just two ingredients: pork and sea salt. Yes, it's high in sodium, but the intense flavor means you'll eat less of it.

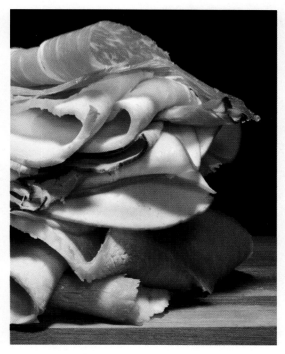

CHICKEN

APPLEGATE NATURAL ROASTED CHICKEN

Health facts: 60 calories, 10 g protein, 360 mg sodium

Flavor: It's made with honey instead of corn syrup for a subtle, sweet taste.

BEEF

BOAR'S HEAD ALL NATURAL CAP-OFF TOP ROUND OVEN ROASTED BEEF

Health facts: 80 calories, 14 g protein, 140 mg sodium

Flavor: This beef comes from cattle raised without the use of antibiotics or growth hormones.

TURKEY

APPLEGATE ORGANIC SMOKED TURKEY BREAST

Health facts: 50 calories, 10 g protein, 360 mg sodium

Flavor: These slices have a smoky flavor that's so good you'll want to roll them up and eat them without bread.

HAM

DIETZ & WATSON ALL NATURAL UNCURED CLASSIC DINNER HAM

Health facts: 60 calories, 10 g protein, 440 mg sodium

Flavor: It's seasoned with sea salt and a touch of organic sugar.

NOTE: *All nutritional data is per 2 ounces.*

Q What's the healthiest choice in the canned tuna aisle?

A: The diversity in tuna options is enough to make your head swim. There's chunk, solid, pouch, can . . . heck, even subtle details, such as light versus white, can be nutritionally significant, says Brian St. Pierre, C.S.C.S., a sports nutrition consultant based in Maine. Albacore, or white tuna, delivers more than three times the omega-3s of skipjack, or light tuna.

But because albacore are typically larger, they also have higher mercury levels. So balance risk and reward, and eat only one 6-ounce serving of albacore a week. (You can have 12 ounces of skipjack a week.) To limit your exposure to BPA, a harmful chemical in the linings of cans, check the label for the words "BPA-free" or opt for plastic pouches. Here are our favorite catches.

BEST GOURMET
Ortiz Bonito del Norte tuna in olive oil

Cooked once instead of twice like most brands, this Spanish albacore has a mellow taste. Add it to pasta with a little of its oil.

160 calories, $17, latienda.com

BEST FLAVOR
Island Trollers Albacore with jalapeño

Caught off the coast of Washington and packed in BPA-free cans, it has a clean taste with a fiery kick.

110 calories, $75 for 12 cans, islandtrollers.com

BEST IN WATER AND BEST IN OIL
Wild Planet Wild Albacore

This albacore in water delivers 1,340 milligrams of DHA/EPA omega-3s in a 2-ounce serving. The oil version has a less intense taste, and the olive oil adds a dose of heart-healthy monounsaturated fats. Because Wild Planet catches small albacore, it says its tuna has less than half the mercury of other albacore brands, so you can eat it more often.

120 calories in water, 190 in oil; $30 for six cans, wildplanetfoods.com

BEST ON-THE-GO
StarKist Flavor Fresh chunk light in water

A three-time MH 125 Best Foods taste-test winner, this tuna comes in an easy-open, no mess, BPA-free pouch.

80 calories per 2.6 ounces. $1.50, starkist.com

Note: *All nutritional data is for 2 ounces unless noted.*

Should I switch from table to sea salt?

A: Your tastebuds will appreciate sea salt's sharp flavor and crunchy crystals, but your thyroid gland will notice something missing. Sea salt contains about 40 percent sodium, just like Morton's finest, but it usually lacks the essential nutrient iodine, which most manufacturers have been adding to table salt since the 1920s.

"Low levels of iodine are associated with thyroid-related issues, including mental fatigue and weight gain," says Sara Blackburn, D.Sc., R.D., a clinical associate professor of nutrition at Indiana University. To hit your quota, aim for 150 micrograms a day; a quarter teaspoon of iodized salt contains about 95 micrograms. To lick this nutrition-versus-flavor dilemma, use standard salt on the table and save the sea salt for sprinkling on grilled fish, meat, and vegetables just before serving. It also kicks up the flavor of chocolate ice cream. The Guy Gourmet's pick: Maldon Sea Salt ($11, williams-sonoma.com).

Are chia seeds worth a try?

A: These tiny seeds won't make you sprout muscle, but they can deliver big benefits. Packed with calcium, iron, and magnesium, they're also high in fiber, omega-3 fatty acids, and antioxidants, says Vladimir Vuksan, Ph.D., a professor of medicine and nutritional sciences at the University of Toronto who has studied the effects of chia in both healthy and diabetic people.

"Chia seeds seem to have cardioprotective properties and can assist in stabilizing your blood sugar."

An ounce of dried seeds is 138 calories and provides 10 grams of fiber, 5 grams of protein, and 5 grams of omega-3s (ALA). Popular in Central America since Aztec times, these nutty-tasting seeds (known botanically as *Salvia hispanica L.*) are now widely available in supermarkets. Try Salba (salbasmart.com), the brand used in Vuksan's studies. Sprinkle the seeds into salads, mix them into yogurt, or blend them into your postworkout shakes.

What's the secret to grilling a great burger?

A: Everyone has a signature burger these days, but the flourishes often come at the expense of flavor. Don't complicate your burgers with elaborate toppings. Instead, focus on the meat to boost your burgers to best-ever status, says David Burke, chef and owner of David Burke Townhouse in New York City.

"The key is to add flavor and texture to the meat itself." This ensures that every bite is consistent and delicious.

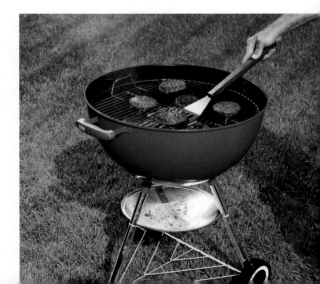

Keep the bun simple (we like Martin's Famous whole wheat potato rolls, toasted), melt Gruyère or aged Cheddar on top of the patty, and tuck a leaf of fresh Bibb lettuce beneath to avoid a soggy bottom bun. Follow these instructions to reach burger heaven.

The meat: Go with grass-fed beef. It typically contains fewer hormones and a heart-healthier balance of omega-3 and omega-6 fatty acids. Ideally, aim for a meat-to-fat ratio of around 80/20, says Pat LaFrieda Jr., owner of Pat LaFrieda Meat Purveyors. "With that mix, you lose just the right amount of fat on the grill, but the burger will still be juicy."

The flavor enhancers: Mix in these boosters to power up your 6-ounce patty, says Burke.

ZESTY:
1 garlic clove, minced

Zest and juice of 1 lemon

1 tsp chopped anchovies

1 tsp grated Parmesan

1 pinch dried basil, chives, red-pepper flakes

TANGY:
1 tsp fresh or pickled ginger

1 tsp soy sauce

1 tsp ketchup

1 garlic clove, minced

BACONY:
3 Tbsp caramelized mushrooms and onions, mashed to a spreadable paste

1 Tbsp chopped cooked bacon

UMAMI:
2 oz cooked ham, finely chopped

2 Tbsp steak sauce

Shape it: Hold on! Don't roll the meat into a ball; it could end up pasty. To keep the burger juicy, simply pull off enough chuck to make the size you want. Then press it down on a flat surface with one hand while shaping it with the other. Keep going until it's round. Another tip: The colder the meat, the better. (It's less sticky.)

Cook it: Season your patties with salt and crank the grill to high. When it's hot, place the burgers on the grate and sear them until a good char develops, about 2 minutes on each side for medium rare. To finish, flip them and kiss them with heat until crosshatched grill marks appear, in 30 to 60 seconds. Add freshly ground pepper and let them rest for about 2 minutes.

The special sauce: Create the super condiment from *Grill This, Not That!* Mix together two parts ketchup, two parts mayo, one part mustard, and chopped pickles to taste.

Note: Consuming undercooked burgers (internal temperature below 165°F) may increase your risk of foodborne illness.

Q My dad thinks bacon is evil. How can I convert the man?

A: In his mind, bacon equals fat, which equals heart attack. So tell him the white coats at Harvard took another look at that equation by reviewing 21 studies on saturated fat and heart disease. Their conclusion: No link. Zip, zero, nada.

Arteriosclerosis is much more complicated than "eat fat, deposit fat in arteries," says John Elefteriades, M.D., director of the Aortic Institute at Yale-New Haven Hospital and an MH cardiology advisor. "Heredity, injury to the wall of the artery by smoking or hypertension, and inflammation play more significant roles."

Next time you're eating breakfast with Pop, tell him he's actually worse off—at least caloriewise—with half a bagel (135 calories) or a bowl of Rice Krispies (126) than with two strips of bacon (84).

Q Are all salad greens nutritional zeros?

A: Steer clear of the iceberg. The deeper the color of your greens, the more phytonutrients and antioxidants they contain, says Susan Bowerman, M.S., R.D., C.S.S.D., an assistant director of the UCLA center for human nutrition. "Stronger flavors—think the broccoli and mustard families—also indicate increased phytonutrients."

To build a better-tasting, better-for-you salad, combine garden-variety lettuce with these high-powered greens.

Kale: A cousin of broccoli, kale is packed with sulforaphane, a phytonutrient associated with reduced risk of colon and prostate cancers. Shred it (to make the fibrous stalks easier to eat) and toss it with olive oil, avocado, and almonds.

Baby spinach: Three cups of raw spinach serves up about a third of the amount of iron men need each day, plus a hit of bone-building calcium. Toss with slices of blood orange, walnuts, and balsamic vinegar.

Radicchio: This spicy-tasting, red-leaf chicory is popular in Mediterranean salads. It's rich in lutein (for eye health) and vitamin K (for bone strength). Toss it with freshly boiled pasta, olive oil, and Parmesan.

Microgreens: Harvested from 7 to 21 days after their seeds go in the ground, these toddler greens are nutrient-dense and diverse in flavor. Look for arugula, beet tops, mizuna, and red cabbage.

Purslane: A lemony-tasting green, purslane is packed with the hormone melatonin, which can function as an antioxidant. It has at least 14 times the melatonin found in any other vegetable tested by researchers at the University of Texas at San Antonio.

PART 3

Muscle Up Fast

Men'sHealth

Power Tools for Your Home Gym

Upgrade your training arsenal with the ultimate home fitness gear.

Trainers like to say that the best gym to join is the one you pass every day. That sets one place above the rest almost by default: your home. Convenience, after all, has a way of inspiring results. So does free membership and not having to wipe someone else's sweat off a bench. And while you don't need a ton of equipment to sculpt a stronger physique, having a few key pieces of gear at your disposal can certainly expand your exercise options and accelerate your results.

That's exactly what you'll find in this chapter: the best tools for building muscle and torching flab from the comfort of anywhere—your home, your office, a hotel room, and even the gym if you're so inclined. Choose the items that best suit your goal—whether it's gaining strength, shedding pounds, or a combination of the two—and then follow our advice to maximize their effectiveness.

You won't find any of these gems hawked on late-night TV—and with our help, you'll also avoid having buyer's remorse. Indeed, you'll be far too busy admiring the leaner, stronger guy staring back at you in the mirror.

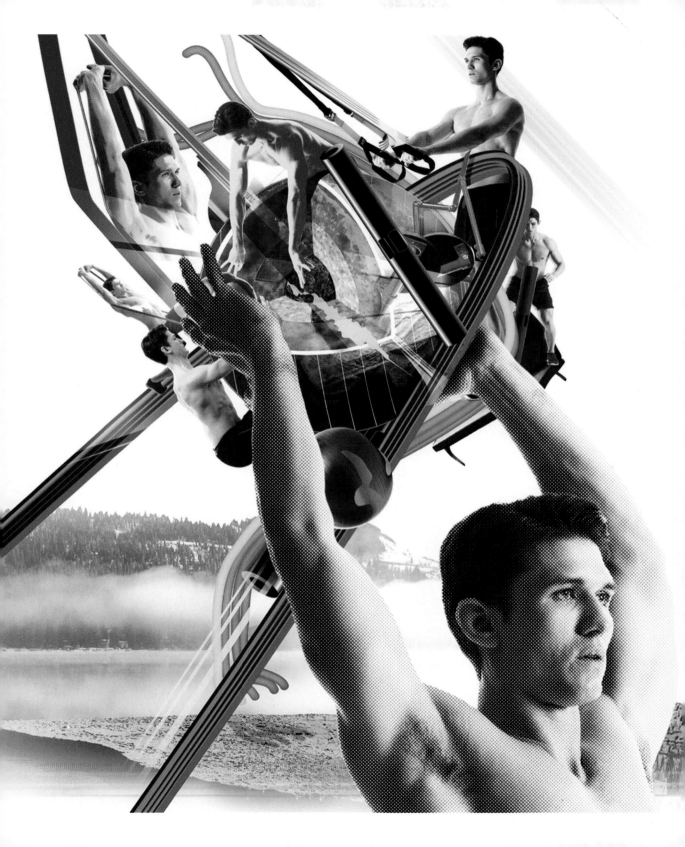

Resistance Band

How can a giant rubber band help you build muscle? Simple: Unlike a barbell or dumbbell, it provides constant tension throughout a lifting movement, increasing the intensity of the exercise and the challenge to your muscles. It's not the best way to add tons of bulk (free weights are still tops for that), but it's a fast, efficient way to gain real-world strength.

Our pick: If you buy one pair, go with the Purple Large Bands from Resistance Band Training Systems; they provide 50 to 75 pounds of resistance. If it's variety you're after, buy the Intermediate Band Package, which has four pairs ranging in resistance from 15 up to 120 pounds, for $100 more. ($45, resistancebandtraining.com)

BEST EXERCISE
Band Overhead Reverse Lunge

Stand with your feet shoulder-width apart, loop the band under your left foot, and press it overhead until your arms are straight. That's the starting position. Keep the band pressed overhead as you lunge backward with your right leg until your front knee is bent 90 degrees and your back knee is an inch or two off the floor. Return to the starting position. Do 3 sets of 12 reps, switching legs halfway through each set.

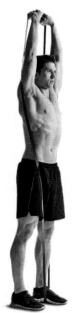
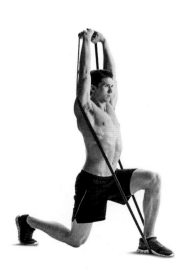

Medicine Ball

Today's medicine balls swap leather for easier-to-grab vinyl, but there's a reason the basic design hasn't changed for decades: It's one of the most dynamic strength builders you can own. It's also one of the few designed to leave your hands. Hurling it against a wall or the ground engages nearly every muscle in your body—especially those in your core.

Our pick: The Dynamax 8-pound Accelerator 1 Ball is designed to absorb impact, so it won't rocket back up into your face when you do medicine ball slams (see below). It's also made from 70 percent recycled materials. If you want room to grow, pick up 12-and 16-pound balls as well. ($85, medicineballs.com)

BEST EXERCISE
Medicine Ball Slam

Grab a medicine ball in both hands and hold it above your head with your feet shoulder-width apart and your arms slightly bent. Now reach back as far as you can and slam the ball to the ground in front of your feet. Grab the ball on the rebound and repeat the movement. Do 3 sets of 12 reps. Want to make it harder? Stand on one leg and try to maintain balance and good form as you do the exercise.

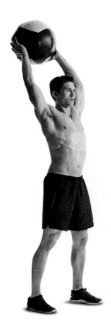
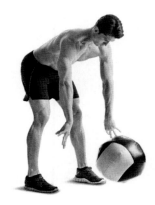

Kettlebell

This Russian import looks like a cannonball with a handle, but that ungainly design is exactly why it's so effective. Unlike a dumbbell, a kettlebell's center of gravity shifts during an exercise, increasing the challenge and building coordination. And because it's intended for total-body moves, it adds a cardio element to what is already an intense strength workout.

Our pick: We like the 16-kilogram First Place Kettlebell (about 35 pounds). There are more-expensive brands with vinyl covers and non-skid bases, but this basic cast-iron bell is all you need to build serious muscle. Want two? Add a 24-kilogram bell (about 53 pounds) to your order. ($70 and $90, performbetter.com)

BEST EXERCISE
Single-Arm Kettlebell Swing

Grab a kettlebell using an overhand grip and hold it with one hand, arm extended, at waist height. Set your feet slightly beyond shoulder width. Now swing the bell between your legs. Keeping your arm straight, thrust your hips forward, straighten your knees, and swing the bell up to chest level as you rise to a standing position. That's 1 rep. Do 3 sets of 20 to 30, switching hands halfway through each set.

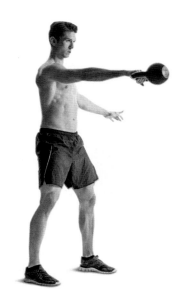
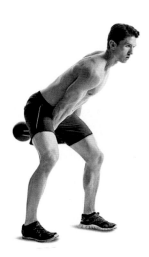

Suspension Trainer

Want to instantly make any exercise more difficult? Take it off terra firma. By adding an element of instability to your workout, a suspension trainer increases the challenge to your core and stabilizer muscles. The greater the challenge, the greater your gains. It's also one of the most portable items on our list; as long as you have access to a sturdy anchor point—a door or a tree limb, for example—you have everything you need for a workout.

Our pick: Try the TRX Pro Kit. Designed by a former Navy SEAL, this suspension trainer features single anchor points, making setup a snap. It's also one of the sturdiest on the market, which is a nice feeling when part of your body is hovering above the floor. ($200-250, trxtraining.com)

BEST EXERCISE
Inverted Row

Hang from the handles with your hands positioned above your shoulders, arms straight. Your body should form a straight line from your ankles to your head. Initiate the movement by pulling your shoulder blades back, and then continue the pull with your arms until your chest reaches the handles. Pause, and slowly lower your body back to the starting position. Do 3 sets of 10 to 12 reps.

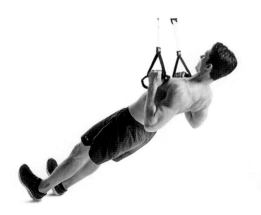
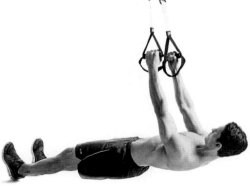

ViPR

It might look like a section of PVC pipe, but look again: This is one of the best fitness tools you probably never knew existed. (There's also nothing else like it on the market, which is why we gave it its own category.) Lift it. Drag it. Throw it. Flip it. Swing it. The ViPR is designed for active, total-body exercises that build balance, agility, and rock-solid core strength. It's also constructed of solid rubber, which means it's virtually indestructible.

Our pick: Start off with the 8-kilogram version (roughly 17 pounds), which is all you'll need for most exercises—trust us. Order heavier models—up to a maximum of 20 kilograms (about 44 pounds)—as your fitness level grows. ($205, perform better.com)

BEST EXERCISE
Lateral Shuffle

Stand with your feet shoulder-width apart and knees slightly bent, and place the ViPR on its end about a foot in front of you. Tug the ViPR so it begins to fall to your right, shuffling sideways to follow it down. As its top nears the floor, grab it with your left hand and tug it so it falls in the other direction. Continue alternating back and forth for 30 seconds. That's 1 set; do 3.

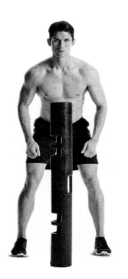
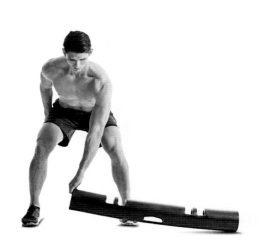

Swiss Ball

Think of a Swiss ball as the opposite of solid ground—a soft, unstable surface that challenges your core and helps you improve your balance and coordination. It's also an excellent substitute for a bench in exercises such as the chest press and the pullover, as long as your goal is to build coordination and stability rather than raw power and strength. Used alone, it's just about the best tool you can own for sculpting a six-pack.

Our pick: Thera-Band Pro Series Stability Ball is available in a range of sizes, depending on your height, but the 65-centimeter model (26 inches) is a good fit for most men. Its latex-free vinyl construction can also support up to 600 pounds. ($29-45, performbetter.com)

BEST EXERCISE
Swiss Ball Jackknife

Assume a pushup position with your arms straight and your shins on a Swiss ball. Your body should form a straight line from your ankles to your head. This is the starting position. Without changing your lower-back posture, roll the ball toward your chest by pulling it forward with your feet. Pause, then lower your hips and roll it back to the starting position. That's 1 rep. Do 3 sets of 8 to 10.

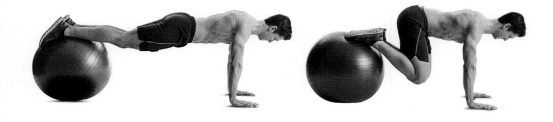

GO-HARD GEAR

If you have the space (and the money), think about upgrading your home gym with one or more of these big-ticket items to fast-track your fitness plan.

KEISER INFINITY FUNCTIONAL TRAINER

Thanks to two independently adjustable arms, the cable crossover machine lets you do hundreds of different exercises, making it one of the most versatile fitness tools you can own. Keiser's Infinity Functional Trainer uses air resistance instead of weights for a smoother, lower-impact workout. ($3,600, performbetter.com)

LIVESTRONG LS13.0T

This sub-$1,500 treadmill proves that a gym-quality machine doesn't have to cost big bucks. Its long (60-inch) belt, speeds to 12 miles an hour, convenient folding design, and suite of interactive features (including a USB drive for tracking your workouts online) make this unit one of the best budget buys out there. ($1,300, livestrongfitness.com)

POWERBLOCK U-90 STAGE II SET

Most selectorized dumbbells max out at 50 pounds, but these Power-Blocks replace an entire dumbbell rack in a fraction of the space, and they allow you to select from 2½ to 90 pounds in each hand. The result: You don't have to worry about outgrowing them. Their urethane coating also makes them extra durable and surprisingly quiet. ($640, powerblock.com)

CORE STIX

Inspired by the demands of farm work, the Core Stix trainer provides one of the best total-body workouts on our lineup. It was designed by an NHL strength and conditioning coach and a former space shuttle engineer, and its flexible rods offer resistance in multiple planes of motion and an almost unlimited number of exercise choices. ($850 to $1,800, corestix.com)

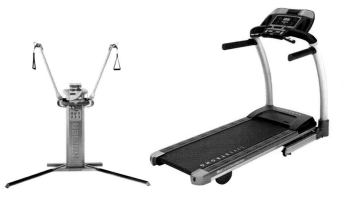
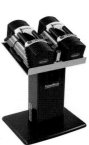
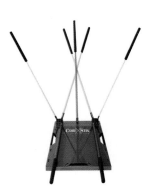

GYM BAG ESSENTIALS

Prefer to sweat in the company of others? No problem. Stash these portable items in your gym bag before you hit the weight room to maximize your workout and accelerate your muscular gains.

GRIP BALLS

A strong grip translates strength from your upper body to the world around you. Hook these onto a cable machine or pullup bar to build your forearms and an iron handshake. ($40, strongergrip.com)

POLAR FT80

Most heart-rate monitors focus on cardio. The FT80 is one of the few with a function for reading your heart rate between sets, so you know when you're ready for your next one. ($320, polarusa.com)

THE HYBRID STICK

Think of this rolling pin as a portable masseuse. Knead your muscles pre- and postworkout to ease stiffness and boost bloodflow. A raised center wheel helps target tight spots. ($45, thestick.com)

STRETCH OUT STRAP

Experts agree that assisted stretching is excellent for boosting flexibility and performance. Don't have a partner? The Stretch Out Strap is the next best thing. ($18, optp.com)

LIQUID GRIP

There's a reason rock climbers, gymnasts, and powerlifters use chalk: It keeps things from slipping out of their hands. Liquid grip provides the same benefit without the dust. ($20, liquidgrip.com)

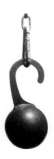 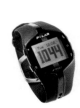 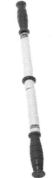 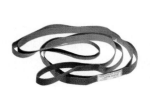 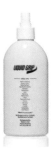

Can't-Miss Muscle

Use movements you've never tried to build the body you've always wanted.

Imagine that the barbell curl came with an autocorrect function, one that instantly perfected your form—no cheating allowed. Yes, you would possibly have to remove some weight. But you'd also slash your injury risk while giving your targeted muscles the maximum challenge. As a result, you'd reap the greatest possible benefit from every set.

Turns out, that autocorrect feature already exists; you just have to choose the right moves. *Men's Health* first learned about these moves, known as self-limiting exercises, from Gray Cook, P.T., whose analysis of human movement patterns is used to enhance his clients' performance and prevent injuries. Cook notes that barefoot running is a self-limiting exercise: If you don't use proper form or aren't in shape to run, the pain in your feet is your body's way of warning you to stop before you injure yourself. Makes sense, right?

By choosing movements that are nearly impossible to do without correct form, you can boost both your strength gains and your fat loss. Here are six self-limiting exercises you should add to your workouts. Now if only your diet had an autocorrect function . . .

TRX Inverted Row

Why it's self-limiting: You're relying on your upper body's weakest link to pull yourself up. If your upper back, arms, grip, or core aren't up to the task, they simply won't allow you to complete another rep.

Attach TRX suspension straps to a chinup bar so the handles are about 4 feet above the floor. Hold a handle in each hand and lie beneath them. Your arms should be straight and your body should be aligned from ankles to head. Brace your core and glutes. This is the starting position. Squeeze your shoulder blades together, pull your upper arms down, and bend your elbows to row your body upward. Pause, and then lower yourself to the starting position.

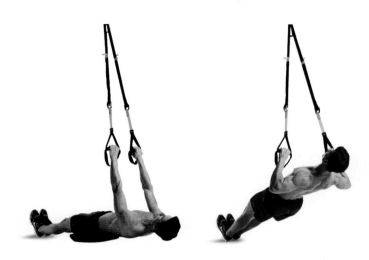

Single-Leg Squat

Why it's self-limiting: Simple: You either have the leg strength to push up from the bottom position, or you don't. (If your heel doesn't touch the floor on each rep, you're not lowering yourself far enough.)

Stand with your left leg on a bench that's about knee height. Your right leg should hang off the side, with your ankle flexed so your toes are higher than your heel. Hold your arms straight out in front of you for balance. This is the starting position. Balance on your left foot as you bend your left knee and push your hips back until your right heel touches the floor. Pause, and push yourself up to the starting position. Finish your left-leg reps before repeating with your right.

Kettlebell Windmill

Why it's self-limiting: If your core or arms tire, you won't be able to hold the weight overhead. It will fall to one side or you'll drop it.

With a kettlebell in your right hand, stand with your feet shoulder-width apart and your toes pointed slightly left. Hold the weight straight above your right shoulder, your left arm at your side. This is the starting position. Keeping your right arm straight, right leg stiff, and eyes on the kettlebell, lower your torso to the left, bending your left knee and lowering your left hand until it touches the floor. Return to the starting position. Finish your left-side reps, and repeat to your right.

Goblet Lunge

Why it's self-limiting: You have no choice but to keep your torso erect throughout the exercise. If you start to lean forward, that means your core is tiring and you run the risk of falling flat on your face.

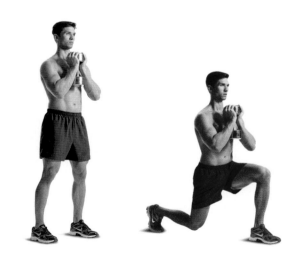

Hold a dumbbell vertically in front of your chest with both hands, cupping the weight by the head (the "goblet hold"). Keep your torso upright and your elbows pointed down. This is the starting position. Take one step forward with your left leg and lower yourself until your left knee is bent 90 degrees. Pause, and then push yourself back to the starting position. Complete the left-leg reps called for in your workout, and then repeat the move with your right leg.

Kettlebell Bottoms-Up Press

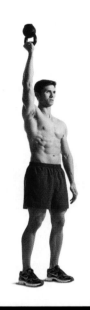

Why it's self-limiting: If your grip, arm, or core tires, you won't be able to push through the lift by overcompensating with any other muscle group; you'll need all three.

Grasp a heavy kettlebell in your right hand and swing it upward until it's next to your shoulder, with your elbow bent and your wrist straight. The weight should be upside down, with the bottom of the kettle-bell facing the ceiling. (You'll have to balance it.) Keep your torso braced and upright. This is the starting position. Press the kettlebell up until your arm is completely straight, and then lower it back to the starting position. That's 1 rep. Finish your right-arm reps before repeating the move with your left arm.

Single-Arm Farmer's Walk

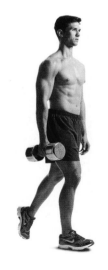

Why it's self-limiting: The challenge is that you have to stay completely upright as you perform this movement. If your core tires, you'll start leaning toward the side holding the dumbbell, creating uncomfortable torque on your spine that will force you to stop the exercise. Or if you lose your grip, you'll drop the weight.

With a heavy dumbbell in one hand, let both arms hang naturally at your sides. Keeping your torso braced and upright throughout the exercise, walk forward for as long as possible before you have to drop the weight. Shift the weight to your opposite hand and repeat. If you can walk for longer than 60 seconds, switch to a heavier dumbbell.

AFTERBURNERS

Here are three smart ways to cap off your workout.

If weightlifting is the fast track to fat-loss—and most experts agree that it is—then why do so many guys in the gym have a gut?

"Too many of them focus on beefing up body parts instead of trying to work as many muscles as possible," says B.J. Gaddour, C.S.C.S., owner of StreamFit.com.

One solution: metabolic finishers—one or two exercises performed at the end of a workout that turn it into a total-body sweat session.

LOWER-BODY FINISHER
5-5 SPLIT SQUAT

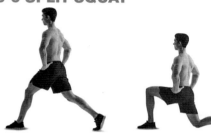

1. Face a wall and assume a split stance with your left foot forward, toes touching the wall. This is the starting position.

2. Take 5 seconds to lower your body until the top of your left thigh is at least parallel to the ground, pushing your left heel into the floor as hard as you can.

3. Hold for 5 seconds, and then explode back up to the starting position.

4. Do 5 reps in 1 minute, and then immediately switch legs and repeat.

5. Rest for 60 seconds and repeat the 2-minute sequence, this time starting with your right foot forward.

"Keeping your toes against the wall more effectively engages your hamstrings and glutes, turning a move that traditionally targets your quads into one that works your entire lower body," says Gaddour.

UPPER-BODY FINISHER
TRIPLE CRUSH

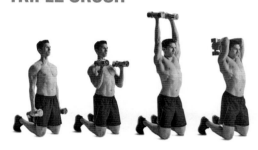

1. Kneel on the floor holding a pair of dumbbells at arm's length next to your sides. This is the starting position.

2. Bend your elbows and curl the dumbbells as close to your shoulders as you can.

3. Next, press the weights overhead with your palms facing each other.

4. Without moving your upper arms, lower the dumbbells behind your head.

5. Now reverse the movements to return to the starting position.

6. Repeat for 90 seconds, and then rest for 30. That's 1 set; do 2.

"You're combining three exercises [biceps curl, shoulder press, triceps extension] into one move," says Gaddour, "and kneeling works your core more effectively than standing."

"Think of them as fast-paced finales that ignite muscle growth and accelerate weight loss," says Gaddour. "Oh yeah, and they're great for melting stubborn belly fat."

To do it, select the finisher below that transforms your typical routine into a total-body workout. If your workout targets your upper body, for example, go with the lower-body finisher. Already doing a total-body workout? Then shift your metabolism into high gear by performing the final two finishers (A and B) as a superset (back to back with 10 seconds of rest between them). Repeat the superset 8 times.

TOTAL-BODY FINISHER A
DUMBBELL SKIER SWING

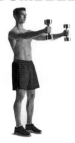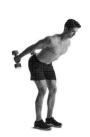

1. Grab two unevenly weighted dumbbells (a 5-pound difference is ideal) and hold them at arm's length in front of your chest. Your feet should be hip-width apart and knees slightly bent.

2. Without rounding your lower back, bend at your hips and simultaneously swing your arms backward.

3. Explosively thrust your hips forward and raise your torso until you're standing upright, letting your momentum swing the weights up to chest level.

4. Continue for 20 seconds. Alternate the heavier weight between your right and left hands in successive supersets.

"This move trains not only your often-neglected hamstrings," says Gaddour, "but also your entire core from shoulders to hips."

TOTAL-BODY FINISHER B
DUMBBELL MOUNTAIN CLIMBER

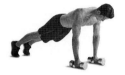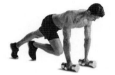

1. Assume a pushup position with a dumbbell in each hand. Keep your palms facing in. Your body should form a straight line from ankles to head. This is the starting position.

2. Lift your right foot off the floor and slowly raise your right knee as close to your chest as you can without rounding your lower back.

3. Return to the starting position and repeat, this time lifting your left knee. Continue for 20 seconds, alternating knees with each repetition.

"You'll target your abs and send your heart rate through the roof," Gaddour says.

The Ultimate Boot Camp Workout

There may be no faster way to gain fitness and transform your body.

If the infomercials are any indication, people spend more money on their abs than on any other muscle group. And why wouldn't they? Your abs play a role in nearly all your movements. But you don't need a credit card to reveal your abs. You need a smart diet—along with this boot camp workout, which will torch your belly fat and work your entire core. Abs still a mystery to you? Here's a blueprint of your midsection muscles.

1. Rectus Abdominis: The rectus abdominis—six-pack—is the best-known ab muscle. Despite the nickname, it's actually eight segments separated by dense connective tissue called fascia. By helping counteract the pull of the muscles that extend your lower back, the rectus abdominis helps your spine stay stable. Its other main duty is to pull your torso toward your hips.

2. Fascia: This tough tissue weaves in and around all your body's muscles to create an interconnective web. In terms of your abs, it's what separates and connects each of the eight segments of your rectus abdominis, giving them their regimented appearance.

3. External Obliques: Running vertically and diagonally, these muscles originate at your rib cage and connect at your hip bone and linea alba (see #5 below). They help bend your torso to the sides and rotate your torso to the left and right. Perhaps most important, they also act to prevent your torso from rotating.

4. Internal Obliques: These muscles lie beneath your external obliques. They assist in side-bending and rotating your torso, as well as in resisting rotation.

5. Linea Alba: This long strip of fascia forms a line of separation down the center of your abdominals. It helps prevent your rectus abdominis from being ripped apart by your obliques.

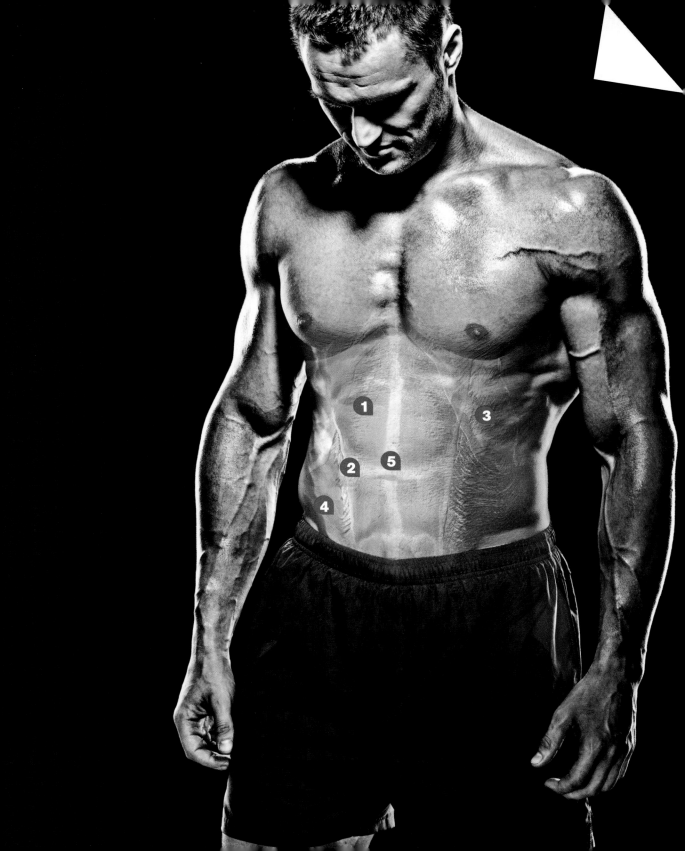

Enlist Muscle, Blast Fat

If you're looking to firebomb fat, pack on muscle, and sweat your way to a six-pack, we have your call to duty: this cutting-edge boot camp workout, designed by fitness expert B.J. Gaddour, C.S.C.S., owner of StreamFit.com.

By moving you through a series of intense exercises at a fast pace, it'll help you burn more calories per minute than a typical weight-training or aerobic workout. Plus, it works every one of your muscles, from head to toe. The best part: Whether you want bigger muscles or faster fat loss, Gaddour shows you how to tweak this workout to achieve your most pressing goal. Now get to work—and that's an order!

Perform this workout as a circuit, completing each exercise in succession.

To blast more fat: Starting with exercise 1, do as many reps as you can in 50 seconds. Then rest for 10 seconds as you transition to the next exercise. After you've done all 10 exercises, rest for 60 seconds. Then repeat the circuit one more time.

To build more muscle: Do as many repetitions as you can in 30 seconds. (You'll need to use a heavier weight than you would for the fat-loss version.) Then rest for 30 seconds as you transition to the next exercise. Do all 10 exercises and rest for 60 seconds; then repeat the circuit once more.

For video instructions and a digital training guide, check out this workout online at mhpersonaltrainer.com. There you'll also find a complete nutrition plan that you can customize for your goals and lifestyle.

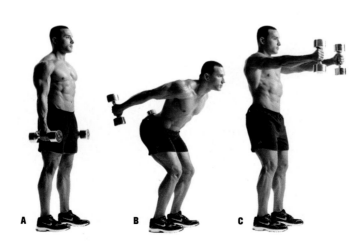

A   B   C

Dumbbell Skier Swing

Holding a pair of dumbbells at arm's length next to your sides, stand with your feet hip-width apart and your knees slightly bent [A]. Without rounding your lower back, bend at your hips as you simultaneously swing your arms backward [B]. Now explosively thrust your hips forward and raise your torso until you're standing upright, while allowing your momentum to swing the weights up to chest level [C]. (Don't actively lift the weight.) Swing back and forth for the duration of your set.

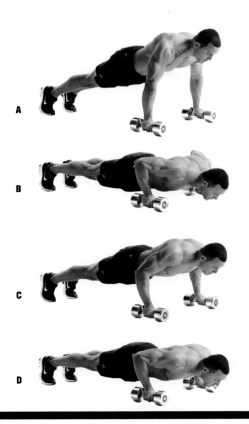

Dumbbell 1½ Pushup

Grasp the handle of a dumbbell in each hand and assume a pushup position with your arms straight. Your hands should be about shoulder-width apart, and your body should form a straight line from head to ankles [A]. Bend your elbows and lower your body until your chest nearly touches the floor [B]. Pause, and then push yourself halfway back up [C]. Pause again, then lower your body back to the floor [D]. Push yourself all the way back up to the starting position, and repeat.

Dumbbell Hot Potato Squat

Grab a dumbbell with your left hand and hold it against the front of your shoulder, your elbow bent [A]. Keeping your back naturally arched, push your hips back, bend your knees, and lower your hips until the top of your thighs is at least parallel to the floor [B]. Then stand back up as you smoothly pass the dumbbell from your left hand to your right [C]. Now immediately repeat the squat while holding the dumbbell in your right hand [D]. Continue to alternate back and forth.

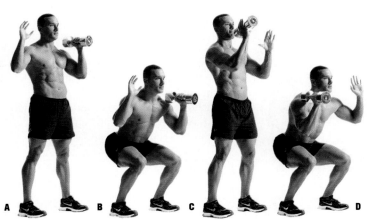

Dumbbell Lawnmower Pull

Hold a dumbbell in your right hand and stand in a split stance, your left foot in front of your right. Bend your left knee and your hips until your torso is about 45 degrees to the floor. Let the dumbbell hang at arm's length [A]. In one move, explosively straighten your left leg and thrust your hips forward [B] as you rotate your torso (pivot your feet) and row the weight to your shoulder [C]. Reverse the move and repeat. Once you've worked for half of your allotted time, switch hands and legs.

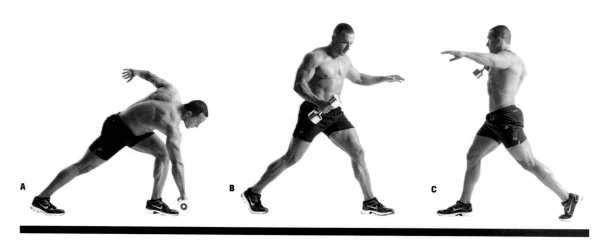

A   B   C

Dumbbell Overhead Shouldering

Use both hands to grasp a dumbbell by its ends and hold it against your chest. Stand tall with your feet shoulder-width apart. Shift the dumbbell to your right shoulder [A]; then press it directly overhead until your arms are straight [B] and lower it to your left shoulder [C]. That's 1 repetition. Continue to move the weight in this manner until you've worked for half of your allotted time. Then switch directions (that is, push the dumbbell up from your left shoulder) and do the rest of your reps.

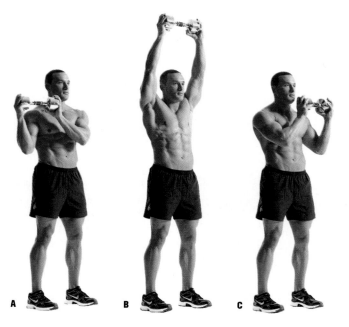

A   B   C

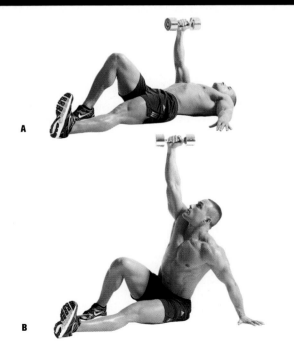

Dumbbell Rotational Deadlift

Stand tall and use both hands to grasp a dumbbell by its ends, letting it hang at arm's length in front of your waist [A]. Now rotate your hips to the left so your left foot is forward and the weight is hanging next to your left thigh. Next, keep your back naturally arched as you bend your knees and hips and lower the weight to the front of your left shin [B]. Push your hips forward, raise your torso, and stand; then rotate your torso all the way to the right to repeat the move on that side.

Dumbbell Bottom-Half Getup

Grab a dumbbell in your right hand and lie on the floor with your right leg bent and your left leg straight. Hold the dumbbell overhead with your arm completely straight [A]. Without taking your eyes off the dumbbell or letting your right arm bend, roll onto your left side and prop yourself up on your left elbow. Now straighten your left arm [B]. Reverse the move to return to the starting position and repeat until the time is up. On your next set of this exercise, do the move with the weight in your left hand.

SPEED UP YOUR GAINS

Certain things fall squarely in the "more is better" category—vacation days, sex—but strength training isn't necessarily one of them.

"There's no reason to spend hours in the gym unless you want to," says Eric Cressey, M.A., C.S.C.S., the cofounder of Cressey Performance in Hudson, Massachusetts, and author of *Show and Go.* "Many of the world's top athletes are in and out in less than 60 minutes."

Learn their secrets and you can do the same. Here's how to stop wishing for more hours in the day to work out, and start building more muscle in the time you have.

DON'T SPIN YOUR WHEELS

If you typically warm up on the treadmill, stop. It chews up workout time and targets only your legs.

"Get rolling faster by focusing on multijoint, total-body movements, like the squat-to-stand with reach," says Cressey. In addition to increasing your bloodflow, you'll jumpstart the signaling between your brain and your muscles, boosting performance from the get-go. The result: a faster warmup and a more efficient workout.

How to do it: Stand tall with your feet slightly beyond shoulder width. Lower yourself into a squat and grab your toes. Keeping your chest and shoulders up, raise your right arm high and wide. Repeat with your left. Now stand up. That's 1 rep; do 8.

Time saved: 5 minutes

MULTITASK YOUR MUSCLES

Ditch the old "one exercise at a time" routine for supersets or trisets—two or three exercises done back-to-back.

"While one muscle group recovers, another is working, reducing the need for rest," says Cressey. You'll also reap a metabolic boost, burning more calories per minute both during and after your workout than you would with a more traditional weightlifting routine with rests, according to Syracuse University scientists.

How to do it: Target noncompeting muscle groups by pairing push and pull exercises (dumbbell chest press and cable row, for example) or upper-and lower-body exercises (dumbbell alternating shoulder press and barbell straight-leg deadlift).

Time saved: 15 minutes

REDUCE THE REPETITION

Instead of doing 3 or 4 sets of 8 to 10 reps each, start off with a few lower-rep sets using a heavier weight.

"It's called a stage system," says Cressey. "The nerves that stimulate your muscles are amped up from the heavy sets, so they're able to lift more weight than normal for a final higher-rep set."

How to do it: Do 3 sets using a weight you can lift only three times in a row, and then lighten the weight by 10 percent and do a final set of 6 reps.

Time saved: 10 minutes

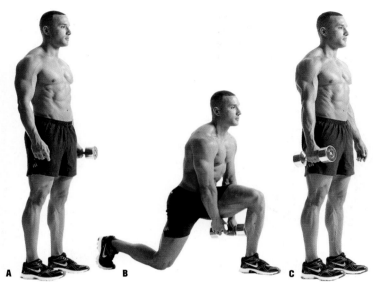

Dumbbell Threaded Lunge

Hold a dumbbell in your left hand and stand tall with your feet hip-width apart. This is the starting position [A]. Keeping your torso upright, take a big step backward with your right foot and lower your body until your left knee is bent at least 90 degrees and your right knee almost touches the floor. While in this "down" position, pass the dumbbell under your left leg to your right hand [B]. Push yourself back to the starting position, and repeat, this time lunging backward with your left leg.

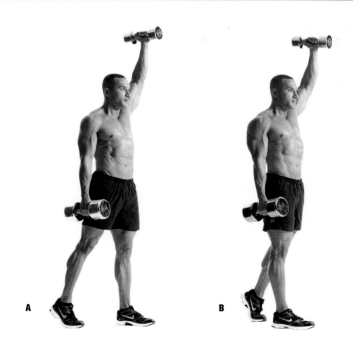

Dumbbell High-Low Farmer's Walk

Grab two dumbbells—a heavy one in your right hand and a light one in your left. (The heavy dumbbell should be about twice the weight of the light one.) Press the light dumbbell over your head, with your arm straight and your biceps in line with your ear. Let the heavy dumbbell hang at arm's length next to your side [A]. With your core braced and glutes tight, walk forward [B] and then backward—and then every which way. Once you've worked for half of your allotted time, switch arms and legs.

Dumbbell Shoveling

Stand in a split stance, your left foot in front of your right. Use both hands to grasp a dumbbell by its ends and hold it at arm's length in front of your left thigh [A]. Explosively loop the dumbbell across your body, up to chest level [B], and then over to your right thigh as you pivot your feet and rotate your hips to the right. Then reverse the move back to the starting position. Continue to move the dumbbell back and forth, as if you're constantly "shoveling" from one side of your body to the other.

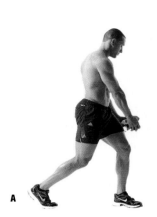

A

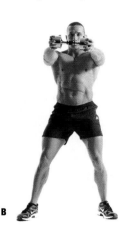

B

INSTANT EXERCISE UPGRADE: HIT THE WALL

Few moves can equal the pushup's do-anywhere power, but it can be more effective if you place your feet against a wall, says B.J. Gaddour, C.S.C.S., CEO of StreamFit.com. Same goes for mountain climbers.

"You'll engage your glutes, stabilizing your pelvis and spine, and focus more attention on your abs."

Here's how to do it: Assume a pushup position with the bottom of your feet planted firmly against a wall or door. (Your toes should still touch the ground.) Now do pushups as usual, trying not to let your hips sag. Keep your core stiff as you lower your torso.

For mountain climbers, alternately keep one foot on the wall as you bring the opposite knee toward your chest without flexing your lower back. Do as many reps as you can of either move in 30 seconds. For an added challenge, elevate your feet. Press back on your heels to prevent them from sliding.

"You'll place more load on your working muscles," Gaddour says, "increasing the difficulty of the move while forcing your core and shoulders to work harder to stabilize your body."

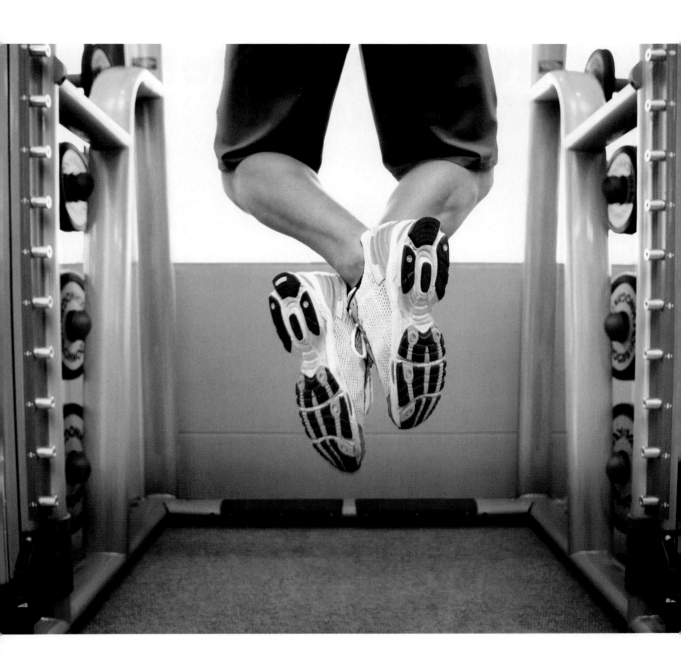

The Stronger, Higher, Faster Workout

Learn the training secrets of the NBA's most exciting player and use this routine to take your game to an all-new level.

Blake Griffin might be the single most explosive athlete in the world today, says Robbie Davis, C.S.C.S., Griffin's strength coach and the owner of Gameshape in Los Angeles. Yes, great genes help. But that title doesn't come without work. That's why Davis has Griffin follow a routine that uses a one-two punch of strength and power exercises. Performing the strength exercise first primes the mind-muscle connection for doing the power move at top speed—the key to improving explosiveness.

The Workout

Do this workout 3 days a week, resting a day between sessions. Perform each pair of exercises (for instance, 1A and 1B, 2A and 2B, and so on) as a superset. That is, do 8 to 12 repetitions of the "A" exercise followed immediately by 3 to 5 repetitions of the "B" exercise with no rest in between. Rest for 60 to 90 seconds and repeat. Do a total of 3 or 4 sets of each exercise before moving on to the next pair and repeating the procedure. For the B (or power) exercises, use a medicine ball that's about 5 to 10 percent of your body weight.

For video instructions and a digital training guide, check out this workout online at mhpersonaltrainer.com. There you'll also find a complete nutrition plan that you can customize for your goals and lifestyle.

Ready to take a page from Griffin's training plan? Then try this workout from Davis. It'll have you soaring in no time.

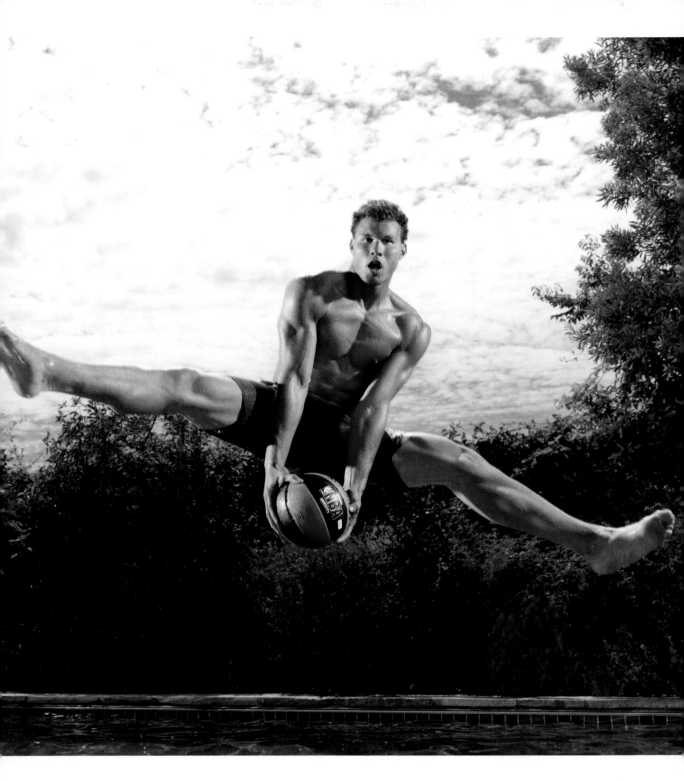

Exercise 1A: Dumbbell Lunge, Curl, and Press

Stand holding a pair of dumbbells at your sides, palms facing each other and feet hip-width apart. This is the starting position [A]. Keeping your torso upright, step forward with your right foot and lower your body until your right knee is bent 90 degrees. Hold that position and curl the dumbbells to your shoulders [B]. Then press the dumbbells directly above your shoulders until your arms are straight [C]. Lower the dumbbells back to your sides, and then push yourself back to the starting position.

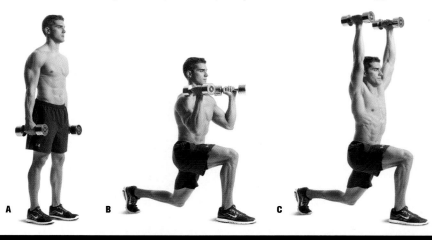

Exercise 1B:
Medicine-Ball Split Jump

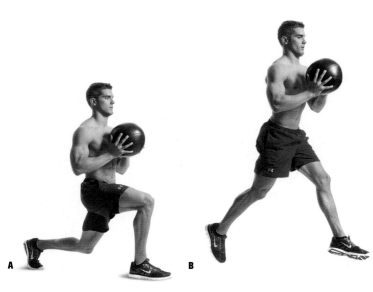

Hold a medicine ball in front of your chest and stand with your feet 2 to 3 feet apart and staggered, your right foot in front of your left. Keeping your torso upright, bend your legs and lower your body into a lunge [A]. Jump with enough force to propel both feet off the floor, and then scissors-kick your legs [B] so you land with your left foot forward. That's 1 rep. Repeat by switching leg positions.

Exercise 2A: Dumbbell Box Squat, Overhead Press, and Calf Raise

Sit at the end of a bench and hold a pair of dumbbells next to your shoulders, with your elbows bent and palms facing each other. Set your feet wider than shoulder-width apart and your lower legs nearly perpendicular to the floor. Brace your core (as if you're about to be punched in the gut), tighten your glutes and thighs, and lean your torso slightly forward [A]. Without moving your torso, stand up [B]. Then in one move, press the dumbbells directly over your shoulders while raising your heels as high as you can [C]. Reverse the moves and return to the bench.

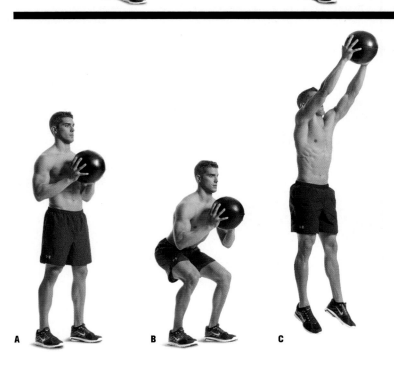

Exercise 2B: Medicine-Ball Backboard Taps

Hold a medicine ball at shoulder height and stand with your feet shoulder-width apart [A]. Dip down into a squat [B], and jump as high as you can while raising the medicine ball above your head and tapping it against a backboard [C]. (If you're not on a basketball court, just try to imagine a backboard.) Land softly and repeat.

Exercise 3A: Basketball-Stance Pushup and Row

Hold a pair of dumbbells and assume a pushup position, but with your knees bent instead of straight and your feet about shoulder-width apart. This is the starting position [A]. (Davis uses it because it mimics the lower-body stance often used in basketball.) Bend your arms and lower your body as close to the floor as possible [B]. Push back to the starting position. Keeping your body steady, row the dumbbell in your right hand to the right side your chest [C]. Lower it and repeat rowing on your left side. That's 1 rep.

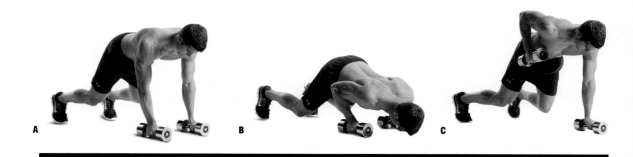

Exercise 3B: Medicine-Ball Chest Pass

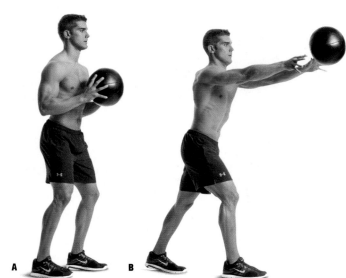

Stand with your feet together a few feet from a wall, and hold a medicine ball in front of your chest [A]. Step forward with your right foot and chest-pass the ball to the wall [B]. Catch the rebound, reset your feet, and repeat, this time stepping forward with your left foot. (You can also pass the ball to a partner instead of bouncing it against a wall.)

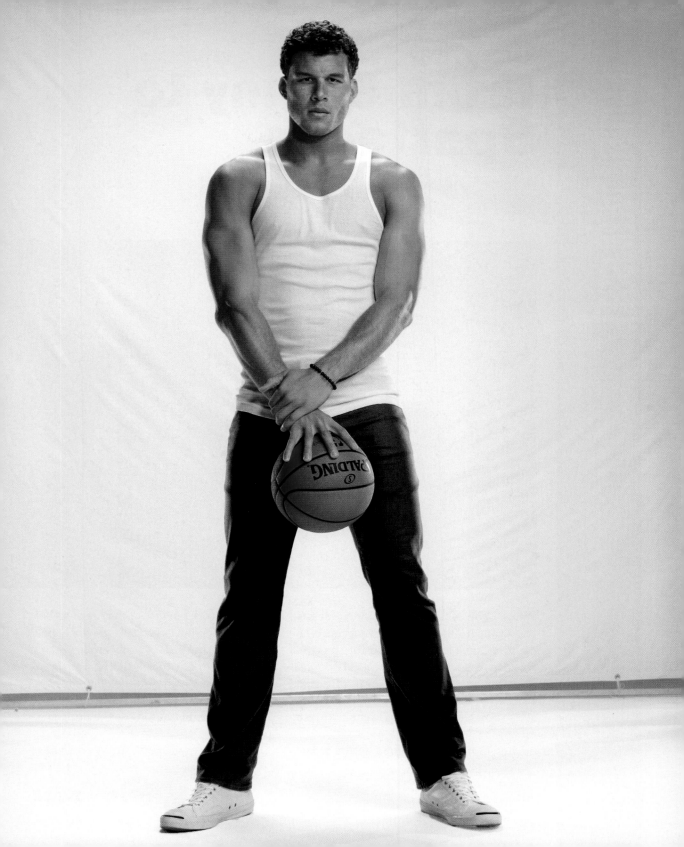

From Skinny to Spartacus

A lanky actor transformed himself into Spartacus. The good news: You can do it, too.

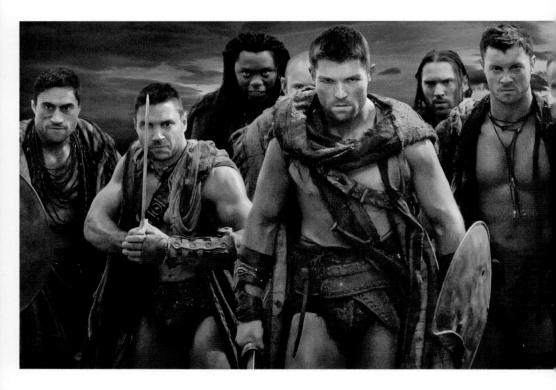

When Liam McIntyre auditioned for the television drama *Spartacus: Vengeance*, he couldn't have looked less fit for the title role. He was fresh off a movie called *Frozen Moments*, playing a man who had awakened from a coma. Skinny made sense for that. For Spartacus? Not so much.

But McIntyre is a good actor, so the Starz network put him at the top of its list, with one major caveat: At go time, he'd better look the part of a rebel warrior.

So he set out to rebuild his musculature. "It was a combination of mental and physical effort," he says. "The body can do incredible things as long as the mind supports it."

We're providing McIntyre's fitness

advice and our own Spartacus workout. Put them both to work, and when you reach go time—beach vacation, high school reunion, first date—you'll be sure to look the part, too.

Spartacus Fitness Advice

The following tips helped McIntyre get warrior ready.

Liam McIntyre set out to rebuild his physique for *Spartacus*. "It was a combination of mental and physical effort. The body can do incredible things as long as the mind supports it."

Create a No-Fail Plan

McIntyre wanted a body like Hugh Jackman's in *X-Men Origins: Wolverine*. It would have been a challenge anyway, but especially so given McIntyre's 13-hour workdays. His strategy: Never miss a planned workout.

Make it work for you. Focus on the means, not the end. University of Iowa scientists found that people are more likely to stick with a weight-loss plan when they concentrate on specific actions instead of the desired result.

"Break your goal into habits that will help you achieve it," says Rachel Cosgrove, C.S.C.S., co-owner of Results Fitness in Santa Clarita, California.

For example, you might set a goal of completing the Spartacus Workout 12 times a month. That's just three workouts a week. But if you reach your 12-workout goal every month, by the end of the year you'll have logged 144 high-intensity workouts. How many gut-busting workouts did you complete last year?

Measure Your Success

McIntyre had never been a gym rat before *Spartacus*. "I didn't treat my body as well as I should have," he says. But with his new role, he needed to perform intense weight workouts 4 days a week—every week, for months. Now McIntyre is stronger and fitter than he's ever been. "When I look back at the photo the *Spartacus* producers took at the start, I think, 'Oh, God,'" he says. "I didn't realize how much weight I'd lost for *Frozen Moments*." Which is a good reminder: Amazing results don't happen overnight, but they do happen over time.

Make it work for you. Because you're not likely to notice a change in the mirror right away, focus on what you can measure: Your performance. "You should be able to do more every workout; lift more weight, do more reps, add more sets," says Cosgrove. "You can bet that if your numbers are improving, so is your body."

Fuel Your Muscles

"You can lift all the time," says McIntyre,

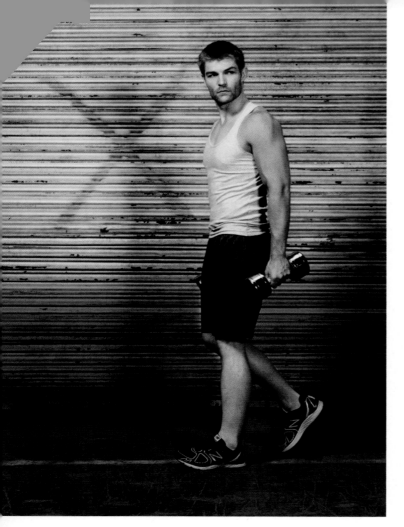

But some guys say it's too expensive; others say they feel like they have to force-feed themselves. So shoot for 0.7 gram of protein for every pound, says Aragon. It's still a highly effective dose for your muscles. The only downside: You might find that you're hungrier and more at risk of binge snacking.

Find a Partner

McIntyre rarely goes to the gym alone. "There are tons of benefits to working out with someone else. You can do a better range of exercises if someone's there to spot you," he says. Plus, others push you outside your comfort zone. "They'll yell at me when I'm not working hard enough, and compliment me when I am."

Make it work for you. Find a workout partner or join a boot-camp class at a local gym, says BJ Gaddour, C.S.C.S., a leading boot-camp expert. "The more people we have training together, the more energy, sweat, and encouragement are in the room."

"but if you don't eat the right foods, you won't have the body you want." The key ingredient for any diet is protein. It provides the nutrients you need for muscle growth and also keeps you satisfied between meals.

Make it work for you. To grow larger and speed fat loss, *Men's Health* nutrition advisor Alan Aragon, M.S., recommends eating 1 gram of protein per pound of your target weight. So if you want to weigh 180 pounds, you should eat 180 grams of protein a day.

Think Beyond Yourself

McIntyre inherited his role as Spartacus from the actor Andy Whitfield, who recently passed away after a long battle with non-Hodgkin's lymphoma. "Andy was amazing at his job," McIntyre says. "I want to do justice to the character he already created. I think of Andy and remind myself that no day is too hard."

Make it work for you. Not in the mood for a sweat session? Keep moving for the people who can't. Says Cosgrove, whose husband is a stage IV cancer survi-

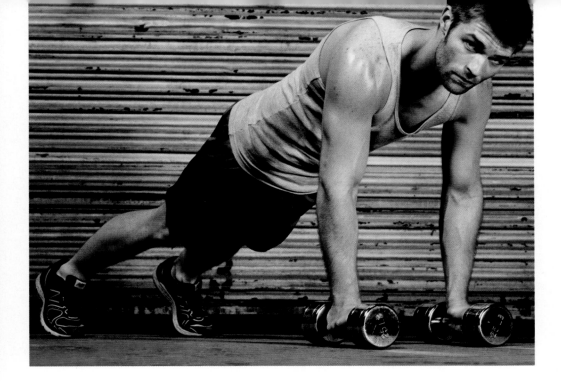

vor and the co-owner of their gym, "Put it in perspective. It's not chemo. When you think about people fighting for their lives, it makes a workout seem like nothing." Honor them by making yourself better. "We owe it to people like Andy to bring our best to everything we do," says Cosgrove. "And that includes taking care of our health."

The Spartacus Workout

Give your body the ultimate fitness challenge. Two years ago we teamed with Starz to create the official *Spartacus* Workout. Its popularity surprised even us: Readers told us it was their favorite *Men's Health* workout ever. So we asked Cosgrove, who created the original routine, to design an all-new version that's even more intense, challenging, and

effective. Like the original, this updated *Spartacus* Workout requires only a pair of dumbbells, a stopwatch, and, well, some serious grit. But try Cosgrove's plan just once and you'll quickly understand why it burns fat, sculpts muscle, and leads to fantastic results.

Do this workout 3 days a week. Perform the exercises—or "stations"—as a circuit, doing one movement after another. At each station, perform as many repetitions as you can in 40 seconds using perfect form. Rest for 20 seconds as you transition to the next exercise. After you've done all 10 exercises, catch your breath for 2 minutes. Then repeat the entire circuit two more times.

If you find that you can't keep working for the entire 40 seconds, then use a lighter weight. If you feel as if you could keep going hard for an additional 15 seconds, progress to a heavier weight.

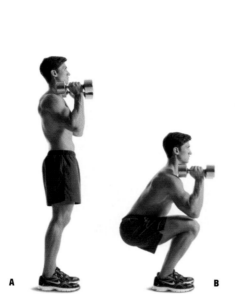
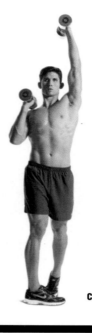

Dumbbell Squat to Alternating Shoulder Press and Twist

Stand with your feet shoulder-width apart and hold a pair of dumbbells next to your shoulders, elbows bent, palms facing in [A]. Push your hips back and squat deeply [B]. Push back up, rotating your torso to the right and pivoting on your left foot as you press the dumbbell in your left hand above your shoulder [C]. Lower the weight and rotate back to center. Repeat, rotating to the left and pressing up the dumbbell in your right hand.

A   B   C

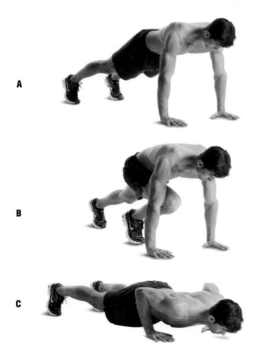

Mountain Climber and Pushup

Assume a pushup position. Your body should form a straight line from your head to your ankles [A]. Without allowing your lower-back posture to change, lift your left foot off the floor and move your left knee toward your chest [B]. Return to the starting position, and repeat with your right leg. That's a mountain climber. Now do a pushup [C].

A

B

C

Dumbbell Side Lunge and Curl

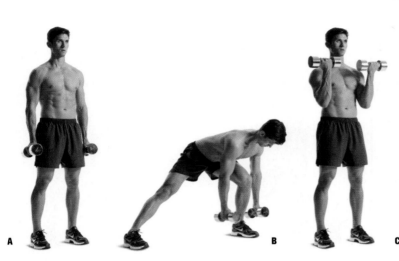

A

B

C

Hold a pair of dumbbells at arm's length at your sides [A]. Take a big step to your left and lower your body by pushing your hips back and bending your left knee. As you lower your body, bend forward at your hips and try to touch the dumbbells to the floor [B]. (Note: Go only as low as you can without rounding your lower back.) Then push yourself back to the starting position as quickly as you can. Perform arm curls [C]. Alternate back and forth, doing a lunge to your left and then a lunge to your right.

Plank Walkup with Dumbbell Drag

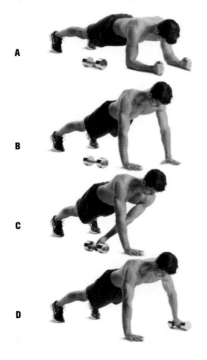

A

B

C

D

Start in a pushup position with a dumbbell on the floor next to your right hand. Lower your body into a plank so you're resting your weight on your forearms instead of your palms [A]. "Walk" back up to a pushup position [B]. Without leaving this position, grasp the dumbbell with your left hand [C] and drag it underneath your chest until it rests on your left side [D]. Repeat, this time dragging the weight with your right hand.

Dumbbell Stepover

Stand holding dumbbells at your sides [A]. Step forward with your left foot and lower your body until your front knee is bent 90 degrees [B]. In one motion, push back up and take a long step back with your left foot into a reverse lunge [C]. Keep shifting between forward and backward lunges with the same leg for 20 seconds, and then repeat on the other side.

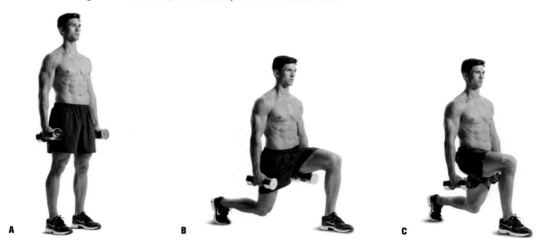

Dumbbell Single-Arm Alternating Clean

Stand with your feet shoulder-width apart and a dumbbell between your feet on the floor. Push your hips back, squat, and grab the dumbbell with one hand [A]. Pull the dumbbell up and "catch" it at shoulder height as you rise to a standing position; keep your knees slightly bent [B]. Pause, lower the dumbbell to the floor, grab it with your other hand [C], and repeat on the other side [D].

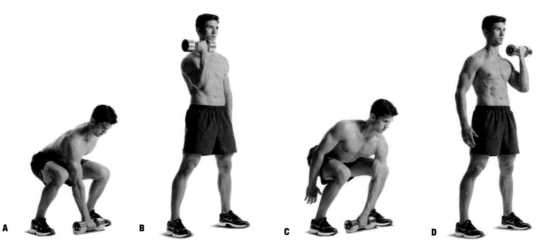

Pushup-Position Row and Squat Thrust

Place a pair of dumbbells on the floor and assume a pushup position with your hands on the dumbbells [A]. Pull the right dumbbell up to the side of your chest [B]. Pause, and then lower the dumbbell; repeat the move with your left arm [C]. While holding the dumbbells, quickly bring your legs toward your torso [D], and then jump up [E]. Once you land, squat and kick your legs back into a pushup.

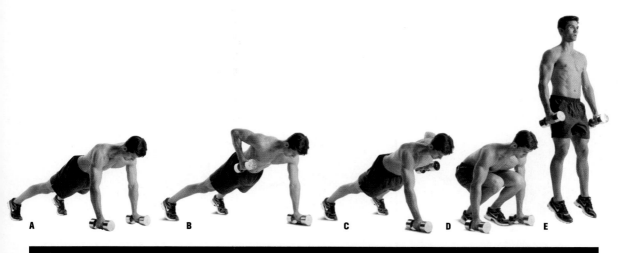

Goblet Squat and Alternating Reverse Lunge

Hold a dumbbell vertically in front of your chest, cupping one end of the dumbbell with both hands [A]. Keep your elbows pointed toward the floor and perform a squat [B]. Then push back up to the starting position [C]. Now step back with one leg—into a reverse lunge—and lower your body until your front knee is bent 90 degrees [D]. Pause, and then push up quickly. Alternate your lunging leg with each rep.

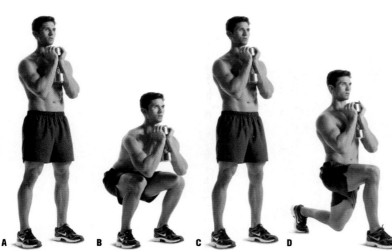

Dumbbell Russian Twist

Sit holding a dumbbell in front of your chest. Lean your torso back slightly and raise your feet off the floor [A]. Without moving your torso, rotate the weight to your left [B] and then to your right [C]. Move back and forth quickly.

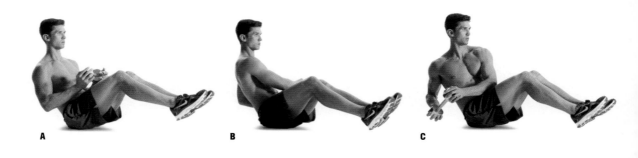

A   B   C

Dumbbell Straight-Leg Deadlift and Row

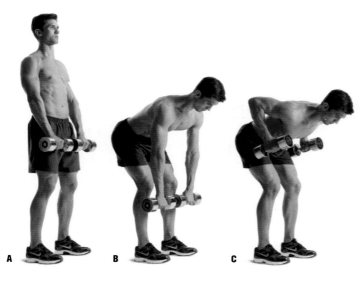

A   B   C

Stand with your knees slightly bent and hold a pair of dumbbells at arm's length in front of your thighs [A]. Without rounding your lower back or changing the bend in your knees, bend at your hips and lower your torso until it's nearly parallel to the floor [B]. Without moving your torso, pull the dumbbells up to the sides of your chest [C]. Pause, and then lower the dumbbells. Raise your torso back to the starting position.

CHILL OUT, MUSCLE UP

Pumping iron is only part of the muscle-building formula. "Recovery is just as important," says Todd Durkin, C.S.C.S., author of The IMPACT! Body Plan.

That's because weightlifting creates microtears in your muscles, and hitting the gym again too hard too soon can undermine the repair process (also known as muscle growth). "Your body needs at least one day of rest between workouts," says Durkin. Follow his four tips to make the most of your downtime.

Feed your muscles.
Lifting weights makes your metabolism race as your body works to replenish energy and repair muscle tissue. "If you don't take in enough calories and protein, you won't have the resources you need to recover," says Durkin. He recommends consuming 300 to 500 additional calories on workout days, and skewing those calories toward protein, the building block of muscle. "Shoot for 1 gram per pound of body weight," says Durkin. See "Muscle Fuel" on this page for three easy ways to help meet your quota.

Roll with it. Here's why you need a regular massage, or at least a foam roller: "Both can help break up the scar tissue that's a natural consequence of lifting," says Durkin. That not only speeds the repair process and reduces soreness but also improves range of motion, reports a study in the *Journal of Strength and Conditioning Research.* "Spend 5 minutes using a foam roller on your quads, hams, glutes, hips, and lower back before a workout and before bed," Durkin says. "If you can, also visit a massage therapist twice a month."

Catch more Z's. Muscle building doesn't shut down when you hit the sack. "Your body repairs a lot of damage as you sleep, so it's critical to get as much as you can," Durkin says. Indeed, a lack of shut-eye can increase muscle loss by up to 60 percent, according to researchers in Brazil. The reason: Your body produces its greatest surge of growth hormone while you're sleeping. What's more, the fatigue that goes hand in hand with too little sleep can torpedo your workout performance. Your goal: 7 to 8 hours of quality slumber every night.

Take a cold one.
Tough workouts don't have to result in aching muscles. Immersing yourself in cold water immediately after intense exercise can reduce delayed-onset muscle soreness (DOMS) by nearly half, say scientists in Ireland. That means a faster return to peak performance and a lower likelihood of missing your next workout. Do this: Fill your bathtub with 50° to 59°F water (cool tap water is usually cold enough) and soak in it for 5 to 12 minutes in order to reduce the inflammation that causes DOMS, the scientists recommend.

Pain-Free for Life

Fact: Active men get HURT. Jordan D. Metzl, M.D., the author of *The Athlete's Book of Home Remedies*, tells in his own words how to heal faster, train smarter, and build an injury-proof body.

My first year of med school, I played soccer for a club team at the University of Missouri. We were having a practice, and it was a beautiful day to be out and moving. I was playing striker up front, and as the goalkeeper cleared the ball, I twisted to reach it and then felt this popping sensation and incredible pain in my right knee. I dropped, screaming, "I tore my ACL, I tore my ACL!"

That "ACL" would be the anterior cruciate ligament, and I knew immediately it was torn. The hospital visit that day confirmed my self-diagnosis. But I was stub-born. I didn't have surgery right away; a funny thing about this kind of injury is that after a couple of weeks you feel pretty normal. In the beginning I was hopeful: Maybe it wouldn't be so bad; maybe the tear would heal on its own. That's denial for you. But every time I twisted my knee after that, even a little bit, I felt it buckle. The joint was totally unstable. Still, that didn't stop me from playing basketball with my brothers. Then one day as I went for a layup, my knee gave out. I hobbled off the court, realizing I had to have this problem fixed.

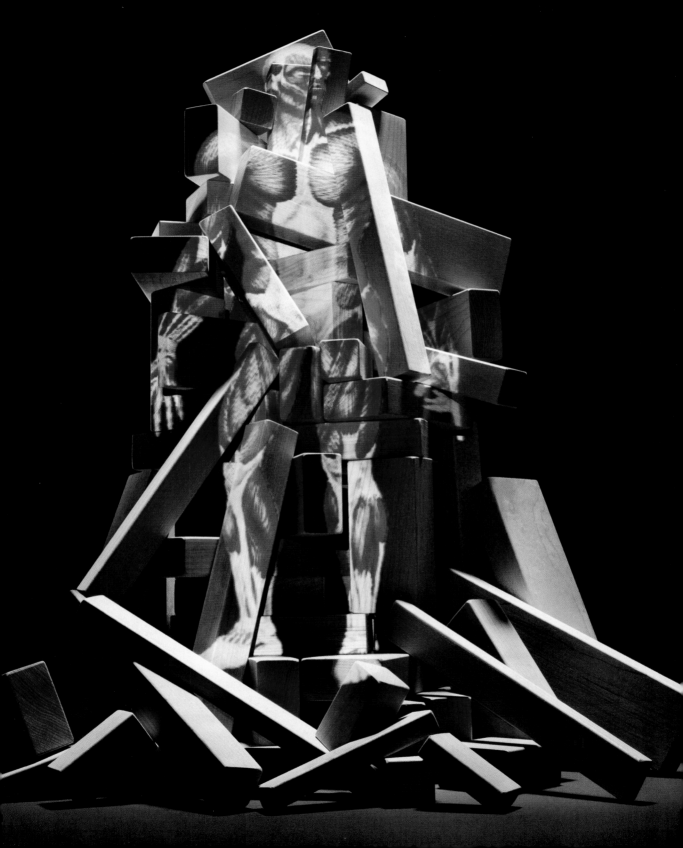

> Make this your mantra:
> Exercise is medicine.
> It's the easiest way to feel
> happy and healthy.

What I didn't know at the time was that I could've been doing a whole host of preventive exercises that might have kept the original injury from happening. Later in life, when I got into plyometrics and strength training, I noticed that my knee felt better when I kept the muscles around it strong. When my hips, glutes, and legs were strong, my knee hurt less.

I had an amazing realization: I can control my pain with strength.

This is crucial information for every active guy, because strength training can not only prevent injuries in the first place, but also ease your symptoms if you do have a joint injury that causes some chronic pain. How? Muscles support and stabilize joints. Despite some meniscus tearing and osteoarthritis, I can now train for the highest levels of endurance competition without a problem. I've completed nine Ironman triathlons and 29 marathons since my injury. Think about that the next time you want to skip a workout or skimp on rehabbing what's hurting.

But I'll never forget how awful that injury felt, not just in my knee but also in my mind. When you're active and that's taken away from you, it's traumatic. That's one of the biggest reasons I went into medicine, and why I wrote this story. If you're in pain and don't know why, or even if you know exactly why, you need to figure out what to do about it. My goal is to help you do that. I want you back in the game ASAP.

Play Around the Pain

One of the first things you hear when you hurt yourself is "R.I.C.E." That's a common sports-medicine acronym for "rest, ice, compression, and elevation." The conventional wisdom for a lot of sports injuries, especially strains and sprains, is to rest your body, ice the injured area a few times a day for the first 48 hours, apply compression (an elastic bandage, for example), and elevate the affected body part above your heart to decrease blood-flow, pain, and swelling.

Most of those work just fine, but I don't throw the term "R.I.C.E." around much. I thoroughly disagree with rest. (More on that in a moment.) Ice? I love ice. Ice is nature's anti-inflammatory. Compression and elevation work, too, but only on certain injuries. (Never compress a nerve-compression injury, for instance.) Put simply, the best treatments aren't always as universal as an acronym.

For me, healing is a two-step process. First, stop what you're doing. Second, keep going. And you're thinking: What does that mean?

It means that if you're hurt, stop the offending activity. And then start the real work. Let's be very clear: An injury does not grant you a vacation from fitness or exercise. You must continue to work out even if you need to take it easy on a particular body part so it can heal. There are specific reasons for this, and I've learned

THE REAL REASON YOU'RE HURTING

If you roll your ankle, you pretty much know what hurts. That's a straightforward sports injury, one that's easy to treat. But sometimes active guys end up with those nagging, debilitating, and ultimately infuriating injuries that won't go away. The problem may be that you're not looking at the right body part. Some of the most common sports injuries can be helped by considering the not-so-obvious.

SHOULDER OR ARM PAIN

Who knows? Maybe you slept on it wrong. But if the pain lingers . . .

The hidden cause: Nerve roots at the top of your spine supply motor and sensory function to your upper arms. When you bend or twist your neck, the nerves can be pinched.

The simple fix: As the pain lessens, stand with your hands interlaced behind your neck. Bend your neck back and squeeze your shoulder blades. Pause and return to the starting position. Work up to 10 reps. Once you're pain-free, build neck strength by doing shrugs.

LOWER-BACK SPASMS

You threw out your back. Herniated disk? Don't go under the knife just yet.

The hidden cause: Weak or tight hamstrings, core muscles, glutes, or hip flexors can mess up your alignment and mechanics, forcing your back muscles to compensate and overextend.

The simple fix: Stay mobile, use ice in the first 48 hours and heat after that, and take NSAIDs. As the pain eases, begin gentle hamstring, glute, core, and hip-flexor stretches. When you're pain-free, add multidirectional lunges, core exercises, and bodyweight squats.

INNER-THIGH PAIN

It feels like (and could be) a groin strain. But groin strains improve.

The hidden cause: You might have a sports hernia—a strain or tearing of muscles or tendons, usually caused by an imbalance between your adductors and abdominals.

The simple fix: Unfortunately, surgery is the only fix for most sports hernias. But you can prevent a hernia in the making. The key is to address the muscle imbalance by training your core. Shoot for 5 to 6 minutes of daily plank time on top of your regular training.

KNEE PAIN

Pain around your knee makes you think arthritis or meniscus tear.

The hidden cause: If your core, hips, quads, and glutes are undercondi-tioned or out of balance, your pelvis will wobble, stressing your knees when you run.

The simple fix: Focus on dynamic rest. As your pain lessens, try squats, jump squats, multidirectional lunges, planks, and glute bridges to stabilize your pelvis. Start slowly and, over several weeks, work your way to 10 to 12 reps and 2 or 3 sets. Do them every other day.

HEEL AND ARCH PAIN

You're ready to blame your shoes or too much running for the pain.

The hidden cause: Your plantar fascia is connected to your heel bone—and so are your calf muscles, by way of the Achilles tendon. Tight calves can stretch and strain the fascia.

The simple fix: Sit on the floor and place a foam roller under your right ankle with your leg straight. Cross your left leg over your right ankle. With your hands flat on the floor, roll forward so the foam is under your knee. Roll back. Repeat for 3 minutes; switch legs.

them firsthand as a doctor and an athlete. There are also smart ways to keep exercising without aggravating the body part that's been hurt.

But first, the why.

Reason one is science based. More and more, doctors are moving away from recommending rest and toward encouraging injured patients to engage in physical activity. I'm one of those doctors. Take osteoarthritis, for example; the most common form of arthritis, it affects almost everyone by the age of 60. Previously, when a patient had a flare-up, we prescribed rest and medication. Now studies show that exercises that build muscle to help support and improve joint function, combined with weight loss, boost quality of life better than medication alone. As I said before: You can control pain with strength.

There's more.

Being sidelined sucks. The feel-good neurotransmitters produced during exercise, like serotonin and dopamine, can act very much like drugs, making exercise our healthiest mind-altering activity. Having that hit taken away can be clinically depressing for people. This was exactly how I felt when I hurt my knee and couldn't exercise. That's why I believe that when you're hurt, rest is more than just unwise; it's medically unhealthy.

You need to work up a sweat to fight all those negatives I've just described. If you do, you'll keep some of your conditioning. You'll get your dose of neurotransmitters. You'll feel better. You'll be more positive. And you'll learn that no injury is the end of the world. Make this your mantra: Exercise is medicine. It's the easiest way to feel happy and healthy.

So how do you exercise while injured? Practice what I call "dynamic rest."

That means two things. The first is rest and rehab. Lay off the injured body part and do what's necessary to nurse it back to health. That could involve specific home remedies, such as ice or stretching, or something prescribed by a doctor, such as targeted physical therapy or exercises.

Second, be dynamic. Stay in motion

WHEN SHOULD YOU CALL A DOCTOR?

A lot of sports injuries can be self-diagnosed and self-treated. But in the following three instances, you should have a pro look you over.

YOU HAVE ANY JOINT PAIN, SWELLING, OR INSTABILITY.

If a joint hurts or swells—especially a knee, hip, shoulder, or elbow— see a doctor. But if the area also turns red and is warm to the touch, head to your doctor ASAP; you could have an infection.

YOUR INJURY INVOLVES LOSS OF CONSCIOUSNESS OR MEMORY.

I'm talking about a possible concussion here, men. Don't be stupid. Even the most minor brain injury needs to be checked out by a doctor—not a buddy, not a coach.

THE PAIN DOESN'T GO AWAY.

Even if you do no self-care whatsoever, just about any strain, sprain, or pain should show some improvement within a week to 10 days. If it doesn't—or actually worsens—then make the call and have the injury checked out.

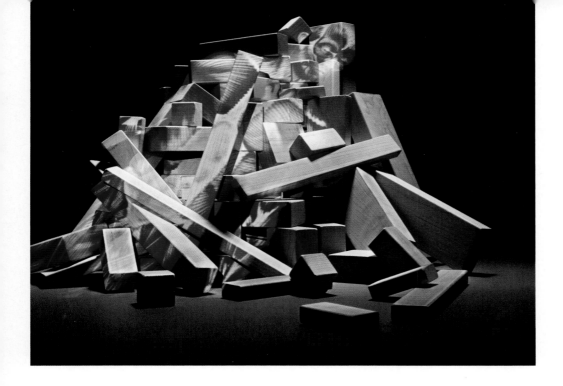

amid all this rest and rehab. Here's how.

Exercise your options. If you sprain your ankle, for example, do something that doesn't load your ankle. Hit the pool. Focus on upper-body weight training. Bad knee? Same idea. Whatever your injury is, don't play through the pain; play around it. Bad shoulder or elbow? Run and do lower-body plyometrics. And here's a big one: Bad back? Simply move. Walk. Shuffle if you have to. Resting a bad back only deconditions the muscles and makes your back weaker. No matter which body part hurts, find something that doesn't aggravate it, and never, ever do "total rest."

Go hard at all times. Whatever your alternate activity is, jack up the intensity. You'll have your heart pounding and lungs heaving as you keep your cardiovascular system in shape. Heck, you might even improve it. You'll also release those giddy neurotransmitters, making you the happiest hurt person on earth.

Build an Injury-Proof Body

To prevent your next injury, I recommend starting now. And my most important advice is to train your entire body. Switch up your activities and hit all the muscle groups, even if you play only one sport. I teach weekend plyometric strength classes that involve functional body motion. I'm a huge fan of this; it trains your body for real-world movement. Back when I was rehabbing my knee, I'd do leg extensions and hamstring curls—isolated movements that have no basis in reality. Now I never use those machines. I do balance work, single-leg work, and plyometric exercises like lunges and squat jumps—movements that hit a lot of muscles at the same time and keep my body in balance.

Why does this work? It's all about your kinetic chain, which is jargon for the series of body parts—including muscles, ligaments, joints, and connective tissue from your neck to your feet—involved in a movement. Your kinetic chain operates interdependently as one system: feet muscles working with ankles working with calves working with knees working with quads, hammies, and hips—all the way up to the top. That's why total-body conditioning helps keep you injury-free: If it's a chain, what do you think happens around a weak link? Exactly. Muscle imbalances eventually cause injuries.

Here are some smart ways to increase your total-body conditioning, as well as hit areas that a lot of guys—even active guys—neglect.

Compound your exercises. Whenever you can, work multiple muscles with a single exercise. If you do a forward lunge, for example, do it holding a medicine ball and add a core twist. And after that forward lunge? Do a reverse lunge and side lunges as well. Hit all directions. That's how you achieve muscle balance.

Stay single. Do single-leg exercises. In my strength and conditioning classes, I have people do single-leg squats, single-leg hops, single-leg lunges—exercises that allow them to use their own body weight while also maintaining their balance. Once you add these exercises to your workout, you'll notice more strength and stability around your ankles, knees, and hips—your most vulnerable points.

Twitch it up. Depending on your sport, you might be doing this already. But if you're not—if you train for steady-state sports such as running or cycling—try adding one or two total-body plyometric and interval (sprint) workouts each week. Neither requires a gym or any special gear. Why do this? It's vital to maintain a balance between fast-and slow-twitch fibers. You become more athletic and less prone to overuse injuries, and you keep your body ready for any type of challenge.

THREE DIY ICE PACKS

Ice is the all-natural antidote for pain and swelling. Make your own ice pack quickly and easily, and then apply to your skin for 10 to 15 minutes.

THE SLUSHIE: Fill a zip-top freezer bag with three parts water and one part rubbing alcohol and toss it in the freezer. The alcohol keeps the mixture from freezing solid, giving you a slushy, pliable ice pack.

THE WET BLANKET: Wet a small towel under the faucet, wring out the excess, and pop it in the freezer. In about 20 minutes, you'll have an icy blanket that's perfect for wrapping around your neck or an injured joint.

THE SIDE DISH: In a pinch, a bag of frozen peas or mixed vegetables makes a terrific ice pack. Then, after they've spent 15 minutes on your aching knee, steam them for dinner!

Some examples of plyometric exercises are squat jumps, lunges, skater plyos (which mimic speed skating's side-to-side motion), and compound movements such as burpees. (Repeat until you can't walk!)

For sprints, choose a time interval that suits your fitness level. That could be anything from 10 seconds on/20 seconds off to 60 seconds on/30 seconds off; listen to your body. Apply it to your normal activity, whether it's running, cycling, swimming, or something else.

Join the women. Yoga and pilates, gentlemen, yoga and pilates. I can't recommend them enough. These disciplines deliver dynamic, movement-based flexibility that can transform your body. Pilates also hammers your core. You'll feel more powerful, and your movement will be easier and more fluid. When you have that going for you, it's harder to get hurt.

Feel kneaded. I'm a big believer in massage. It feels great, of course, but you're also keeping your muscles supple. Plus, a good massage therapist can feel where your muscles might be chronically tight and setting you up for potential problems down the road. Shoot for two massages a month.

Rehab in your sleep. If you take nothing else from this chapter, know that sleep is the most important activity of your day. This is a huge blind spot for so many people, especially if they're training hard. Sleep gives your body an opportunity to repair and rejuvenate itself as it rebuilds muscle, strengthens bone, restocks red blood cells, and engages in other crucial processes that take time. And good sleep means better athletic performance and less chance of taking a bad step in the first place.

PAIN-FREE FOR LIFE

Read more in *The Athlete's Book of Home Remedies* by Jordan D. Metzl, M.D., with Mike Zimmerman, available at athletesbookofremedies.com.

GET A 30-MINUTE MAKEOVER

Forget the excuses: Just half an hour of weekly interval training can improve your health, say researchers at McMaster University.

When people with type 2 diabetes did 10 minutes of intervals 3 days a week for 2 weeks, their metabolism spiked, and their blood-sugar levels fell.

Intense intervals might stimulate muscle changes that help shuttle sugar from your blood, the researchers think.

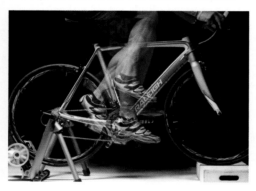

UPGRADE YOUR ROUTINE TO BOOST YOUR STRENGTH

By doing just a few more sets, you can gain a lot of extra strength, a study from Australia suggests. Lifters who performed 8 sets of squats twice a week were about 20 percent stronger after 6 weeks, while those who did just 4 sets were only 14 percent stronger. Lead study author Paul Marshall, Ph.D., recommends starting your workout with heavy sets of squats, bench presses, or deadlifts.

LIFT WEIGHTS TO BLAST BP

Back in the day, docs kept guys with high BP (blood pressure) out of the gym. But no more: Weight training might help lower high blood pressure, say researchers in Brazil. When a group of men with hypertension stopped their meds and lifted

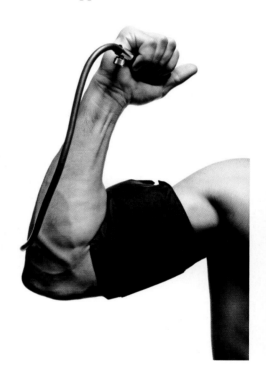

weights 3 days a week for 12 weeks, their blood pressure dipped 11.5 percent.

"We think weightlifting directly improves blood vessel or nervous system function," says study author Ronaldo Araujo, Ph.D. The best part: The men's blood pressure stayed lowered for a full 4 weeks even after they quit pumping iron.

DON'T CHEAT YOUR MUSCLES

Watch your form, because doing an exercise correctly builds stronger muscles, say Brazilian researchers. Compared with men who performed curls using only a partial range of motion (that is, they didn't bring the weight all the way down and back up), lifters who used a full range of motion were about 10 percent stronger. Why? They stressed their muscle fibers more.

LACE UP TO LIFT MORE

Squats and deadlifts, similar to houses, need a strong foundation. Shoes with rock-hard soles can help you squat more effectively, the *Journal of Strength and Conditioning Research* reveals. Why? They allow you to exert more vertical force on the ground. You can achieve a similar effect with a firmer-heeled shoe that mimics the feel of solid ground. Try Converse

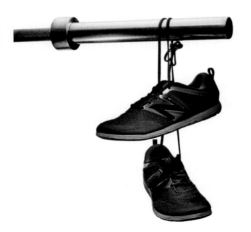

Chuck Taylor All Star or New Balance Minimus MX20 shoes.

Over time, lifting in flat-soled footwear can help improve ankle mobility, says Eric Cressey, C.S.C.S.

GIVE YOUR WORKOUT A TUNE-UP

It's not your imagination: Hearing your favorite music may boost your athletic performance. A study in the *Journal of Strength and Conditioning Research* found that men who listened to their own playlists had more power in the weight room than when they lifted in silence. The men also reported feeling more energetic while they lifted, which the researchers believe may have led to the improved results.

For the perfect lifting mix, check out our "100 Best Workout Songs" at Mens Health.com, keywords "100 best workout songs." We promise it will be Bieber-free.

SHORE UP YOUR SHOULDERS

Warning: Lifters, especially those who do behind-the-neck lat pulldowns and presses, are more likely to suffer chronic shoulder instability, according to a Nova Southeastern University study. This can lead to serious injuries. The fix? Strengthen your rotator cuffs, says study author Morey J. Kolber, Ph.D. Find out how at MensHealth.com, keyword "shoulders."

ADD SPRING TO YOUR SQUAT

Build powerful legs in leaps and bounds: A jumping warmup can instantly make your legs stronger, say scientists in England. Men squatted nearly 18 pounds more after doing depth jumps—hopping from a bench to the floor and then immediately leaping vertically.

"The jumps alert your nerves, helping you recruit more muscle fibers during your next activity," says study author Paul Comfort. Try four depth jumps 4 minutes before squatting.

When squatting, lower your body until the top of your thighs is at least parallel to the floor.

TAKE A DOSE OF EXERCISE

Ever feel happier after a good workout? You should, because studies show that exercise has a significant antidepressant effect, and European researchers might have figured out why.

1. Long, intense exercise stresses your body, and it responds by releasing hormones, including cortisol, from your adrenal glands.

2. The increase of cortisol in your blood revs up a molecule of your endocannabinoid system called anandamide.

3. Anandamide signals regions of your brain to release a substance called BDNF, which can protect your neurons and act as an antidepressant.

SPICE UP YOUR ROUTINE

Use the condiment of champions. Mustard might help you build bigger muscles. When scientists at Rutgers University fed rats a steroidlike hormone that can be found in mustard seeds, it triggered an anabolic response: The rats' muscle fibers increased in size and number. More research is needed to determine if this effect exists in humans.

HANG IN THERE

Hate intervals? Hang in there. The pain of interval training may subside after just six sessions. In a new study from California State University, cyclists had higher power output and less leg pain by their sixth day of high-intensity intervals. Over time, interval training boosts muscle stores of glycogen and phosphocreatine, two fuels for intense exercise. As your body adapts, your perceived effort declines, says study author Todd A. Astorino, Ph.D.

PAY ATTENTION

Ever start to feel stronger while your buddy is yelling encouragement? There's a reason for that: Hearing someone assess your lifts can make you more powerful. In a New Zealand study, men generated up to 3 percent more power while hearing comments on how well they were performing an exercise. "It's easy to lose focus and motivation when lifting, and that can decrease performance," says lead study author Christos Argus, Ph.D. "We think providing feedback keeps people on track."

GO LIGHT

Next time you do the bench press, try this: Take half the weight you normally use, but do twice as many sets. A study in the *Journal of Strength and Conditioning Research* found that men who used this approach produced more power and force than when they did a more conventional routine. Further research is needed to determine if this strategy can translate to better gains.

CALM DOWN

Stress can really disrupt your recuperation. Anxious exercisers don't recover as fast, a study *in Medicine & Science in Sports & Exercise* found. Just an hour after they'd exercised, stressed-out people generated less force in the leg press than their chilled-out counterparts did. The scientists think stress blunts an anti-inflammatory chemical that's linked to muscle repair. To leave your stress behind, get a full night's sleep and spend time with friends.

REORGANIZE YOUR WORKOUT

If you bike or use a treadmill before you hit the weights, you might want to reorga-nize your routine. According to a new study in the *Journal of Strength and Conditioning Research*, doing cardio prior to lower-body strength training can limit the number of reps you can pull off. Lifters who averaged 9 reps per set of back squats one week averaged only 71/2 reps when they preceded the squats with 45 minutes of pedaling the following week. Bottom line: Start your workout with iron.

ROLL WITH IT

DES there's a spot image here of a roller if you want to add it. ED

The secret to better exercise might be molded in foam. A foam roller can help increase your range of motion, which can bolster your form and reduce your risk of injury, say researchers in Canada. When men spent 2 minutes foam-rolling their quads, the scientists found that the men's knees bent nearly 13 percent more afterward.

"We think foam-rolling warms the connective tissue around the muscle, making it more conducive to stretching," says study author Graham MacDonald, M.Sc.(c).He recommends rolling your quads, hamstrings, calves, glutes, and hips 2 minutes apiece before your workout.

Q **Is there one exercise that will blast my whole body?**
A: There is, but it's brutal. In fact, the name alone can make your muscles twitch: It's called "the death crawl."

Our guest torturer, Todd Durkin, C.S.C.S., author of *The Impact! Body Plan*, explains: "The death crawl, combined with a dumbbell jump squat, works your chest, shoulders, triceps, back, and biceps. It also pounds your core and smokes your legs."

And there's an endurance element that'll make you think you're starring in *Saw: Jigsaw's Gym*. Still want to do it? Grab two 10-pound dumbbells. Or go with 25-pounders if you want the same challenge that Durkin gives his elite clients—NFL stars like Drew Brees and Darren Sproles.

Step 1: Position yourself in the up phase of a pushup, grasping the dumbbells in your hands. Lower your body to the floor, pause 2 seconds, and push yourself back up.

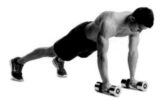
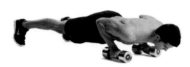

Step 2: Row the dumbbell in your right hand up to the side of your chest. Then lower it to the floor. Do the same with your left arm.

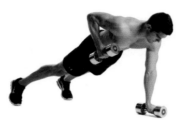
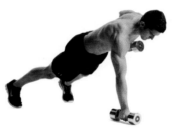

Step 3: "Walk" the dumbbell in your left hand forward one step, followed by the one in your right. Next, bring your left foot and right foot forward. Move ahead three steps with each hand. Keep your core tense and back straight.

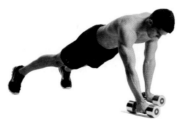
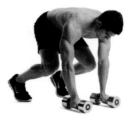

Step 4: Stand up and do three dumbbell jump squats. Holding the dumbbells at your sides, bend your knees and squat; then jump up explosively. That's 1 rep of the death crawl. Aim for 2 or 3 sets of 5 to 10 reps, with 2 minutes of rest between sets.

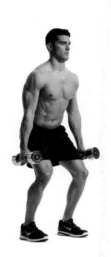 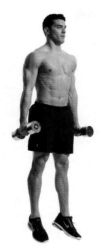

Q **My buddy claims his core is stronger than mine. What's the best way to settle this?**
A: Okay, we need to say it: Do not punch each other in the gut. Here's a more objective (and less injurious) method that measures the strength of your abdominal muscles in three directions, courtesy of Bill Hartman, P.T., C.S.C.S., owner of Indianapolis Fitness and Sports Training. Recruit a judge, head to the gym, and try these three timed tests.

Plank

Assume a pushup position but with your weight on your forearms. Brace your abs, clench your glutes, and keep your body straight from head to heel. Start the timer. When you lose alignment, stop the clock.

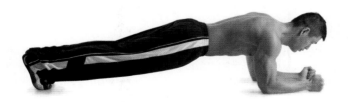

Side Plank

Lie on one side with your legs straight, and prop up your upper body on your forearm. Raise your hips so your body forms a straight line from nose to toes, and hold. Start the timer. Once you sag, stop the timer. (For bonus points, raise your top leg.)

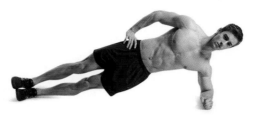

Back Extension

Position yourself facedown on a Roman chair with the pads set at hip level and your ankles braced. Bend your torso back by contracting your hamstrings, keeping the natural arch in your back. When your body is straight, pause. Start the timer. Hold that position as long as you can.

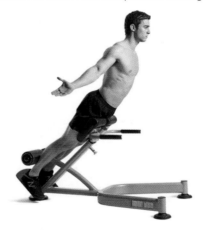

Q I'm bored with planks. What's a more exciting way to strengthen my core?

A: Climbing. Swap horizontal for vertical. Indoor climbing twice a week can improve your core and hand-grip strength, according to new German research. No rock wall at your gym? Do 2 sets of 5 to 10 hanging leg raises twice a week, suggests David Pearson, Ph.D., C.S.C.S., a professor of exercise physiology at Ball State University. Hang from a chinup bar using an overhand grip, and then simultaneously bend your knees and scoop your thighs up to your chest. You can also do these on a dip station, resting on your elbows.

Q What exercise can I do to build a bigger chest?

A: First we'll tell you one move not to do: pec-deck flys. These hit only a portion of your chest, and you increase your risk of injury by doing them. You're better off doing three dumbbell exercises that target different parts of your chest muscle, resulting in better definition and size, says Craig Ballantyne, M.S., C.S.C.S., of TurbulenceTraining.com. "The dumbbell bench press allows you to use a heavy, muscle-building weight safely. The neutral-grip incline press targets the upper chest area. And the fly is the perfect exercise to finish with because it works a full range of motion." Use dumbbells to do the prescribed sets and reps twice a week, resting at least 2 days in between.

Dumbbell Bench Press

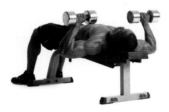

Lie on a flat bench with your feet on the floor; hold a pair of heavy dumbbells above your chest, with your arms straight and your palms facing forward. Slowly lower the weights to the outside of your chest. Pause, and push them back up. That's 1 rep. Use the heaviest dumbbells that allow you to complete 3 sets of 6 repetitions. Note: Keeping your shoulder blades tight stabilizes your shoulder joints, helping you lift more weight.

Neutral-Grip Incline Dumbbell Bench Press

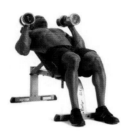

Lie on an adjustable incline bench set to 45 degrees. Hold a pair of dumbbells above your chest, with your arms straight and palms facing each other. Lower the weights to chest level, and then slowly press them above your chest. At the top position, squeeze the dumbbells together. Lower and repeat. Do 4 sets of 8 reps—your upper chest needs that extra set for max growth, says Ballantyne.

Dumbbell Fly

Lie faceup on a flat bench. Start by holding the dumbbells above your chest, with your elbows slightly bent and palms facing each other. Without changing your arm position, take 3 seconds to lower the dumbbells until your upper arms are parallel to the floor. Pause, and then raise the dumbbells back to the starting position. Do 3 sets of 12 reps. Slowly lowering a weight a dozen times activates more muscle, says Ballantyne.

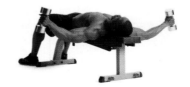

What's the fastest way to big biceps?

A: Some guys swear by preacher curls. We think they must've had divine intervention. The problem with preachers is that they limit the amount of weight you can pile on your biceps, says Tony Gentilcore, C.S.C.S., co-owner of Cressey Performance. His pick? The cable row.

"It allows you to lift serious weight—upwards of 100 pounds—and it smokes your biceps because they help pull the weight to your chest." Gentilcore recommends doing cable rows twice a week, alternating your sets. On the first day, perform 2 sets of 12 to 15 repetitions; this forges endurance and muscle definition. On the second day, do 3 or 4 heavier sets of 4 to 6 reps; this builds size and strength.

The Cable Row

Attach a bar handle to a cable row machine and sit with your feet braced and knees slightly bent. Using an underhand grip, grab the bar with your arms extended. Keep your back straight and squeeze your shoulder blades together as you pull the bar toward your upper abs. Return to the starting position. That's 1 rep.

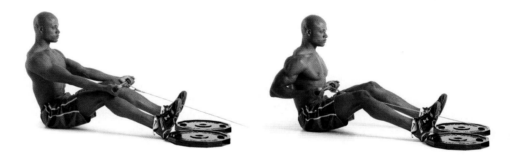

How can I build cut triceps like the guys on your cover have?

A: The key to looking cover-cut isn't Photoshop—it's fat blasting.

"Your muscles can never be defined if they're covered in a layer of blubber," says Mike Robertson, C.S.C.S., co-owner of IFAST gym in Indianapolis. "Focus on reducing your body fat to around 10 percent." (Try our workout program at MensHealth.com/deltafit.) Then grow your tris with the close-grip barbell bench press.

"You can use a heavy weight, which provides a lot of stimulus to the muscle," Robertson says. "And using the close grip targets your triceps."

Close-Grip Barbell Bench Press

Grab a barbell and lie on a bench. Using a shoulder-width, overhand grip, hold the barbell above your sternum with your arms straight. Lower the bar to your chest and push it back up. Do 3 sets, increasing the load every set. Do 8 reps the first set, 6 reps the second set, and 4 reps the third set.

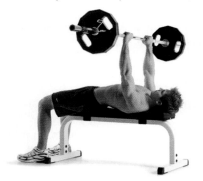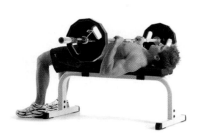

Q **What's the best body-weight exercise to work my back?**
A: In the old days, you'd get your workout trying to move a mule, budge a tree stump, or drag a barge down a canal. What do all these efforts have in common?

"The best body-weight exercises to train the muscles in your back are pulling exercises," says *Men's Health* contributor Alwyn Cosgrove, C.S.C.S. He recommends scouting out a sturdy branch or a pullup bar in your local park, or buying a TRX Suspension Training Kit ($200-250, performbetter.com). The TRX system is quick to set up, anchors to a doorway, and is more versatile than a door-mounted pullup bar. You can do hundreds of different exercises for your whole body. One of the best for your back is an inverted row.

Inverted Row

Hang from the straps with your body in a straight line and your heels touching the floor. Pull yourself up until your chest is level with your hands; pause and return to the starting position. Do 3 sets of 8 to 12 reps, resting 30 seconds between sets, 3 days a week. For more of a challenge, try it with your feet elevated on a medicine ball, or do a single-arm version.

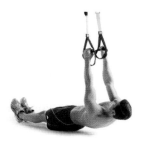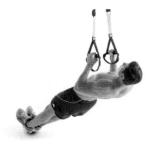

How long should I rest between sets?

A: Time is muscle. If you rest too long, your muscles won't tire enough to stimulate growth; if you rest too little, they'll be too fatigued.

To find your stopwatch sweet spot, decide what you want out of your workout, says Hartman. "Do you want to burn fat, build muscle, or forge strength?" Find your answer below.

Burn fat: Rest 30 seconds between sets of 12-plus reps: By taking shorter rest times, your heart rate stays in overdrive, cranking your metabolism and melting more fat.

Build muscle: Rest 1 to 2 minutes: This lets you pump out multiple burn-inducing sets of 8 to 10 reps with heavy weight. You're balancing between exhausting the muscle and resting long enough to recover.

Increase strength: Rest 2 to 5 minutes: To build strength, you must go all out every lift for sets of 3 to 5 reps. That requires using near maximum weight, which recruits the most muscle fibers. They use more energy to contract and need more time to recover.

Everyone at my gym is talking about amino acid shooters. Should I bother?

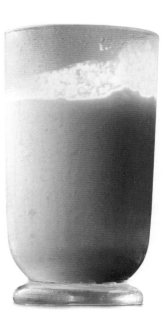

A: Your workout is a muscle-growth party, and pounding a branched chain amino acid (BCAA) drink kick-starts it. BCAAs are protein building blocks that fuel your muscles and help them grow, says Mike Roussell, Ph.D., author of *The Six Pillars of Nutrition*. In fact, a recent study from Sweden found that drinking BCAAs during resistance training activates key enzymes used in building muscle more than exercise alone does.

We like Champion Amino Shooter Core, which provides 6.5 grams of amino acids ($25 for 18 servings, bodybuilding.com).

But you'll have to watch what you eat at mealtime, too. Roussell cautions that shooting BCAAs won't help you if you aren't eating enough calories and protein. His advice: Eat 500 extra calories on workout days, including 1 gram of protein per pound of your target body weight. Drinking a shake with 20 to 40 grams of protein and 40 to 80 grams of carbs after working out makes it easier to hit that target.

Q Will drinking a few beers after my workout sabotage my muscle gains?

A: Well, that depends on your definition of "a few." While it's true that alcohol can lower your testosterone levels, you'd have to really binge to experience a significant reduction. Smaller amounts of alcohol—less than six brews for a 180-pound guy, for example—were shown in a *Strength and Conditioning Journal* review to have no significant effect on testosterone.

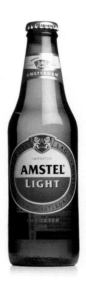

"Just having a round or two after a workout won't reduce your T levels enough to cripple your gains or stall recovery," says Martin Berkhan,
a nutrition consultant and author of leangains.com. However, Berkhan recommends sticking to a light beer because some craft brews can contain upwards of 300 calories. Our beer of choice: Amstel Light, with only 95 calories and 5 grams of carbohydrates.

PART 4

Look
Better
Instantly

Men'sHealth

The Good Life, Guaranteed

You can benefit from the finer things in life without going broke. Here are five smart ways to tap the power of carefully chosen luxuries.

For most of his life, Sean Wilson, a former Marine now in medical sales, didn't see the point of spending lots of time and money on his appearance. Then his wife bought him a $1,500 bespoke suit. It changed his life.

"I was hooked," Wilson says. "I felt more confident and closed more deals."

Extravagant purchases—tailored suits, pricey watches—may not seem sensible in our current economy. But research suggests that certain luxuries might contribute to career advancement, creativity, perceptions of attractiveness, and even problem-solving skills. According to a 2011 study in the journal *Evolution and Human Behavior*, displays of luxury brands can net you preferential treatment in everything from job interviews to charity fundraising. Scientists attribute this to the "costly signaling theory," which posits that outward displays can reliably convey desirable inner qualities. So we tapped our experts to find the five upgrades you're most likely to benefit from—and show you how to snag them without going broke.

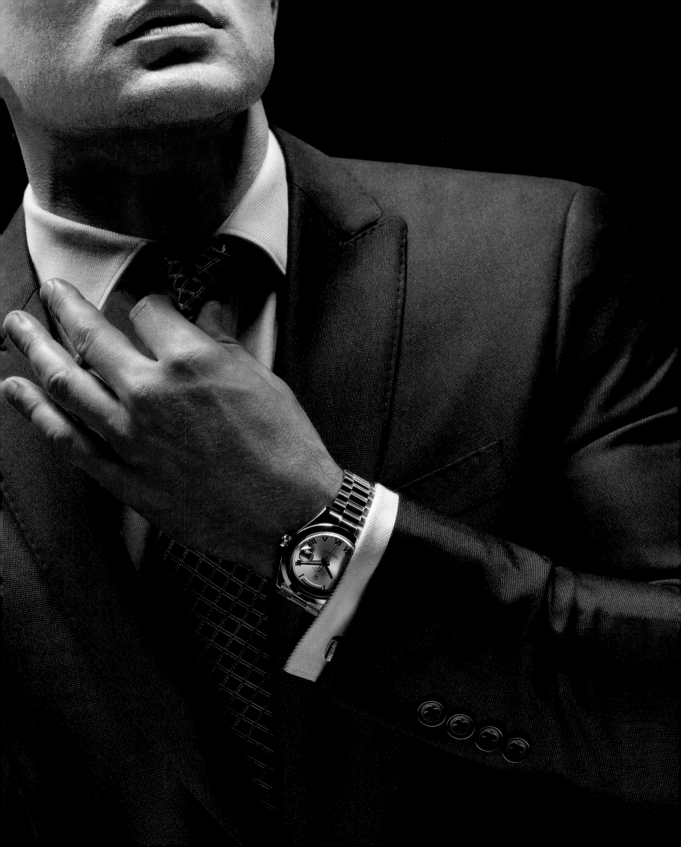

PREMIUM WRISTWATCH
The Secret Handshake

Younger guys might be forgoing watches in favor of their cellphones, but that could be a big mistake. The right timepiece, glimpsed at the right time, can telegraph important signals about you, studies show.

Certain branded luxury goods, such as watches—particularly those from premium but less widely known brands—remain discreet but powerful status signifiers to those in the know, according to a 2010 study in the *Journal of Marketing*. Of course, the barrier to entry is high. Expect prices to start around $1,000—and rise from there.

Upgrade Tactic

Go gray market. Buying from an authorized dealer will land you a manufacturer's warranty but not necessarily the best deal, says watch critic Ariel Adams. But buying from a nonauthorized retailer—such as through eBay, which has done well weeding out fakes, Adams notes—can often score you a new, authentic watch at a steep discount.

"Then find a good repair shop, which, if needed, may be faster and cheaper than manufacturer service," Adams says.

So how do you pick a watch? Read watch blogs and magazines, and browse. Adams suggests finding one you love and then

BEAT YOUR WORST FINANCIAL HABITS

We surveyed financial advisors to ask where their clients make the most money mistakes. Use their tips to keep tabs on all your loose change—and start banking some coin.

Cut memberships. Unused club affiliations and movie services can add up, especially if auto-billing is in play, says Ronald Van Surksum, CFP, of Advanced Asset Management. Check your statements for these charges—some of which you might have forgotten about—and start canceling.

Make fewer withdrawals. Some men tend to toss receipts, use all their cash, and hit the ATM again and again, says Cheryl Sherrard, CFP, of Rinehart Wealth Management. Save your ATM receipts for a month, subtract 20 percent from the total, and use that as your budget for the next month.

Don't overpay for investments. An actively managed mutual fund might charge more than 1 percent—so over decades, a lot of your return goes to the manager, says Joe Alfonso, CFP, of Aegis Financial Advisory. Consider index funds or index-based ETFs, which charge only around 0.2 percent.

Fire the handyman. Instead of paying a pro for repairs or upgrades, do them yourself. "If a tax lawyer can paint a house, anyone can," says Martin Shenkman, P.C., of Shenkman Law Firm. Look at it this way: Since you pay your handyman in posttax dollars, you'd have to earn about $750 to cover a $500 repair.

Stock a fridge. Buying a sandwich at lunch is convenient but also a huge daily expense, says Philip Lee, CFP, of Modera Wealth Management. If you don't like the morning prep, stock the work fridge with a few staple items and prepare a sandwich at work. You could save $150 a month.

Look Better Instantly **MH**

looking at others for a few weeks. "Just before you're ready to buy, come back to the first watch," he says. "If you still feel the same way about it, it's a keeper."

LUXURY CAR
Your Ticket to Ride

As much as men love cars, they might find it hard to justify a real indulgence in one—especially once the sticker strays north of, say, $35,000.

On the other hand, a luxury car can make you seem more handsome. It's true! When women in a British study were shown a photo of a man in a luxury car and then another shot of the same guy in an econobox, they thought he looked better in the luxury car. The real benefit, however, might lie in your own perceptions once you climb behind the wheel. Makers of premium autos fold in design and technology features—sound dampening, smooth acceleration—that conspire to influence how you see yourself, says Sven Beiker, Ph.D., executive director of the center for automotive research at Stanford University.

"It makes you want to fulfill the image," he says. "You may actually feel pressure to live up to the status of your car."

Upgrade Tactic

Focus on your total ownership cost, factoring in depreciation, maintenance, insurance, and fuel efficiency in addition to the purchase price. Kelley Blue Book rates Audi, Lexus, and Cadillac as the luxury brands with the lowest total cost of ownership.

> Luxury vehicles influence how you see yourself. You might actually feel pressure to live up to the status of your car.

Or go vintage—sort of. Some contemporary classics, such as the 2003 Mercedes-Benz SL500 (which listed for $86,000 new), can now be picked up in the mid-20s. And they'll still net you the style points. Because such cars are older than conventional "late-model used" vehicles, consider an extended warranty, which will add $500 to $2,000 to your outlay.

EPIC VACATION
A Refresher Course

Think those fantasy getaways should stay in your dreams? We say pack your bags. A trip abroad can be one of the most effective ways to broaden your perspectives, new research from Northwestern University finds.

Exploring an unfamiliar culture—and no, we don't mean the nightlife in Acapulco—improves your professional creativity and "self-clarity," says study coauthor Adam Galinsky, Ph.D. "The key is understanding and adapting to a local culture," he notes. "That process leads to increased creativity."

Furthermore, bumping up your services and accommodations to a more luxurious

If your confidence on the job is slipping, perhaps you should fully unleash the super-fan lurking in your subsconscious.

level creates an experience that allows you to move completely outside your normal life. "You achieve a psychological distance that lets you see your life in a new light," Galinsky says.

Upgrade Tactic

Travel in the off-season—and without the kids. You'll be able to upgrade (first-class seats, swankier digs, better restaurants, and cooler activities), Galinsky says, and leave behind the routine stresses and activities that seem to follow your kids wherever they go. And by going in the off-season, you'll fully experience the local community. People are more eager to engage when the tourist hordes are gone, leading to deeper cross-cultural interactions.

CUSTOM SUIT
A Maker of Men

Sean Wilson isn't the only man who thinks his wardrobe enhancement enhanced his bottom line. A study in *Human Resource Development Quarterly* found that workers who were dressed to kill felt more authoritative and more competent

than those in less formidable attire.

With custom tailoring, you end up with a suit that fits perfectly, and you can specify details and stylistic elements, such as a cellphone pocket or a unique collar design. Surprisingly, bespoke clothing isn't all that much more expensive than off-the-rack designer duds: At Michael Andrews Bespoke in New York, custom shirts start at about $200 and suits at $1,000.

Upgrade Tactic

Do some homework. If you're a standard size, you could get away with a tailored off-the-rack suit. But be aware that the fit of an off-the-rack item in the United States might not be as good as that of its counter-part in Europe, where men are typically more slender and clothes are more fitted to start with.

Made-to-measure, in which an existing pattern is altered based on your measurements, is an economical middle ground. Visit a few custom shops and make sure you like the people there. You'll have a long relationship with them—suits can require multiple fittings and months to reach completion.

SEASON TICKETS
MVP Status

If your confidence on the job is slipping, perhaps you should finally unleash the super-fan lurking in your subconscious. Sports enthusiasts who own season tickets or who are otherwise "highly identified local fans" feel greater self-esteem and well-being than less committed fans, says Daniel Wann, Ph.D., a psychologist at Murray State University who studies fan behavior.

He notes that season ticket holders bounce back from defeat faster than fair-weather fans. That's because the more intense their fandom is, says Wann, the more likely they are to have developed heightened coping skills for dealing with defeat. "A fan like this blames referees, remembers a past that's more glorious than it was, and overlooks bad performances," Wann says. "These techniques, perhaps surprisingly, have positive applications far beyond the playing field and may account for some of the success sports enthusiasts have in their careers."

Upgrade Tactic

Season tickets in most cities can be hard to come by. But add your name to the waiting list anyway: Most teams grant people on the list special access to purchase face-value tickets and offer other perks, such as access to practices. They might also sell special multigame packages. Failing all that, start watching the games in sports bars or clubs where you can gab with equally rabid aficionados, Wann says—or hey, host parties yourself and share the joy!

The Life-Altering Power of Faking It

No, not that way. We're talking about faking it at work, at home, among friends and lovers. We're talking about faking it as the fast lane to a better life. Does that actually work? (And, okay, what about faking it in bed?)

Can you really fake it till you make it? It's a big cliché, to be sure, and big clichés often have a kernel of truth rattling around inside. But we always sort of hoped it was just an empty phrase that was tons of fun to say and nothing more. Because if it were true, well . . . that would suck.

The world already has plenty of fakers, thank you. Nobody's doing any hand-wringing over a shortage of insincere flatterers, frenemy coworkers, heavily cologned auto salesmen, liar-liar bosses, corporate spokesprevaricators, bad toupees, Ponzi schemes, or fanciful match.com profiles. We don't need to be encour-aging slick, phony behavior. We need to encourage authenticity. Especially now in the digital age, when it's easy to pretend you're cooler, more popular, or less married than you actually are.

So it was upsetting—very upsetting—to find out that, yes, fakery has its uses. Not just uses, but advantages. It can make you happier and healthier; you can be more effective at work and more loved at home. This is based on laboratory experiments; apparently there's no shortage of experimental psychologists who are also interested in faking it.

And so, very much against our will, we

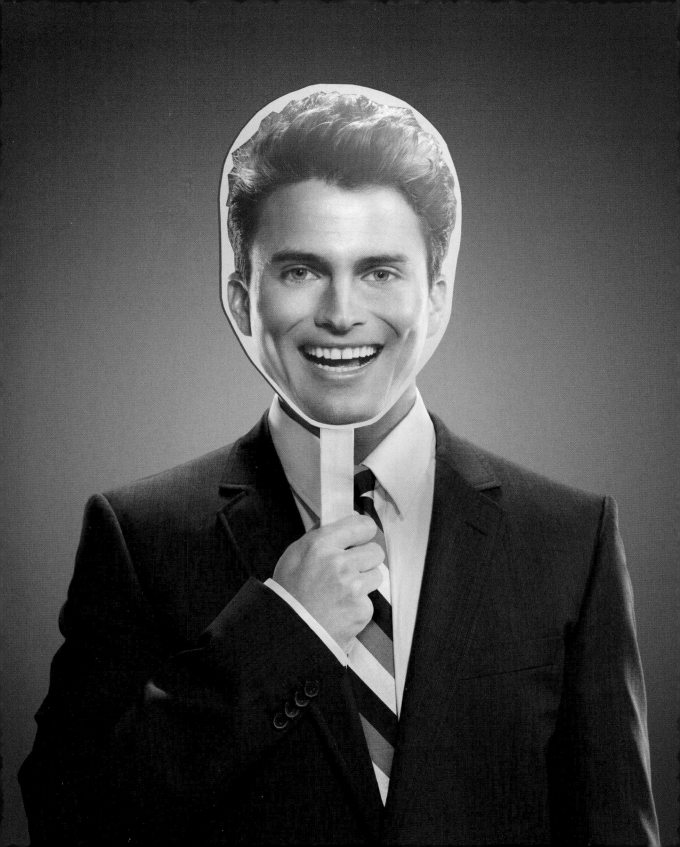

> "Act as if you were confident and outgoing. You'll rise to the occasion and become a happier person."

present to you the official *Men's Health* guide to faking it. Read it and weep along with us. Then we can all start faking more, and succeeding more, because evidently, one follows the other . . . like water into wine (or at least a convincing red-colored liquid).

Let's Begin with a Forced Smile

Back in the late 1980s, psychologists at the University of Illinois recruited 92 undergrads to take part in an experiment in which the members of one group held felt-tip markers between their teeth while rating cartoons. Those clever researchers were simply forcing the students to smile. And as it turned out, the cartoons were funnier to those students than to others who hadn't been forced into felt-tip smiles. It seems our facial muscles send signals to our brains telling us we're happy (which makes you wonder how brainy our brains really are). This is known as the "facial feedback hypothesis."

Researchers have also discovered that what's true for the face is true for the rest of the body as well. No, your body doesn't smile, but it does radiate nonverbal messages of confidence or weakness. Two different psychology labs recently conducted experiments involving body postures and came up with the same result: If you "put on" a powerful body posture, you will think and behave with more power.

At the Kellogg School of Management at Northwestern University, professor Adam Galinsky, Ph.D., and his colleagues conducted an experiment in which 77 undergrads sat for 3 to 5 minutes in either an "expansive" position (taking up maximum space with their bodies; one arm on the back of the neighboring chair and legs crossed widely, one ankle on the other knee) or a "constricted" one (hands under thighs, shoulders dropped, legs together). The students then performed word-completion tasks. Those who sat like arrogant masters of the universe were more apt to complete "l__d" as "lead," for example, rather than the shriveled favorite, "load."

In the next experiment, Galinsky recruited 77 more undergraduates and had them assume the same body postures. Then everyone played simulated blackjack. Guess what? The hotshots were more likely (81 percent, versus 58 percent) to take an extra card from the dealer.

Galinsky thinks the recent work on body posture is even more important—and practical—than the research on facial feedback.

"For one thing, it's easier to fake posture than it is to fake a smile," he says. "It literally changes us, and it changes how people perceive us."

Galinsky's research verifies findings produced by Dana Carney, Ph.D., and grad student Andy Yap, both of Columbia University, along with Amy Cuddy, Ph.D., of the Harvard Business School. They had 42 people assume either power poses (feet on desk, hands behind head; or standing, one hand on desk, leaning forward) or wimpy ones (sitting, arms held close and hands folded; or standing, arms and legs crossed tightly). As predicted, the more widely spread postures led to more widespread feelings of being in charge. And this was after only 2 minutes of posing.

But the experiment took matters a step further. The researchers swabbed saliva from the participants before and after the posing, and used the samples to gauge hormone levels. The finding? After a mere 2 minutes of posing, the people who'd assumed the take-charge stances had more testosterone and less cortisol (a stress hormone), whereas the converse proved true of the milquetoast impersonators. So yes, the effects of body posture are measurable in the body at a molecular level.

Fair warning: Power poses don't work when you're supposed to be showing deference. If you're at a job interview, for example, don't spread out. You won't look confident. You will look like an asshat.

Otherwise, faking it works. Carry yourself like a maestro, wave the baton, and you just might fool everyone—or at least yourself.

WHEN SHE WANTS YOU TO FAKE IT

In the game of love, it pays to cheat once in a while. But not that way! Done right, a little dash of fakery can spice up your relationship—and your sex life, too.

THE PROBLEM: Your mate asks you what you think of her decidedly pudgy body.

The fake: Her question has an emotional subtext, says psychiatrist Paul Dobransky, M.D., of menspsychology.com. It's not about her weight; it's about the depth of your regard for her. So answer the question she's really asking.

The payoff: When you say, "Your body is one of the wonders of the world" and back it up with a lustful stare, she'll try to live up to that—at the gym.

THE PROBLEM: She wants to go to a ballet, museum, or some other thing you're not into.

The fake: Don't let on that you think it's a snooze, says Patricia Covalt, Ph.D., the author of *What Smart Couples Know.* "Show support and go along." Ask specific questions, such as which painting was her favorite. That shows you care.

The payoff: She'll support your oddities next time, Covalt says. And by making an effort to be interested, you'll relate to her better.

THE PROBLEM: It feels as if your relationship is in need of a five-alarm wake-up call.

The fake: Compliments can reignite your love. Even if it feels phony compliment her about something new every day says Paul Rose, Ph.D., chairman of the department of psychology at Southern Illinois University at Edwardsville.

The payoff: Your relationship will feel fresh as you discover her new qualities, Rose says. And she'll be happy you're paying close attention.

THE PROBLEM: Her favorite sex act is as arousing for you as a pair of granny panties.

The fake: Give it a go, Dr. Dobransky says. Even if you hate it at first, try it three times before you give up. "Focus on how you're making her feel," Dr. Dobransky says. "That is a Rosetta Stone for what men and women want in the bedroom."

The payoff: You might end up liking it after all, Dr. Dobransky says. And her turn-on is likely to stoke your fires. Bonus: your turn!

So how about faking negotiating? What if fakery landed you a better deal from, say, one of those heavily cologned car salesmen? They're so full of tricks themselves that we're totally down with any bit of subterfuge. (Oh. Your dad sells cars? Except for him.) You're just leveling the playing field.

Okay, Then. Can You Fake Anger?

The role of anger in negotiations was first explored by Gerben van Kleef, Ph.D., now an associate professor of social psychology at the University of Amsterdam. In a 2004 research paper, he proposed what every car salesman already knows: Emotion is a tool you can use for getting what you want. He had 128 students each negotiate the price, warranty, and length of a cellphone contract with a buyer via a computer. The students gave up more when the opponent was angry than when he was happy. (Head fake: There was no human opponent. They were haggling with a software program. A very angry software program that would say things like, "This is really getting on my nerves" and "This negotiation pisses me off.")

In subsequent experiments, Van Kleef and colleagues discovered that anger has its limits. Anger won't get you very far if you're the one with less power in the negotiation. In fact, your anger might backfire. An opponent who holds the advantage might demand more from you if he thinks your anger is inappropriate. Van Kleef's latest experiments, published in the *Journal of Applied Psychology* in 2011, suggest that anger on the buyer's part works because it implies a threat—that the buyer is about to walk away from the negotiating table, for example. So why not just threaten to bolt? Good idea: In fact, that tactic works better than anger. Delivering a take-it-or-leave-it ultimatum in a calm, matter-of-fact way shows that you're confident and in control. Your threat is perceived as more credible. And that "cold" strategy yielded the biggest concessions from the hundreds of students who were brought in to act as sellers.

In related research, scientists at the University of Pennsylvania tested the role of emotional transitions in negotiations. They replicated Van Kleef's setup but had certain "buyers" make a shift in mood—either from happy to angry or angry to happy. The students tended to concede more to a happy-to-angry buyer because they either "caught" the happiness (in a process known as "emotional contagion") and therefore became more acquiescent, or figured they had done something to spark the shift to anger. But if a buyer displayed only anger, the students tended to dismiss him as a hothead.

As for the buyers who shifted from angry to happy? The students conceded the same small amounts to them as they did to buyers who displayed only happiness.

Bottom line: The next time you buy a car, you don't have to get mad. Just threaten to walk. Whether you mean it or not. And whatever you do, don't go to one of those dealers who brag about being so gosh-darn nice, and oh, everyone's so happy in here! You could succumb to emotional contagion and, despite your best intentions, start acting nice! And even though they won't budge on price, you'll refuse to lose your cool and won't threaten to walk out, so you'll reach a deal that is way more than what you should have paid. Way to go, Mr. Nice Guy.

Remember these three words, buried in the conclusion of one of Van Kleef's scientific papers: "Happiness elicits exploitation." If you're happy and you know it, fake a frown.

Let's Move on to More Uncomfortable Terrain

Let's talk about faking it with our friends. And girlfriends. Let's suggest that you should be a little more caring than you actually are. What if you could become a close compadre, or the love of her life, simply by saying the right (false) words at the right time? Are you capable of being that icky?

We're taught to think that our steadfastness in intimate relationships is cemented by the moments when we're with someone in times of crisis. ("Honey, I was there for you when things went wrong!") But in reality, people feel a teeny-weeny bit uncomfortable when you're there as they hit bottom. There's no surer signal than your sympathy to indicate to them that they're losers. Sympathy is wonderful and all, but how do they move on from that big-L-stuck-to-forehead loser

A guy who blows his top in negotiations often comes out on top.

mentality? Do they always have to feel inferior to you?

It might be much more important to be there when things go right, according to studies from UCLA and the University of Rochester. When someone tells you about something terrific that just happened to them, do you light up and show some love? Great! In that case, they actually perceive the event as more important, and your enthusiastic response promotes a bond of trust between you and the other person. But if you're only quietly supportive, that's not so valuable. It's really problematic if your response is either active-destructive ("Jeez. Why would management pick you for that project?") or passive-destructive—that is, you ignore what they just said ("Hey! Guess who retweeted me today!").

Gentlemen? Have you ever been guilty of such a callous or clueless response?

But can you truly fake enthusiasm? Yes, says Todd Kashdan, Ph.D., an associate professor of psychology at George Mason University.

"When we give an enthusiastic, interested response, even if we pretend, the same benefits occur," he says. "People feel more excited about the good thing that happened, and they feel more invested in you."

Times like this separate you from the other people who are on the periphery of that person's life.

Kashdan's latest research experiment illustrates the importance of proper reactions in a relationship. He brought 180 couples into his lab, and then he had one member of each couple share something positive that recently happened in his or her life. Six months later, Kashdan discovered that those partners who had not provided spirited responses were more likely to be in Splitsville.

"People want to feel their life is cool," Kashdan says. "So throw them a bone."

Even if you're not really excited for them at first, your enthusiasm will usually kick in given some time. And, all things considered, isn't it better to be a faker than to be a jerk?

Let's Summarize What We've Learned

Faking it makes you more confident, helps you connect with your friends, and gives you an edge in negotiating with your enemies. Where's the harm, you say? A few moments of artfulness for specific situations, you say. It's not like anyone's suggesting that we make a habit of faking it. It's not like anyone's promising a better life, a life of health and wealth and lollipops.

Oh yes they are.

In what has to be one of the most intriguing psychology experiments ever conducted, Harvard psychologist Ellen Langer, Ph.D., once recruited 16 elderly men and took them off to a monastery in

BE A PHONY

It's the shortcut to success—if you fake it the right way. Here's how.

Fake on a new job. If you want to be seen as a superstar, start playing the role. The strategy: Volunteer for a new leadership position, especially one you might be underqualified for, says Gina Bellavia, Ph.D., a career coach at Breakthrough Coaching. "It's like giving yourself that extra push and saying, I can do this," she says. You'll learn new skills and maybe excel in your new position. If you fail, you'll be more ready next time.

Buy a killer suit. To be a big shot, dress like one—even if you're a pipsqueak. "We've all seen TV shows where people get makeovers," Bellavia says. "It works because people feel so differently about themselves when they change their wardrobe."

Be a phony at 10:35 a.m. Schedule your fakes into your daily planner. "Enter a motivational quote, or even a reminder like 'Be an extrovert today' every day for 3 weeks," Bellavia says. After 3 weeks, it'll sink in and help you make your new ways into new habits.

Amp up your ambition. Set deadlines that are more ambitious than ones you think you can pull off, says Richard Griffith, Ph.D., an executive coach and associate professor of industrial organizational psychology at Florida Institute of Technology. "Ambitious goals are a harmless form of deception and can have a real benefit in overall performance." Crazy goals become self-fulfilling prophecies as you work smarter to achieve them.

Look Better Instantly **MH**

New Hampshire for a week. Half the men spent the time reminiscing about the year 1959; the rest actually pretended it was 1959. They watched Ed Sullivan and Jack Benny on black-and-white television; they listened to Perry Como and talked about bomb shelters. They lived as if the "nifty fifties" were happening all over again.

At the end of the week, all the men scored better on measures of grip strength, memory, and hearing, but the eight who'd spent the week faking it scored well in other areas, too. Sixty-three percent showed improved intelligence test scores, versus 44 percent of the control group. Before-and-after photos of the let's-pretend men were shown to a random group of observers, who said the men all looked noticeably younger by the end of the study.

Langer used that study as a springboard for her 2009 book *Counterclockwise*, which recounts her other studies over the years, all of which prove the same general point: When people think they're healthier, they actually become healthier.

And what if you pretend to be happy? Will you become happier? That's a popular notion in American culture, and it's been around for a long, long time. Just listen to this bit of advice, doled out more than a century ago by William James, the father of American psychology: "Thus the sovereign voluntary path to cheerfulness, if our spontaneous cheerfulness be lost, is to sit up cheerfully, to look round cheerfully, and to act and speak as if cheerfulness were already there."

Update the lingo and you have one of the core messages of today's positive-psychology movement. One of its leading

Caution: Anger works best if you hold more power in the discussion.

lights is Sonja Lyubomirsky, Ph.D., a professor of psychology at the University of California at Riverside. In her 2008 book *The How of Happiness*, she breaks down the pursuit of our national longing into 12 activities. They are a sensible and scientifically validated dozen: expressing gratitude, avoiding overthinking, practicing acts of kindness, savoring life's joys . . . all good stuff. But there, at the end, nestled in "Happiness Activity No. 12: Taking Care of Your Body" is "Acting Like a Happy Person." Her advice: "Act as if you were confident, optimistic, and outgoing. You'll manage adversity, rise to the occasion, create instant connections, make friends and influence people, and become a happier person."

And if you're happier, according to a hundred different studies, you'll be more likeable, creative, accomplished, and successful. Plus, you'll catch fewer colds.

Really? All that just by faking it? We called Lyubomirsky on it—literally. "It's maybe the least powerful of the 12 strategies in my book, but it's still a tool," she says. Look at it this way: We're social creatures. For most of us, happiness and success in life hinges on how well we interact with others. If you're glum you'll get no traction, and the reason is very simple. As Lyubomirsky puts it, "We don't like to approach people who look unhappy."

Okay, okay, she's right. If your authentic

Introverts are less satisfied in life than extroverts, studies show.

self is Eeyore, maybe a little fakery could do you good.

Just ask William Fleeson, Ph.D.

Fleeson has taken an interest in the Eeyores of the world. As a psychology professor at Wake Forest University, Fleeson has spent the past decade wondering why some people are introverted and others are extroverted, and whether there's really much difference between the two types. From his studies with students who recorded their actions and feelings on an hourly, daily, or weekly basis, he has concluded that extroverts sometimes act introverted, and introverts sometimes act extroverted.

In other words, he finds that extroversion and introversion are not so much fixed traits as momentary states, with so-called extroverts rating themselves as "talkative," "active," "energetic," "assertive," and "adventurous" relatively more often than introverts do. And Fleeson also corroborates what other researchers have concluded: Extroverts are happier than introverts.

But he wondered whether introverts could be happy, too, if they acted like extroverts. Or, as the subtitle of one of his research papers put it, "Is Acting Extraverted as 'Good' as Being Extraverted?" Are you with us here? Fleeson actually conducted an experiment on whether you can fake it till you make it! He had 47 students meet in small groups; each student was randomly assigned to act either introverted or extroverted during a 10-minute group discussion. When the time was up, participants rated their own behavior and mood before joining another group discussion and acting the opposite way. The result: Nearly everyone was happier when acting extroverted. Including the introverts.

As Fleeson puts it, "Tell people to be extroverted, and 10 minutes later they're having a blast."

But he was bothered by the idea that his results might encourage people to be inauthentic to their true selves—the kind of pretense that eventually takes a toll on mental health. So he recently conducted four more studies—three in his lab with college students who took part in activities such as Twister or debates about medical ethics, and one with a broader range of participants (ages 18 to 51) who rated their behavior several times a day as they went about their lives. Here's what he found: Although introverts thought they would feel most authentic while acting introverted, their responses were actually quite different when they were caught in the moment and quizzed about whether they were being true to themselves.

"Introverts were not 'faking it' when they acted extroverted," Fleeson says. "All the participants said they were more true to themselves while they were playing the role of an extrovert, even if they were introverts." Furthermore, it's not that hard for them; it doesn't wear them out or make them anxious to be extroverted. When introverts act less shy/lethargic and more assertive/energetic, "they are becoming more authentic, not less so," he says.

The world is still full of manipulative phonies, but sometimes this advice is smart and genuinely helpful: Fake it till you make it. There was a kernel of truth rattling around in there after all.

Still With Us?

We almost forgot. The only reason you're still reading this article is to learn something about faking it in the sack. And why is that? Because you're already faking it? (Yes, a quarter of men have done so.) Or because you suspect that she's faking it? (At least half of women plead guilty.)

The world's foremost authority on this topic, Erin Cooper, is still working on her Ph.D. in clinical psychology, but already she has interviewed close to 1,500 young women, ages 18 to 32, who admit to play-acting at orgasm on occasion. Asked why, the various answers can be grouped into four categories: (1) She wants to spare your feelings, a ploy Cooper calls "altruistic deceit"; (2) She doesn't want you to think there's something wrong but

The shyness cure? Pretend you're extroverted; reap the rewards.

doesn't know how to talk about it, and a cluster of similar reasons that Cooper labels "fear and insecurity"; (3) She wants to go to sleep already. But get a load of reason 4: She's actually turning herself on by doing so.

Cooper's contribution to the sum of human knowledge regarding female orgasm is answer 4. Nobody thought of that before. Nobody considered that faking it could actually be a good thing.

The women who cite that final reason "are faking an orgasm to increase their arousal in the moment," says Cooper. "It's a tool women use to make sure they have a good time. My guess is that, for some, they're literally faking it till they make it."

Which doesn't help you much, but . . . wait. What the hell are we saying? Of course it helps you! Nothing is so arousing as an aroused mate! And if you suspect that's what she's doing (Can you tell? No, says Cooper, you probably can't), pretend you don't know anything. Be clueless. In this case, it's working for you.

Trends

Here are the latest trending styles, from the top style gurus.

People usually think of magazine editors as folks who are up to date on the latest fads. But we'll be honest with you: We hate fads. What we care about are trends.

At first, fads and trends sound like the same thing. You're following a fashion fad if you're wearing something trendy, right? Well, sort of. But there's a huge difference between the two. Think of a trend as a long, drawn-out bend in a river; fads are just ripples in the water flowing down that bend. A fad is last night's scores; a trend is the win/loss record for the season. Sometimes fads point in the direction of the trend (the Heat wins again!), but at other times they're just weird blips that run counter to the long-term trend. Here are some style trends you can count on.

Tactical Cool

Try the classic military look, updated—no woods or desert required. You don't have to look hard at all to see camouflage anymore.

"The military inspiration has been a style basic for a while, but now we're seeing it reinterpreted with a modern twist," says designer and camo fan Tommy Hilfiger. A little goes a long way, so stick to one accent at a time.

FOR WORK

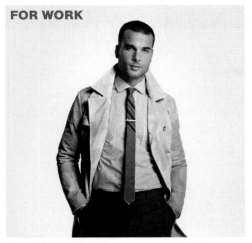

SUEDE OVERCOAT: It's only fitting that camo can hide. "A light-colored print gives it a more sophisticated feel," Hilfiger says. "This way you can easily mix in a pop of camo with your daily wardrobe." Wear it over a tailored suit to amp up your work look.

FOR TRAVEL

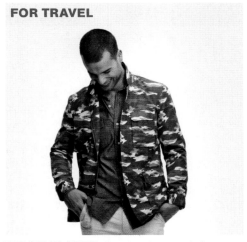

NYLON BLAZER: Stay true to camo's functional roots with this nylon jacket. Perfect for a swagged-out vacation, it's loaded with useful pockets, and the tailored shape can be dressed up or down. We suggest pairing it with a casual denim shirt. If your office is casual, you can also wear it with a tie at work.

FOR A DATE

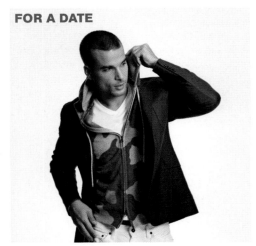

CASHMERE HOODIE: Rich purples, blues, and greens—plus the lush cashmere—allow this hoodie to transition from a casual weekend setting into something you'd wear out. Layer it under a fitted blazer with a pair of crisp white jeans for a clean, sharp style.

FOR TRAVEL

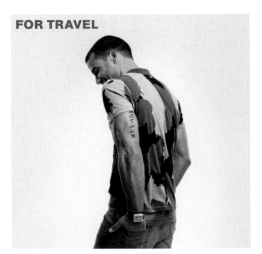

COTTON POLO: Camouflage goes contemporary with this less traditional pattern. The deep shades blend in unassumingly, but the look is still plenty bold. Balance the dark colors by pairing the polo with a light pair of jeans.

BOOT FORCE

We dragged five boots through hell to find the toughest ones.

Boots are supposed to last. So with help from Edward Shimunov, owner of Manhattan's Cobbler Express, we devised this torture test to attack their weak spots: (1) assault the soles with carpenter's pincers; (2) baptize the boots in the East River; (3) batter them on the streets of New York City; and (4) simulate wear with a wire-bristle paint-stripping tool.

We scored comfort, style (trail-to-sidewalk versatility), and value (do the materials and construction justify the price?) each on a 5-point scale; then we assigned up to 10 points for durability.

COLUMBIA BUGABOOT PLUS

Here's a boot dressed in proprietary technology. The full-length Techlite shell makes it the lightest pair we tested. Multidirectional Omni-Grip treads help on the hills, and Omni-Heat linings keep your feet warm. The sole gave way with little effort, but the rubberlike sidewalls held up to the wire brush nearly as well as leather did. The Bugaboot also emerged from the soak test only slightly heavier than when it went in. ($115)

Comfort: 3
Style: 2
Value: 4
Durability: 8
Total: 17

L.L. BEAN'S WATER-PROOF TRAIL MODEL HIKERS, MID-CUT

See that price? Bean kept costs down by using its own materials instead of Vibram soles and Gore-Tex linings. Much of the upper boot is soft synthetic material, but metal eyelets (supported by an external rib cage of leather straps) withstood the stripping tool. The boot emerged from our test broken but still functional. ($90)

Comfort: 5
Style: 2
Value: 5
Durability: 6
Total: 18

HELLY HANSEN LYNX

With high rubber sidewalls and faux fur linings, these bad boys look ready to stomp the Batmobile's gas pedal. In our test, Thermolite wicking dried them quickly of river water. Our wire bristles bounced right off the rubber siding and only slightly frayed the leather overlay. "Rubber punctures easier than leather," Shimunov says. "But it's still sturdier than plastic or some cheap synthetic material." ($150)

Comfort: 4
Style: 4
Value: 3
Durability: 7
Total: 18

ECCO NAMCO MID GTX

A boot with sole power, the Ecco has a tough polyurethane midsole and a rugged Vibram outsole that wouldn't tear off. Vibrams are "tougher than the soles that companies make themselves, and the multidirectional tread provides very sturdy footing," says Shimunov. The uppers are made of supposedly tough yak leather, but they frayed just as cow leather did with the stripping-tool abuse. ($225)

Comfort: 5
Style: 3
Value: 3
Durability: 8
Total: 19

VASQUE TAKU GTX

The body: thick nubuck. The sole: Vibram. The liner: Gore-Tex. Every component is of the highest quality, making this the boot Shimunov correctly predicted would hold up best. It's also fairly priced and stylish enough to wear on or off the trail. These boots should withstand years of serious wear and tear, looking great along the way. ($165)

Comfort: 4
Style: 5
Value: 4
Durability: 9
Total: 22

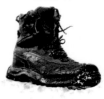 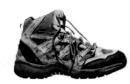 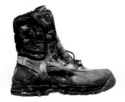 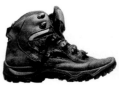 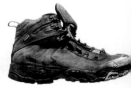

Look Better Instantly **MH**

Green: The New Black

Sustainable clothing, from organic cotton to repurposed leather, is ready to refashion your fall wardrobe.

Somewhere between Woodstock and Portlandia, ecofriendly fashion moved beyond hemp and into the mainstream. Today, "there's a general mantra in the industry that any act of sustainability needs to be invisible," says Lynda Grose, a designer and associate professor at California College of the Arts. In other words, organic clothes are now as stylish as everything else on the rack. You can't tell they're different just by looking, which means you can shrink your carbon footprint while dressing as sharply as ever.

Save More, Shop Less

Americans throw away more than 13 million tons of clothing and textiles a year, the EPA says. That's the antithesis of shopping sustainably. The idea is to make stuff last—in your closet, not the dump.

Age-proof your suits. Don't let that suit hit the floor. "As soon as you take it off, hang it up on a proper suit hanger, not a wire hanger," says Jerry Pozniak, managing director of the New York branch of Jeeves dry cleaners. Suit hangers relax wrinkling and help the shoulders keep their shape. When necessary, have a dry cleaner steam-press the suit to remove smells and wrinkles.

"I clean my suits only when there's a stain or I've worn them three, four, or five times, or if I notice any odors," Pozniak says.

Age denim gracefully. To delay your jeans' fading, "put ½ cup of vinegar in the washing machine when you wash them for the first time to help set the dye," Pozniak says. After that, wash them sparingly. And use cold water because excessive heat breaks down the fabric and color.

Cobble it together. Don't go strutting around in your new dress shoes just yet. "The first thing I do is put rubber half-soles on them," Pozniak says. "And as soon as the soles or the heels start to wear down, replace them." Preventive cobbling and early repairs can save big money later.

Mend the details. "If you wear out the lining of a favorite or an expensive suit, you don't necessarily have to replace the whole suit if the outside fabric is in great condition," Pozniak says. "Have the lining replaced, and you've got a suit that will last another 10 years."

Quick fixes—from replacing loose buttons to repairing broken zippers—can give old pieces new life.

WRIST MANAGEMENT

Sure, your cellphone can tell you the time, but a stylish man still wears a watch.

Despite the cool economy, the watch industry is heating up. According to *The New York Times*, sales of watches in the $150 to $1,000 range rose 15 percent in 2011. And sales of luxury watches ($10,000 to $25,000) jumped 33 percent. Still, expensive doesn't necessarily mean better or cooler.

"Some people come in looking for a specific brand or piece, but it doesn't fit with their style or look," says Michael Gordon, store director of Tourneau on Madison Avenue.

So think: Which of these five styles is right for you? Your choice will be an investment that pays dividends long after you've recycled your cellphone.

KEY:

$: Entry level

$$: Moderate

$$$: High end

EVERYDAY

These babies are the watch world's workhorses, straddling office and weekend.
The message: "I'm straightforward and reliable."

Breitling Montbrillant ($9,000), breitling.com **$$$**

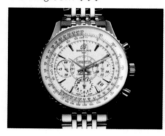

Victorinox Swiss Army Alliance ($475), (800) 442-2706 **$$**

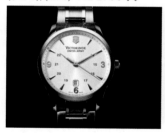

Kenneth Cole New York Classic Stainless Steel ($95), (800) 536-2653 **$**

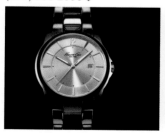

TRENDING

Like any fashion item, watches follow trends. Once you have the basics, grab a piece in today's look: all black.
The message: "My gold one's at home."

Bell & Ross BR03-92 Phantom ($4,200), (888) 307-7887 **$$$**

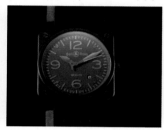

Oakley Gearbox Titanium ($900), (800) 403-7449 **$$**

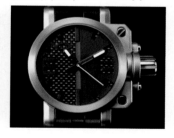

Diesel DZ1543 ($160), watchstation.com **$**

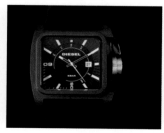

FITNESS

Watches are tools to measure heart rate as well as time. Many runners and cyclists can't live without them.

The message: "I take care of my body."

Suunto Quest ($275), (855) 258-0900 **$$$**

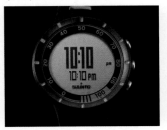

Polar FT7 ($120), (800) 227-1314 **$$**

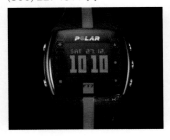

Timex Personal Trainer ($70), (800) 448-4639 **$**

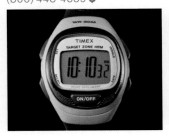

GOLD

Inherently flashy, a gold watch can be artfully downplayed with a leather strap instead of a bracelet.

The message: "My portfolio is doing just fine."

Officine Panerai Radiomir Oro Rosa ($19,100), panerai.com **$$$**

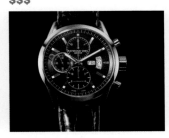

Raymond Weil Freelancer ($13,700), raymond-weil.com **$$**

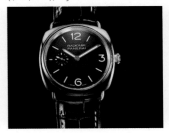

Bulova 97A104 ($400), (800) 228-5682 **$**

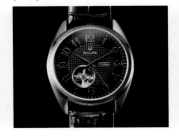

SQUARE

Watches with square cases call attention—the good kind—to your wrist.

The message: "Look again. I'm not like the other guys."

Jaeger-LeCoultre Reverso Squadra Chronograph ($11,600), Jaeger-LeCoultre Beverly Hills **$$$**

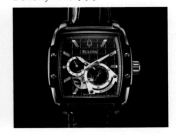

Tag Heuer Monaco ($3,300), us.tagheuer.com **$$**

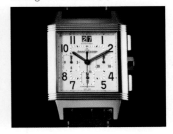

Bulova 98A118 ($450), (800) 228-5682 **$**

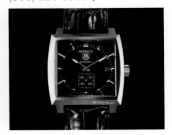

Perfect Fit

Why buy off the rack when you can have custom clothes for the same price–or less?

If the thought of custom clothing triggers a chorus of cha-chings in your head, set those cash registers to mute. Bespoke options aren't reserved for royalty anymore. They're popping up everywhere, from casual weekend gear to formal attire, at prices you can afford. And the low cost isn't the only draw. Here are three more reasons to embrace the tailored trend.

To Achieve the Perfect Fit

For muscular guys, off-the-rack clothes can present a classic Clark Kent dilemma: trying to fit broad shoulders and a slim waist.

"Hard-to-fit men have trained themselves to live with ill-fitting clothes," says Lloyd Boston, TV host and author of *The*

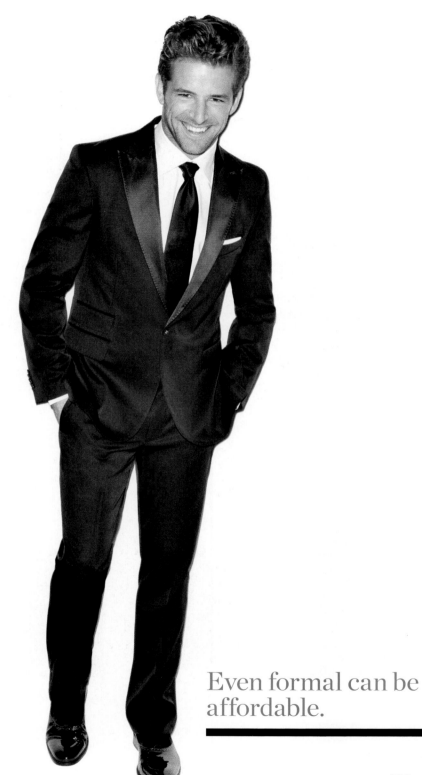

Even formal can be
affordable.

Style Checklist. "So much so that they overlook the sometimes obvious flaws, which scream out to onlookers."

Don't settle for a sloppy fit. Instead, invest in items that are tailored to your specific proportions.

"Custom clothing is what separates well-dressed men from men who are just dressed," Boston says.

To Reclaim Your Weekends

If you dread the idea of scouring racks at the mall on a Saturday afternoon, worry no longer. Many custom clothiers will fit you online (with simple instructions for measuring yourself), or even send a tailor to your home.

You can go far beyond the custom suit. Let your typing fingers do the walking at these custom-clothing sites.

To Dictate the Design Process

Be as bold or as conservative as you like in the details of your clothing, from the number of buttons on your cuffs to the location of the monogram. If you ever wanted a purple-lined suit, now's your chance.

Visit the following sites to buy custom clothing at your fingertips.

J. Hilburn
jhilburn.com

Price: $90 to $630 (various)

Turnaround time: 4 weeks

Special features: Style advisors come to your home or office anywhere in the United States with a large selection of high-end fabrics from Italy, where the clothing is later made. Also available: ready-to-wear jeans, sweaters, and ties.

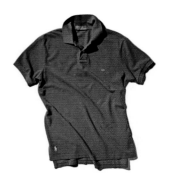

Ralph Lauren
polo
($95, ralphlauren.com)

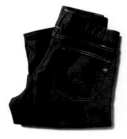

INDI
jeans
($180, indicustom.com)

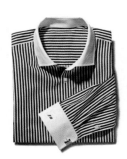

ALFA
shirt
($45, worldofalfa.com)

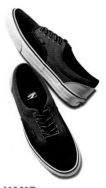

VANS
sneakers
($60, shop.vans.com)

Service includes style advisor visits with no minimum purchase; $90 to $160 (shirt), $125 to $225 (trousers), $395 to $630 (suit jacket/sport coat).

Suitsupply
suitsupply.com

Price: $600 to $1,900 (suit)

Turnaround time: 4 to 8 weeks

Special features: Suits from the Blue Line collection are customized with a variety of fabric and pattern choices. The Suit Up collection is a full custom program featuring wool, flannel, and cashmere. Also available: ready-to-wear suits, dress shirts, and ties. Fittings available in New York City only.

Bonobos
bonobos.com

Price: $890 (tuxedo)

Turnaround time: 4 to 6 weeks

Special features: Choose the piping and lining of your tux for a unique spin on special-occasion dressing. This online-only retailer also customizes casual options, like chinos, and offers a wide selection of ready-to-wear clothing. Fittings available in New York City only.

Alfa
worldofalfa.com

Price: $29 to $75 (dress shirt)

Turnaround time: 2 to 4 weeks

Special features: A 3-D design page brings your shirt to life. Monograms are available, and you can also design your own suits and ties.

Ralph Lauren
ralphlauren.com

Price: $95 to $155 (polo shirt)

Turnaround time: 2 to 4 days

Special features: Personalize your polo by choosing the colors and adding a monogram in place of the pony. Options include long- and short-sleeve shirts, as well as adding city names, custom flags, and bigger or smaller ponies.

Vans
shop.vans.com

Price: $60 to $70 (sneakers)

Turnaround time: 4 to 6 weeks

Special features: Pick the shape of your sneakers—from slip-ons to old-school lace-ups—and customize 10 different areas in 48 colors and patterns. You choose everything from the fabric on the top to the colored line above the rubber sole.

Indi
indicustom.com

Price: $175 and up (jeans)

Turnaround time: 5 weeks

Special features: The site's Jean Builder streamlines the design process, letting you create your perfect pair in minutes. Select one of three fits and 10 rinses, ranging from raw to vintage. Other options include pocket and leg styles.

Time Stoppers

Put up a good front, from hairline to chin, with our decade-by-decade plan.

A dab of lotion on your mug can't counter years of abuse. So follow a multipronged plan to prevent and treat your skin as the decades unwind. These strategies, from dermatologist Brad Katchen, M.D., will help you face the passage from your college years to middle age.

YOUR TWENTIES

THE PROBLEM:

Acne now, sun damage later.

THE PRESCRIPTION:

Sunscreen: In the morning, apply an SPF 15 (or better) moisturizer to prevent dryness and shield ultraviolet rays.

Cleanser: Discourage blemishes with a cleanser. Avoid harsh scrubs; these can actually stimulate oil production if you rub too hard. An exfoliating cleanser with glycolic acids does the job without the elbow grease. (Anthony Logistics for Men Glycolic Facial Cleanser, $21, anthony.com)

The plan: Now's the time to prevent wrinkles. Try sleeping on your back so your skin won't crease from the pressure of your head. And don't squint; wear glasses if you need them and always wear sunglasses.

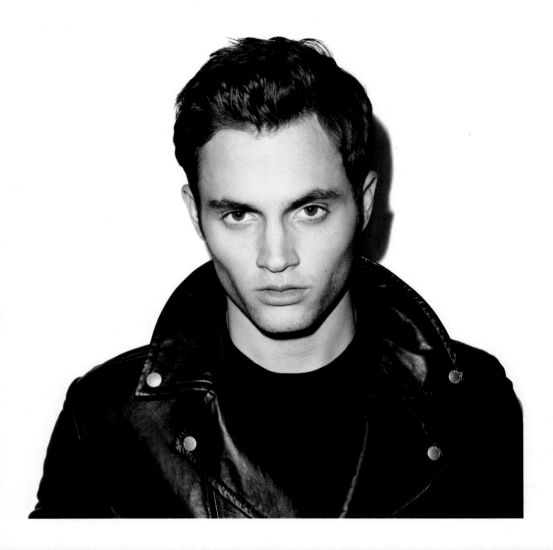

HUMIDITY, IN YOUR FACE

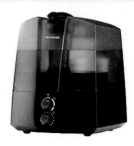

Here's a skin care solution for all ages. The condition of your skin and the onset of wrinkles depend largely on the air around you, says Neal Schultz, M.D., a Manhattan dermatologist. He suggests using a cool-air ultrasonic humidifier at home—especially at night, when skin tends to become dehydrated. Try the AOS 7145 Cool Mist Ultrasonic model by Air-O-Swiss. ($140, airoswiss.net)

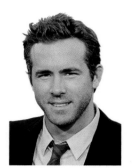

YOUR THIRTIES

THE PROBLEM:

Your career is taking off—and so are your wrinkles. (Coincidence?) Expect blotches and fine lines.

THE PRESCRIPTION:

Eye cream: Every morning, use a cream with sirtuins and other ingredients that can stimulate cell growth and collagen production to bolster the fragile scaffolding of skin around your eyes. (Lab Series Skincare for Men Max LS Instant Eye Lift, $44, labseries.com)

Exfoliating pads: Evening is the best time to treat pigmentation and lines. Swipe your face before bed; the fruit acids can gently clear off old cells and reveal fresh skin. (Origins Brighter by Nature, $40, origins.com)

WAKE UP YOUR FACE

Wild night? Here's how to hide the evidence.

Even if you're in no shape to talk about your evening, your face says it all. Whatever the cause—brews with the guys, an all-nighter with a colicky newborn—don't let bleary eyes, dry mouth, and puffy skin ruin your morning. Put your best face forward.

DEHYDRATED SKIN

The damage: Sleep deprivation reduces skin clarity, says Boston dermatologist Jeffrey S. Dover, M.D. It spikes production of the stress hormone cortisol, which damages your skin's primary structural protein.

The fix: Smooth on a serum or cream with retinol, tretinoin, vitamin C, and peptides. Try Task Essential New Time Serum for Men ($76, groominglounge.com).

ACNE FLARE-UP

The damage: An outbreak could mean you didn't wash your face well before bed. Carb-rich cocktails with high glycemic loads could also be to blame.

The fix: Restore balance with a clean sweep from Neutrogena Men Skin Clearing Acne Wash ($6, neutrogena.com). Its mild salicylic acid formula wipes away dirt, opens oil-clogged pores, and dries zits.

COTTON MOUTH

The damage: Excessive salt or alcohol consumption dehydrates your mucous membranes.

The fix: To dislodge the gunk, vigorously brush your tongue after you scrub your teeth. Then rinse with a mouthwash that contains hydrogen peroxide, which keeps the odor-causing bacteria countdown. (Just don't swallow the stuff.) Afterward, pop a mint.

CHAPPED LIPS

The damage: Your cadaverous-looking lips are tip-offs to skin dried out by booze or neglect.

The fix: Remove dead skin with a paste of baking soda and water, rubbed in lightly with your finger. When the dry patches are rinsed away, seal in moisture with a protective coating like Every Man Jack Lip Balm ($5 for two, everyman jack.com) to bring your smackers back to life.

The plan: Scale back your favorite dehydrating habits from your 20s (sodium intake, excessive alcohol). Fewer late nights should reduce the dark circles under your eyes.

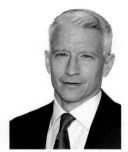

YOUR FORTIES

THE PROBLEM:
Wrinkles deepen, and skin loses elasticity. The fine lines from your 30s become crevices.

THE PRESCRIPTION:

Antioxidants: Sunscreen remains key, and a cream with vitamin C can protect against damaging free radicals generated by sun and pollution. (Kiehl's Powerful-Strength Line-Reducing Concentrate, $58, kiehls.com)

Overnight serum: A lightweight serum added under a lotion (or worn alone) can keep your skin cells reproducing as you rest. (Dermalogica Overnight Repair Serum, $63, dermalogica.com)

The plan: Visit your dermatologist for treatments and cancer screenings. Exfoliating treatments—from chemical peels to Fraxel laser resurfacing—can return the luster to your face.

MOBILIZE FOR MORNING

Prevent tomorrow's problems tonight with these five tips.

Don't drink on an empty stomach. Eat a full dinner to slow alcohol absorption and lessen the potential for hurt tomorrow.

Sleep on an extra pillow. This will elevate your head and keep fluids from pooling around your eyes.

Before you hit the sack, slather on a night moisturizing cream. Cover your face to stave off dehydration.

Apply lip balm before bed. It'll be absorbed in the night, and the swelling will fuse any skin cracks before they form.

Sleep with a glass of water by your bed. This way you'll be more likely to drink it if you wake up in the middle of the night. Also, frequent urination helps flush the toxins from your system sooner.

PICK HER UP

A pickup strategy that works: We all know that the funny guys often win the women in bars, but a study in the journal *Personality and Individual Differences* found that men still underestimate the degree to which women value humor in pickup lines. (More important, men overestimate the appeal of sexually loaded remarks.)

Try this: Open with a funny line about the music or the bartender, and then carry on the exchange for 5 minutes before offering your name. The key is using the wisecrack to leapfrog past the awkward introduction mode.

"Men and women operate off scripts in the mating game," says psychiatrist Paul Dobransky, M.D., of menspsychology.com. "Acting as if you're already acquainted speeds up the intimacy process."

LIGHT A FIRST-DATE FIRE

There's a scientific reason why sweating together is sexy. A new study in the *Journal of Experimental Social Psychology* suggests that moving in sync with her could enhance your connection. When people's body movements were similar in style and flow, they rated their interactions as more positive. Matching your movements—by, say, exercising together—can create closeness, helping you bond. Plan active dates, such as hiking or rock climbing, that have you moving in sync, says study author Tanya Vacharkulksemsuk, Ph.D.

HARD TRUTH

70

The percentage of guys who feel anxious approaching women in bars.

DON'T GIVE HER THE EYE

Your "seductive" look might actually be a turn-off. In a University of Michigan study, women perceived men with lowered eyelids to be more promiscuous, less caring, and poorer as potential fathers. As a result, they were shunned not only as prospective husbands but also as casual sex partners.

"Lowered eyelids are a signal of mating interest but not mate quality," says study author Daniel J. Kruger, Ph.D. Rethink your online dating pics: Skip the seductive gaze and just smile, says Kruger.

SHOW HER A GOOD TIME

Looks like the fun guys win at love: In a Penn State study, women rated "playful" and "fun-loving" as highly desirable qualities in men—more than good looks and intelligence. Playfulness is the opposite of aggression, so it gives women a sense of safety, notes study author Garry Chick, Ph.D. So work more lighthearted stuff—sports, games, fun foreplay—into your downtime.

DIY

Ninety percent of women prefer a long-term partner who earned his money rather than inherited it.

"Women associate self-earned wealth with reliability, self-sufficiency, intelligence," says study author Peter Jonason, Ph.D. If you have family money, play up your generosity—say, donate to charity. That shows you don't take wealth for granted.

GO TO BAKERIES, NOT BARS

Starbucks might be the ultimate pickup spot. Pleasant smells could help you score her number, according to research from France. Women were more likely to give men their phone numbers when approached at delicious-smelling places—bakeries, coffee shops, pastry shops—than when they were chatted up in clothing stores or banks. Enticing scents might lift her mood, making her more receptive to your advances.

CHECK YOUR TOOTHPASTE

What's good for your teeth could be bad for your ticker: When University of California at Davis researchers exposed cardiac cells from mice to triclosan—an antibacterial ingredient in some toothpastes—the cells stopped contracting properly. One theory is that the chemical impairs signaling between calcium channels in those cells. More research is needed to determine if this poses any risk to people.

SAVE YOUR SKIN

Those big guns could save your life: Having strong muscles can keep melanoma from killing you, according to a study from the University of Michigan. Researchers who examined the muscles of people with an advanced form of the deadly skin cancer found that those with denser muscle tissue were 45 percent less likely to die of the disease. Dense muscles are a sign of better health—and perhaps a stronger immune system, says study author Michael Sabel, M.D.

COMB FOR CLUES

How are your LDL, HDL, and triglycerides? How about hair color? A salt-and-pepper look may signal heart trouble, say scientists in Turkey. They found that just a 1-point increase on a 5-point scale of hair whiteness raised a man's risk of coronary artery disease by almost 30 percent, regardless of his age. Gray hair has been tied to DNA damage, which also contributes to narrowing arteries, says study author Sinan Altan Kocaman, M.D. Dyeing your do won't help, but de-stressing might; chronic stress can accelerate DNA damage, say researchers at the University of California at San Francisco.

Q The toothpaste aisle always has something new. What actually works?

A: It depends on what you're looking for. Toothpaste that merely cleans your teeth is passé.

"Companies are trying to cash in on the buzz about how good oral hygiene can help you fend off a host of health problems, including heart disease," says Kenneth Young, D.D.S., a private-practice dentist in New York City and *Men's Health* dentistry advisor. "This has led to increasing specialization in toothpaste."

In fact, a staggering 67 new toothpastes hit store shelves in a single year. To help you choose a tube that's right for you, we checked with a panel of dentists, including Dr. Young; Mark Schlesinger, D.D.S., a clinical associate professor of dentistry at New York University; Paul Levi, D.M.D., an associate clinical professor of periodontology at Tufts University school of dental medicine; and Jennifer Jablow, D.D.S., a Manhattan-based cosmetic dentist.

Sensitivity: Most sensitivity formulas contain 5 percent potassium nitrate, which blocks receptors that translate hot and cold signals into pain. We like Sensodyne ProNamel iso-active ($5) because it's also pH balanced to help prevent acid erosion. To maximize the pain blocking, says Dr. Schlesinger, spit after brushing, but then wait 20 minutes before rinsing.

Gum health: The best way to kill the germs that cause gum disease is to use a toothpaste with the antimicrobial triclosan, such as Colgate Total ($4.50). In a University at Buffalo study, it outgunned a stannous fluoride product. Just brush at a 45-degree angle, says Dr. Levi. This helps the bristles reach up under your gum line, where bacteria burrow.

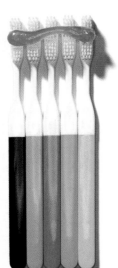

All-around: Only one brand, Crest Pro-Health ($4), is accepted by the American Dental Association in six categories. It whitens, reduces sensitivity, and helps prevent cavities, gingivitis, plaque, and bad breath. One caveat: Its stannous fluoride can cause tooth staining. If you notice brown spots, alert your dentist, who can easily remove them.

Natural: Go natural to avoid artificial flavors and colors, but make sure the brand you choose has cavity-fighting fluoride. The Natural Dentist Anticavity ($6) has fluoride as well as xylitol (which makes plaque less sticky) and aloe vera (an inflammation fighter). Plus, it's free of sodium lauryl sulfate, which is a foaming agent that may cause canker sores.

Whitening: Most whiteners are not powerful enough. For real results, pick a product with hydrogen peroxide, such as Supersmile Professional Whitening System ($36, supersmile.com). Bonus: Two tubes keep the toothpaste separate from the whitening gel, the best way to maintain bleaching power, according to Japanese research.

Q My girlfriend has one of those sonic face scrubbers. Should I use it?

A: On your golf balls? No. On your face? Go for it.

Sonic scrubbers contain microbristles that pulsate hundreds of times a second to clean your pores, says Adnan Nasir, M.D., the *Men's Health* dermatology advisor and an adjunct assistant professor of dermatology at the University of North Carolina at Chapel Hill.

"They're especially great for men with oily, flaky, or clogged skin because they clean deeper than your fingers or a washcloth can, and they easily remove acne-causing grime from your skin." He likes the Clarisonic Plus ($225, clarisonic.com) because it has three speeds; that way you can vary the intensity of your scrub. Use it with a mild face wash, such as Cetaphil Gentle Skin Cleanser ($7, drugstore.com).

Just two caveats: Men with sensitive skin or eczema should skip the scrubber, says Dr. Nasir, and if you share a device with your girlfriend, make sure you buy a separate brush head so you don't gunk up hers.

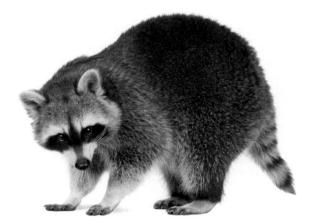

Q How can I eliminate the dark circles under my eyes?

A: Keep your paws off your peepers. Every time you rub the skin under your eyes, you open up little packets of soft pigment that are deposited into your skin to give it a darker appearance, says Bruce Robinson, M.D., an assistant clinical professor of dermatology at Mt. Sinai Medical Center. Plus, rubbing increases pressure in the blood vessels under your eyes, making them more visible. That's what not to do.

Here's what you should do to look bright-eyed.

In the morning: A facial moisturizer with sunscreen, like Neutrogena Men Sensitive Skin Oil-Free moisturizer SPF 30 ($7, neutrogena.com), can protect the delicate skin under your eyes.

At night: Lay off the tequila shots. Excess alcohol and salt can make your cells retain extra water, leading to the A.M. puffiness that makes dark circles look even more pronounced.

At bedtime: Use a cream with vitamin C, like La Roche-Posay Active C Eyes ($43, laroche-posay.us), or caffeine Olay Professional Pro-X Eye Restoration Complex ($40, olay.com).

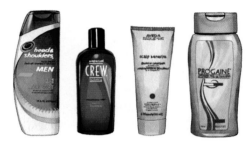

Q Are there any real differences in shampoos?

A: Every potion for your pate is designed to remove oil, dead skin cells, and grime from your scalp, says Paradi Mirmirani, M.D., a dermatologist with Kaiser Permanente. "The biggest difference is the strength of the cleanser." If you have an oily scalp (and greasy hair), you need a strong shampoo; a dry scalp (and wispy hair) requires gentler stuff. But don't confuse dryness with dandruff, which is caused by a fungus.

Now, if you're running out of hair to shampoo, you need a formulation that creates the illusion of thicker hair. We've identified four categories and tested a slew of shampoos in each to find the best. Top off with conditioner for a covetable coif.

Dry scalp: Look for mild cleansers called betaines high up on the ingredient list, says Zoe Draelos, M.D., a consulting professor of dermatology at Duke University school of medicine. These don't bind to oil as well as harsher cleansers do, so they leave some of your natural moisture. (*MH* picks American Crew Daily Moisturizing Shampoo, $7)

Thinning hair: Minoxidil is the only proven OTC way to stimulate hair growth. But the shampoo you use can make each strand appear thicker. Look for volumizing formulas with plumping polymers (like quaternium) that bind to each strand, says Jim Hammer, M.Ed., a cosmetic chemist. (*MH* picks Progaine Volumizing Shampoo, $7)

Oily scalp: Control greasiness with a shampoo that contains anionic surfactants, such as sulfates, sulfoacetates, or sulfosuccinates. An Italian study review found that these detergents, which contain negatively charged particles that bind to oil, are the strongest cleansers. (*MH* picks Aveda Scalp Benefits Balancing Shampoo, $14)

Dandruff: Eliminate the itch by using a product containing either zinc pyrithione or selenium sulfide, which fight the flake-causing fungus and soothe inflammation, says Dr. Draelos. Alternate that with a salicylic acid shampoo, which exfoliates to remove dead skin cells and flakes. (*MH* picks Head & Shoulders Active Sport 2-in-1, $6; Selsun Blue Naturals Island Breeze, $9)

Q Which sunscreen is the best?

A: We'll start by naming the worst: that half-empty bottle left over from two summers ago. Not only is there a good chance it's expired, but it also may not meet new FDA guidelines for UV protection. Today any sunscreen labeled "broad spectrum" must block out the UVA and UVB rays that cause cancer and burns. With the help of *Men's Health* advisor Dr. Nasir, we picked three sunscreens that'll cover you in any situation—if you combine them with common sense.

"You need to follow a strategy that includes a broad-spectrum sunscreen, protective clothing, and shade," says Dr. Nasir. Read on for the rest of your solar survival plan.

Oily skin: To avoid acne, use an alcohol-based product, such as Neutrogena Wet Skin Sunblock Spray, SPF 30 ($9, neutrogena.com). It'll also protect your scalp if you have thinning hair.

Dry skin: Fight scaliness with a moisturizing block, such as Clarins Sunscreen for Face Wrinkle Control ($30, clarinsusa.com). Its aloe hydrates, and titanium dioxide blocks the sun's harmful rays.

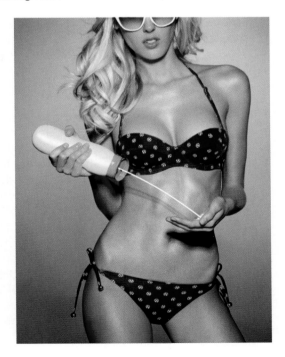

Sweaty skin: Often, lotions end up in the eyes of active guys. Go for a solid, like Coppertone Sport Stick SPF 55 sunscreen ($11, cvs.com). It won't blind you when the ball heads in your direction.

Slather on 300 percent more. A recent study in the journal *Photochemistry and Photobiology* found that people applied just 25 percent of the recommended amount of sunscreen. How much is 100 percent? For your whole body, that's enough to fill a shot glass. And don't stop at one shot. "Apply a new coat every 2 hours," says Dr. Nasir. "Sunscreen's UV-fighting active ingredients degrade rapidly."

Watch your blind spots. Apply sunscreen before you get dressed to ensure complete coverage, says Dr. Nasir. If you do smear it on after dressing, make sure you hit where your clothes end and bare skin begins, especially at your collar line and sleeve openings. And don't overlook the tops of your ears, your lower lip, your eyelids, and the tops of your feet. For extra eye protection, wear wraparound 100 percent UV-blocking sunglasses; we like Kaenon's. If you can handle a hat, go with a wide brim. The combo of hat and glasses can reduce your risk of melanoma by 41 percent, according to University of Minnesota research.

Be smarter about shade. Take at least one 15-minute shade break for every hour you're in the sun, says Dr. Nasir. People using a similar tactic reduced their risk of severe sunburn by 31 percent, a study in the journal *Cancer Epidemiology, Biomarkers and Prevention* found. But don't count on a beach umbrella: Researchers in Spain found that canvas beach umbrellas block only 66 percent of UV radiation, probably because the sun's rays reflect and penetrate from the sides. Your defense: Seek shade in areas where you can't see light shining off water or other surfaces.

Eat for your epidermis. Foods rich in omega-3 fats, monounsaturated fats, and antioxidants can help you fend off sun damage and inflammation, Dr. Nasir says. "The research is strongest for the Mediterranean diet." And load up on the antioxidant lycopene. A recent study in the *British Journal of Dermatology* found that people who ate 2 ounces of lycopene-rich tomato paste every day for 12 weeks showed fewer signs of deep skin damage than people who went without it.

Q I can't dance. Help me before I hurt someone!

A: First, learn a basic move so you don't have to concentrate on your own feet. Yuriy Datsyk, director of the Fred Astaire Midtown Dance Studio in New York City, recommends the box step: It's easy to learn, and it works whether you're dancing with a partner at a wedding or grooving solo at a club. Cue the music: Step forward with your left foot and then bring your right foot forward and to the right. Move your left foot next to the right. Now step back with your right foot, then back and to the left with your left foot. Bring your right next to the left. If you're making moves solo, let your body's natural movement dictate the swing of your arms. If you're dancing with someone, hold her with your right arm at her left shoulder blade level—this creates an intimate common space for the two of you. Join your left hand with her right hand at chest level. Now focus on your partner, not yourself.

"Your job is to showcase her; you are her foil," says Datsyk. That also means protecting her from collisions.

Q How many ties should I have in my quiver?

A: Even if every day is casual Friday, arm yourself with at least eight. Wearing one when it's not required will keep your colleagues on their toes and score points with the boss. Bonus: Women notice, too. For inspiration, use this guide from Andy Stinson, fashion historian and codesigner at Stinson R. Ely.

POWER TIES (KEY MATERIALS: SILK, WOOL, CASHMERE)

The basic pinstripe: Red, blue, and gold mean business.

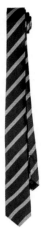

The solid: It's a go-to solution for that tough-to-match patterned shirt.

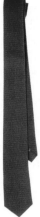

The discreet polka dot: Key word: discreet. Avoid contrasting colors.

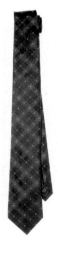

The black silk: A good, safe option for a wedding or funeral, it's an essential that flatters most men.

CASUAL TIES (KEY MATERIALS: SILK, COTTON, LINEN)

The floral: It takes confidence to break out the blooms—wear it on a date with a black jacket.

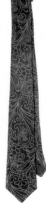

The skinny: Stick with solid colors or bold stripes for this 3-inch-wide (or skinnier) noodle.

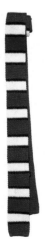

The seersucker: Wear it with a linen sport coat for a cool, casual look.

The wool blend: It's more laid-back than 100 percent wool. Wear a classic solid with a corduroy blazer.

What stylish dress shoes will hold up best in rainy and snowy conditions?

A: Back when Mad Men roamed the earth, "sharp shoes" and "dry feet" were mutually exclusive. But thanks to modern waterproofing technology, that's no longer the case.

"Oxfords, wingtips, and toe boots are all available with membranes fused to the inner linings that repel water but have micropores that allow your feet to breathe," says *Men's Health* Fashion Director Brian Boyé, whose picks appear below. Another option—which Boyé utilizes because his favorite dress shoes aren't waterproof—is Swims Classics ($95, swims.com). These seamless, lightweight rubber galoshes slip over your shoes, protecting the soles and uppers. Plus, they're insulated and have grippy soles to help you keep your footing on slick surfaces.

Split toes: These Geox Rubbiano Amphibiox shoes repel slush thanks to their burly tread and waterproof leather uppers. ($200, shopgeox.com)

Boots: If you're trudging through snow, you need ankle-high protection. The waterproof Ashmont Plain Toe Boots from Johnston & Murphy provide that coverage and have full-grain leather uppers and a sheepskin lining. ($165, johnstonmurphy.com)

Oxfords: Rockport's Ellingwood waterproof oxfords are made of durable full-grain leather and have a polyurethane outsole. ($110, rockport.com)

Which antiperspirant best stops sweat and stink?

A: Stop gaping at the marketing messages on the front label, and squint at the concentration of active ingredients on the back. According to David Pariser, M.D., a dermatologist who studies excessive sweating, "Antiperspirants work by blocking your sweat glands, and those containing higher levels of aluminum chloride or an aluminum-zirconium compound are most effective."

The numbers to look for: 12 percent aluminum chloride or 20 percent aluminum zirconium. Two products that hit sweat-block bingo are Certain Dri and Dove Men + Care Clean Comfort Clinical Protection.

An antiperspirant won't work if you're already sweating, so the best time to apply it is at night, says Dr. Pariser. Don't worry, showering in the morning won't wash off your protection. Now, if you don't sweat much, all you need is deodorant to kill odor-causing bacteria or mask stink. Thai research found that deodorants containing the antimicrobial triclosan, such as Arm and Hammer Ultramax, are effective. If you prefer something unscented, look for a stick that uses zinc ricinoleate, like Tom's of Maine. Want maximum power? Dr. Pariser says a double-barreled approach is better than a 2-in-1 combo, so apply antiperspirant at night and then deodorant in the morning.

Q How can I stop slouching?

A: Your body adapts to the position that you most often assume, which for most guys is hunching in a chair. To break your slump, adopt these three habits, says Bill Hartman, P.T., C.S.C.S., *Men's Health's* Muscle Guy. (1) Set your work e-mail to ping every 15 minutes to remind you to sit up straight with your shoulders back. (2) Twice a day, perform this diaphragm-strengthening drill: Lie facedown on the floor with your forehead resting on your palms. Breathe in through your nose and drive air into your belly while keeping your chest relaxed. Exhale through your mouth. Repeat 10 times. (3) Last but most important, strengthen your back so it's as strong as your chest. These exercises can fix an imbalance.

Thoracic Rotation

Kneel on all fours and place your right hand behind your head with your elbow pointing out to the side. Brace your core and rotate your right shoulder toward your left arm. Then reverse the movement and follow your right elbow with your eyes until it points toward the ceiling. That's 1 rep. Do 12, and then switch arms and repeat. Do 2 sets before every workout.

Incline Y Raise

Grab a pair of light dumbbells. Set an adjustable bench to a low incline and lie with your chest against the pad. Let your arms hang straight down, palms facing each other. Raise the dumbbells until your arms are at a 30-degree angle to your body and form a Y. Pause for 2 seconds, and then slowly lower the weights back to the starting position. Do 10 to 12 reps. Do 3 sets at the end of your upper-body workout.

PART 5

Work Smarter, Grow Wealthier

Men's Health

Your Financial Fresh Start

Recover from Your Financial Hangover.
Take two aspirin and read these 25 tips before calling
your broker. You'll feel much better.

Check out a financial story online or read a newspaper and you might feel a little light-headed. Things became a little fuzzy. You feel like you have the worst hangover ever. You're not entirely sure, but you think you might have spent your 401(k) on Jagermeister and a 1999 BMW. Don't worry about that for a while. Just lean back and take your physical and fiscal recovery one step at a time.

Where to start? How about with a reminder that you're not alone? We're all feeling buoyed by an economy that appears to be on the rebound, so now is the perfect time to use a little groupthink to stay focused on maintaining that successful financial momentum.

"With your friends, family, the media, and now social media talking about making changes and setting goals, it's easier to be part of a group instead of striving alone," says Kathleen Gurney, Ph.D., CEO of Financial Psychology Corporation and the author of *Your Money Personality: What It Is and How You Can Profit from It*. Take comfort from the fact that times are challenging for everyone, and let yourself be motivated by social pressure. After all,

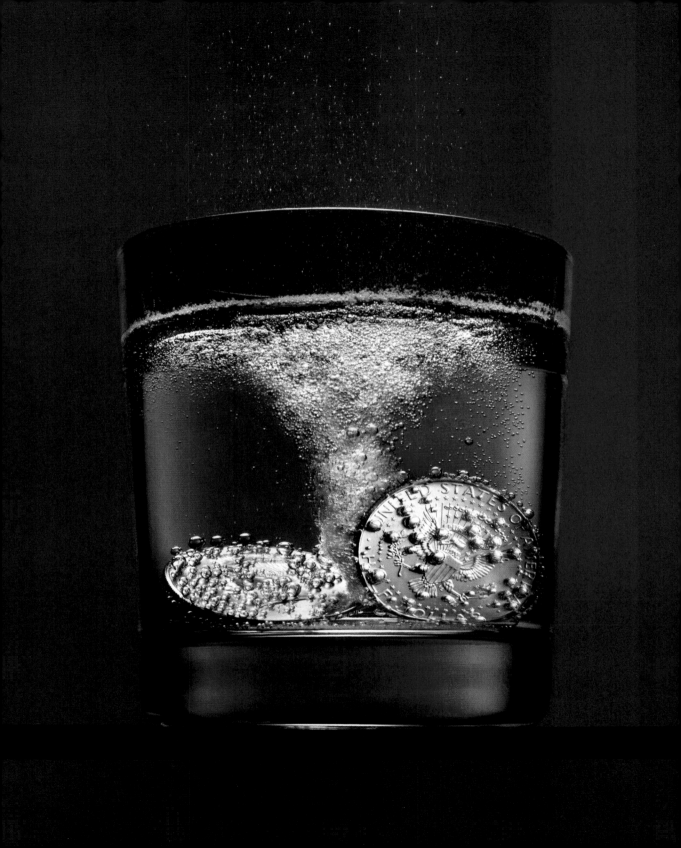

you don't want to fail while watching someone else succeed.

Every journey begins with a few small and possibly hungover steps. Use our 25 expert ideas—helpfully organized by your level of financial incapacitation—to hardwire your year for financial success.

The Just-Shoot-Me Hangover

You're still on the couch and can barely function.

Open your eyes—to money. Because you can't sit up, you might as well lie there and think about stuff, such as why you even care about money. This is important, because your dominant motivation affects all your decisions, making you potentially overly conservative, too optimistic, or excessively altruistic.

Start by considering the three things that money primarily achieves, says Joe Duran, CEO of United Capital Financial Advisers. It gives you security, makes you feel good, and helps you take care of your loved ones. Now figure out how you respond when your finances fluctuate.

"If your money views are influenced by fear, for instance, then when the market dips, you might move everything to cash, which isn't necessarily the right thing to do," says Duran. "If you're optimistic, you might not even want to watch as your 401(k) balance goes down, and that's bad, too."

The key is realizing your bias and compensating for it by considering other financial choices you might not ordinar-

ily make. To see which biases could be influencing your financial decisions, visit honestconversations.com and take Duran's Money Mind quiz.

Make some quick cash the easy way. Grab your laptop and visit fiverr.com, a global marketplace for buying and selling services. The site lists about a million jobs in 200 countries, and most of them can be completed in a few minutes. These could include writing 30-second pitches or offering craft lessons online. Fifteen percent of users say they've earned over $1,000 since joining, and 14 percent say it's their primary source of income, according to the site.

Spot your moneymakers. Almost everything you can see from the couch—or the other parts of your house if you ever stand up—can be rented out for extra money. For example, you can use Airbnb to rent that spare bedroom. With Zilok (us.zilok.com) and NeighborGoods.net, you can rent appliances, lawn equipment, and just about anything else you have lying around the house. RelayRides.com lets you rent your car, and it even pays your renter's insurance. Those bucks add up!

Show your kids how it's done. Instill basic finance skills by teaching them to count change, says Craig Everett, Ph.D., an assistant professor of finance at Pepperdine University and the author of *Toby Gold and the Secret Fortune*, a novel that teaches financial literacy to children. His favorite game: toy store. Set up a bank of coins and bills, and line up some of their toys. Buy a toy for $2.85. Pay for it with a twenty, and show them how to count up from $2.85 until they give you the right change. Math and financial knowledge imparted! You're an awesome dad.

Change your attitude. Many men hold unconscious negative associations about wealth, says Brad Klontz, Psy.D., a financial psychologist and the director of research at H&R Block Dollars & Sense. Instead of clinging to the belief that people get rich by taking advantage of others, he suggests rewriting your internal script. Here's how it should go: "While some rich people are greedy, many gain their wealth by making an honest living and then give to charity to help make the world a better place." By focusing on positive role models instead of harboring resentments, you come away with a more contented and productive attitude. Feeling less nauseated now?

Turn your mate into a financial ally. Agree with your partner that you won't spend more than a specific amount of money—$100, say—without consulting each other first. This isn't about permission, Klontz says, but about slowing down and thinking a purchase through.

The Head-Pounding Hangover

You're off the couch but still need to take it slow.

Ditch the budget. Instead, try a spending plan, Klontz suggests. Establish a goal and create a plan that will enable you to afford it. Say you want to buy a motorcycle. Print a picture of the one you want and slap it on the fridge. Then create a graph to track how close you are to your savings goal. Nail down the total cost of the bike and divide that by the number of months until the road trip you want to break it in on—or set your purchase date based on what you can easily save each month. You'll see your progress, which will take your mind off the austerity measures, Klontz says.

Teach kids patience. Help them learn delayed gratification—which can be a valuable financial skill—with the "cookie game," says Everett. Give Junior one cookie. Tell him that if he waits 5 minutes to eat it, he will get a second cookie. If he doesn't wait, he gets only the one. (No, you can't have the other cookie if he cracks.) In a similar test involving marshmallows decades ago, it was found that children who were able to defer gratification were more competent and scored better on their SATs when they grew older.

Trim that mane. Be a haircut model at your local hair academy, salon, or any place where people are learning to cut hair, says Rob Grader, creator of the *Cheap Bastard's Guide* series, and you'll never pay for a cut again. Or shave your head. A recent study from the University of Pennsylvania's Wharton School showed that a close-cropped or shaved head suggests masculinity, dominance, and possible leadership potential.

Stay in season. If you buy fruits and vegetables that are out of season—such as tomatoes in January—you'll pay much more for your produce than if you buy in-season items. If you just can't live without those tomatoes, do a little planning: Buy extra when they're cheap and freeze them to use in winter.

Temper family expectations. Get

this one out of the way as far from the holidays as possible. Tell your kids they're only going to receive three (or some reasonable number) presents next year. Reset expectations now, says Ellie Kay, the author of *Living Rich for Less*, and you'll create less greedy kids tomorrow. Not to mention a smaller hit to your credit cards next year.

The Glimmer-of-Hope Hangover

You're kind of woozy, but you can take a little bit of action.

Find a money mentor. Now that you're up and about, make a new friend. Find a financial mentor who is operating in the world you want to join, advises Klontz. Ask for some time to pick the brain of your boss, a neighbor, or a successful individual you don't know personally. You will be surprised at how willing successful people are to share their stories with a motivated protégé. Start off your session with a few smart questions ("What do you most attribute your success to?" "What would you do differently?"). Explore the specifics as they come up. Eventually, shift the conversation toward your specific goals, and see what advice your mentor may have to offer, Klontz says.

Snag a massage. You've earned it, sort of. If you volunteer at a professional massage school, you can expect a ridiculously cheap or free rubdown, says Grader. Upside: Free massage! Downside: Your masseuse might be a masseur, and a

sweaty one at that. But hey—free massage! To find a school, go to massageschools guide.com.

Spread some knowledge. You know stuff. Lots of stuff. You may as well start sharing it with the world. You can earn as much as $20 an hour in your spare time imparting your vast knowledge to people who are studying for the SATs and other exams. Start by contacting a test-prep school, such as Kaplan, to receive some sanctioned experience before heading out on your own.

Boost your number. FICO scores aren't just about qualifying for credit anymore. They are used to set auto and homeowners insurance rates and even determine if you need to pay a deposit when you sign up for utility services. If you can't pay your cards off each month, pay at least $5 or $10 more than the minimum, Kay says. "Even these small overpayments show up on your credit report as a sign that you're paying off your principal," says Kay. This directly improves your score.

Fill those coffers. If you don't have an emergency fund with a minimum of 3 months' worth of living expenses, stop contributions to your IRAs and 401(k)s until you have that buffer fully stocked, says Curtis Chambers of the Chambers Financial Group. This is the most important step in escaping a paycheck-to-paycheck mentality, he says.

Show your kids how to save. Give your kids a food allowance the next time you take your family out to eat, says Kay. Tell them they can spend it on whatever they want and that they're allowed to keep whatever they don't spend. "Some kids are natural spenders; some are natural savers," Kay says. "When the spenders see that the savers walked out of that restaurant with dollars in their hands, they will become savers very quickly."

Hit the books. Stop off at the library on your way home. It probably has lots of free classes, lectures, movies, and museum passes, says Grader. And most libraries have embraced the electronic age and now offer downloadable e-books free of charge. Don't forget: Women dig well-read guys.

The "What Hangover?" Hangover

You're feeling fit, rested, and ready for more!

Earn your ticket. Dying to see a show but gagging at the ticket cost and broker fees? Volunteer. If the theater needs people to hand out fliers or do other jobs, you could snag free admission, Grader says.

Hit the road. If you're hankering for a road trip but don't have a car, consider Auto Driveaway (autodriveaway.com). It'll hook you up with a vehicle that needs to be relocated. You'll receive a tank of gas and a certain number of days to complete the trip.

Trim the fat. Study your monthly bills—cable, phone, credit card. You'll be horrified by the amount you're spending on features you don't use. Do you really need 2,400 minutes of talk time when you average 800? Are you still being billed for a website you stopped updating years ago? Save hundreds of dollars by cutting out all the stuff you're not using, says Leah

If you can't pay your cards off each month, at least pay more than the minimum. This directly improves your credit score.

Ingram, founder of the Suddenly Frugal blog (suddenlyfrugal.com).

Score restaurant discounts. Buy some gift certificates to local eating spots at restaurant.com, suggests Kay. You'll grab $25 gift certificates for only $10.

Press "pause." Institute a mandatory 24-hour waiting period before pulling the trigger on any big-ticket purchase—that 90-inch television, the stainless-steel gas grill, the new car. A "gotta have" item can turn into a "glad I didn't" near miss while you're sound asleep, Klontz notes.

Pick the right day to buy. Research by Extrabux, a cash-back shopping site, shows that online retailers vary their prices throughout the week. The variations aren't big, but the savings can add up. Buy computers on Monday (you could save up to $46), TVs on Wednesday (about $20 in savings), and books on Saturday (about $2 less per book).

Grab some bites. Crash happy hour for some free snacks, but go with the right mindset, says Grader. Do it only if you're intent on meeting people and expanding your social circle. Otherwise, you just look like you're there for the food, you hungry drunk.

For Richer or Poorer

Read the following five myths about marital finances before you sign on any more dotted lines together.

Marriage is a union of love, not business. (Well, we hope . . .) But if you don't treat your marriage as something of a vocation—with as much impact on your financial security as on your happiness—then you're compromising the future you'll share. And even if you manage your finances with the same enthusiasm you lavish on your fantasy football league, you might still be making major missteps.

Read on for five marital finance myths that show that traditional marriage money arrangements might not lead to "happily ever after."

MARITAL MONEY MYTH #1

We should have joint credit cards and cosign our loans.

This is the default position for most married couples, and it can cause some very big credit score headaches, says Anthony Sprauve, a spokesman for myfico.com. After all, there's no such thing as a "joint" credit score. Each score reflects all the debt the person is responsible for, and with joint accounts, both spouses' scores

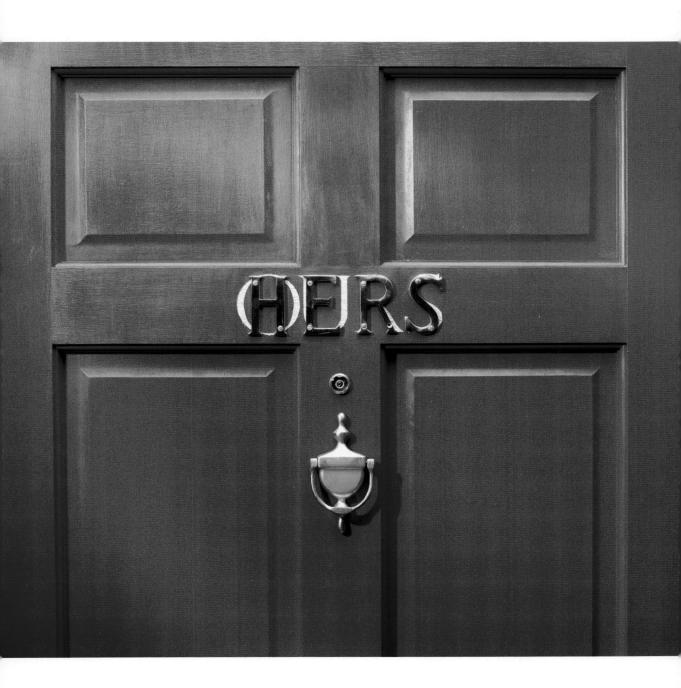

Even when a husband and wife both work full-time, she still spends more time on household chores than he does. As a result, her stress levels may increase.

are impacted by 100 percent—not just 50 percent—of the debt. This can drag down your scores, and it can also compromise your ability to secure more credit if one of you loses a job or otherwise ends up in financial trouble.

Make It Work

If you can qualify for a credit card on your own, take that route, says Sprauve, and keep as much control over your own credit score as you can. Consider alternating who signs smaller loans, such as those for cars or home improvements. Don't worry about things such as legal ownership; having one person's name on a loan doesn't make that person the sole owner of any purchased property. Ownership is determined by the names on the deed or title or by your state's community property laws.

full-time, she still spends more time on household chores than he does. As a result, her stress levels may increase, according to a 2011 study in the *Journal of Family Psychology*. And no, she's not having fun doing the laundry: A marriage in which the wife works full-time and the husband doesn't help much with chores is 44 percent more likely to fail than a marriage in which the man helps out more, a 2010 London School of Economics study found.

And securing outside household help can make you more productive at work, potentially raising your household income. For example, a 2010 Stanford University study found that women in academic science positions who had outside household help published more papers.

Make It Work

Cleaning-service companies are a good place to start, but websites such as care .com and sittercity.com will let you comparison shop for individual housekeepers. They also provide the benefits of background checks and references, says housekeeping consultant Marta Perrone, the author of *Help!! How to Find, Hire, Train & Maintain Your Household Help*.

Be sure to confirm that your cleaning company is bonded and pays all employment taxes and workman's comp insurance.

MARITAL MONEY MYTH #2

We shouldn't pay for household help if we can do it ourselves.

Even when a husband and a wife both work

MARITAL MONEY MYTH #3

We should file our taxes jointly.

For most couples, "married filing jointly" produces the softest tax hit. But "married

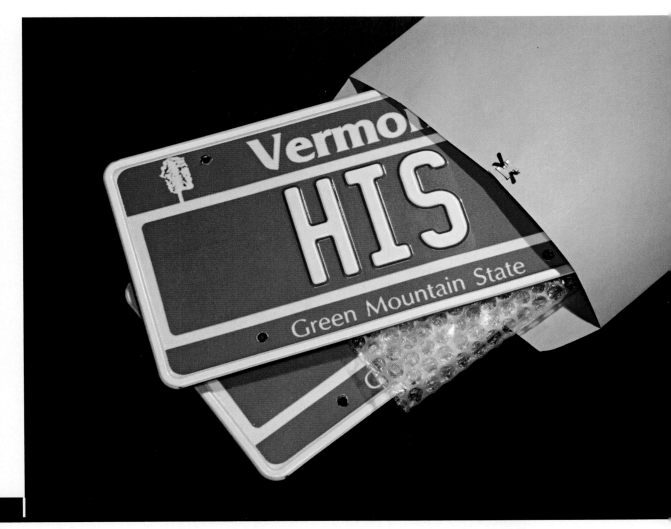

PROTECT YOUR FINANCES FROM A BREAKUP

No couple is immune from this threat. If it does happen, here's your plan.

Before you marry: Make copies of your investment accounts and document your property, advises accountant Tracy Stewart, CFP, PFS, who specializes in counseling divorcing couples. This establishes the value of the assets you'll want to recoup if you end up divorcing.

While you're married: Share the financial workload, says Andrew Hoffman, a certified divorce financial analyst. "If divorce comes, it'll be harder to hide assets or lie about what each person earns or owes." This minimizes conflict, which can mean lower legal fees.

If divorce looms: Stay cool and don't dump marital assets— property, investments—without her specific agreement, says Seth Kaplan, a certified divorce financial analyst. If a decision you made alone harms your spouse financially, she may demand recourse.

Who has a traditional marriage anymore?

filing separately" might make more sense, says Mark Steber, chief tax officer at Jackson Hewitt Tax Service. The reason: potential tax benefits. These typically come when one spouse earns far less than the other and has significant deductible expenses. Some deductions can be applied only if they're larger than certain percentages of your income. For instance, medical expenses and unreimbursed job expenses—assuming they were paid by the person filing for them—kick in only if they total more than 7.5 percent or 2 percent, respectively, of adjusted gross income (AGI). So if your joint AGI is $150,000, you two will need more than $11,250 in medical expenses to be able to itemize them. But if you each file separately, the lower-earning spouse with income of $50,000 needs medical expenses of only $3,750, or unreimbursed job expenses of $1,000, in order to access the tax benefits of itemizing. One caveat: If your spouse itemizes deductions, you have to do the same.

Make It Work

Use your tax program to calculate your taxes both ways. Remember that state taxes have different rules for filing separately, Steber says. If the state rules aren't favorable, you could lose the gains you made on your federal return. Weigh all the pros and cons before splitting up your forms.

We should own our home together.

Most married couples own their home under a form of ownership called "joint tenancy with survivorship." That simply means you two own the property together, and if anything happens to one spouse, the other spouse becomes the sole owner. For traditional marriages, this might work just fine. But who has one of those anymore?

"Second marriages, third marriages, or marriages between U.S. citizens and noncitizens can make things more complicated," says Steven Carr, an estate and trust attorney with Pabian & Russell in Boston. Alternative structures ensure that the property can be passed on to your heirs (as opposed to your spouse), if that's how you want it. It also helps minimize or delay taxes on your estate, and having clearly defined inheritances helps avoid probate court, which can tie up a property for years.

Make It Work

If you want to pass a home on to someone other than your spouse but you want her to have the right to live in it if something happens to you, Carr suggests a revocable living trust.

"The house would pass to the trust upon your death, and then to your beneficiaries upon your spouse's death, all without going to probate," he says. If you're a U.S. citizen and your wife is not, she will have to pay taxes due on the entire estate immediately upon your death. (Of course, the same holds true if you're the noncitizen and she dies.) Set up a qualified domestic trust. Estate taxes won't have to be paid until the noncitizen survivor dies or takes some of the principal out of the trust.

MARITAL MONEY MYTH #5
If her job doesn't pay well, she should quit to raise the kids.

If your wife's take-home cash barely covers child care and commuting costs, you'd think she'd be better off staying home with the kids. That might be true in the short term, but over the long term this plan could spell disaster. If you find yourself laid off, sick, or hit by a bus, your family could be just months from financial ruin. Unless you two have a large nest egg (and if you're a typical couple, you don't), your wife would have to start job hunting from scratch in the midst of a family emergency.

There are also mental health benefits to working outside the home even if it can mean some short-term financial strain. A 2011 *Journal of Family Psychology* study found that women who worked part- or full-time in the years before their children started school reported fewer symptoms of depression and better overall health than moms who stayed home.

Make It Work

If you both plan to work, you'll need quality child care and equally shared parenting, says Kerstin Aumann, Ph.D. a senior research associate at the Families and Work Institute.

"The good news is that men are becoming more involved in parenting," she says. In fact, a recent Institute report shows that men with children in dual-earner homes are now reporting more work-life conflict than women are. And people seem to be more creative about child care, says Paul Busceni, Ed.D., dean of the school of education at Kendall College in Chicago.

"Families are banding together to create a sort of time-share for child care," says Busceni. Each parent takes a day to serve as caregiver for all the kids. Check your community social media networks to see if other parents would be interested in such arrangements—or launch a time-share yourself!

The Money Habits That Hold You Back

Dig into your psyche to see why you keep making the same financial mistakes—then stop!

Building wealth is never simply about making the number work, just as health is never merely an exercise in calorie counting, and love is never a simple mix of pheromones. The truth is that a dollar, like a cheeseburger (or a woman), can really mess with your head.

"Money has a multitude of meanings, and we're always in a dialogue with it about what we think we deserve and what we're capable of," says David Krueger, M.D., a former psychiatrist and the author of *The Secret Language of Money*. "The mistake we make is when we try to use money to reach non-financial goals—to

regulate our moods, to adjust our self-esteem, or to control people."

Read on to find out how to uncover some of the deeply ingrained beliefs that might be limiting your wealth-building potential. Once you knock those pups down, you'll be on your way to riches.

BAD MONEY HABIT #1
You're looking for scapegoats.

The Great Recession took its toll on

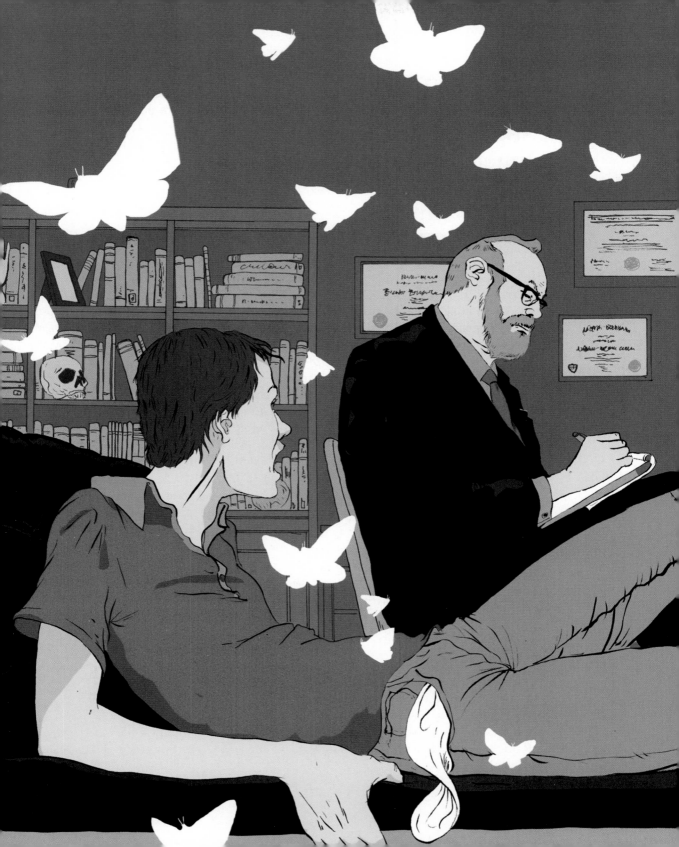

It's time to stop blaming the shady lenders, Wall Street titans, and government agencies that might or might not be standing in your way.

everyone; now it's time to stop playing that card. It's also time to stop blaming the shady lenders, Wall Street titans, and government agencies that might or might not be standing in your way. Somewhere in your own financial past, you signed on some dotted lines. Quit stewing about all of this and focus on yourself.

"You need to take an honest inventory of your role in your own financial situation," says Brad Klontz, Psy.D., coauthor of *Mind over Money: Overcoming the Money Disorders That Threaten Our Financial Health.* "Unless you admit that your distress has something to do with you, you're doomed to repeat your mistakes."

BAD MONEY HABIT #2
You don't know where your financial values came from.

Michael A. grew up in small-town California, where his parents strived to live on the "right" side of town and have the "right" friends. When he moved to San Francisco as a young adult, he felt uncom-

fortable in the urban setting. But he had a pretty good idea of how to find the right friends: He bought them. "I was springing for dinners and signing on for pricey trips to buy people's attention," he recalls. "Eventually I ran up over $100,000 in credit card charges and was fending off debt collectors." His troubles led him to Debtors Anonymous, an outgrowth of Alcoholics Anonymous.

Our attitudes about money are indeed forged in the dramas of youth, Klontz says. Occasionally our parents will teach us a dysfunctional lesson—that money is the root of all evil, or of all happiness. More often, though, we infer our own messages. If your family was poor and unhappy, you might conclude that money can buy happiness. If your home was rich and unhappy—maybe your dad was always at the office—you might conclude that pursuing wealth leads only to misery.

The ideas might be childish, but they can survive in your unconscious well into adulthood. Work to remember how your parents talked about money. What were some of the most memorable experiences you had with the stuff? How did they make you feel? Confronting those questions clearly and working through the answers can help you move beyond the hangups, Klontz says.

BAD MONEY HABIT #3
You don't challenge your beliefs.

These early experiences with money shape the scripts we give ourselves, Klontz argues. In other words, we might fall into beliefs and never really challenge them. Often we're not aware of those beliefs because of the taboo our culture places on talking about personal money matters.

To uncover your money scripts, Klontz suggests filling in the blanks: "Rich people are . . ." or "Poor people are . . ." Or think about your early life experiences relating to money and answer this question: "The moral of my story is . . ."

Your scripts might seem unsophisticated, but don't shy away from them. "Even the craziest money beliefs might make sense if you see how they're rooted in past experience," Klontz says. In other words, if your father sent your family to the poorhouse with his gambling, it makes certain sense to grow up believing that even the safest investing is just another gamble. Writing this script down means you can more easily start to revise it, Klontz says.

BAD MONEY HABIT #4
You use money as a drug.

Dan Nainan was a spindly, bespectacled nerd in school, and he was bullied mercilessly for it. So when he got his first credit card in college, he spent his way out of his

RICH HABITS

We asked advisors how their wealthiest clients got that way.

Go shopping—sort of. The reason many of us aren't getting rich is that we follow crowd logic, not our own instincts.

"People have the opposite psychology when they invest than when they shop for clothes," says David Kudla, CEO of Mainstay Capital Management. "If they see an item at half off and they like it, they buy it. With stocks, people wait until prices are up and everyone feels great." If you like the stock when it's low, go for it.

Build a pyramid. You're the pharaoh, and your investment portfolio is your pyramid. Build it up steadily over time, and limit your risk to the very tip—the top 10 percent, says Scott Tiras of Tiras, Pennington,

and Associates. That's the money you can throw into hunches and instincts. Everything else should be in well-managed mutual funds that spread investments over dozens of stocks.

Maintain, then gain. Once you have some wealth built up, protecting it becomes as important as accumulating more. Instead of investing in the next big vaccine or computer breakthrough, allocate more of your assets to CDs, bonds, and treasury securities, says Tiras.

Once you have pulled together a decent portfolio, then start subtracting your age from 100 to determine what percentage should be invested in stocks.

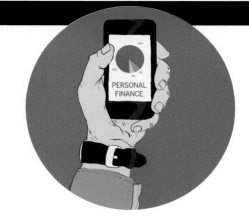

Run toward fire. Hold on to the kayak no matter how rough the financial white-water becomes. Historically, declines have always turned into recoveries. Jump on a few stocks that seem to be in distress or that are being abandoned by other investors, says Stephan Cassaday, president and CEO of Cassaday and Company. So run toward a few fires. That's where the opportunities are.

> Our attitudes toward money are forged in the dramas of youth. Occasionally our parents will teach us a dysfunctional lesson—that money is the root of all evil, or of all happiness.

shell: He sprang for contact lenses, took women on killer dates, and bought stylish clothes and new cars. Eventually he found himself hiding his Volvo from the repo guys.

"I was powerless as a child, and money made me feel more like a man," admits Nainan, now a comedian based in Manhattan.

Some of us buy stuff for the same reason we get drunk or turn to drugs, according to Karen McCall, author of *Financial Recovery: Developing a Healthy Relationship with Money.*

"It fills a void in our lives," she says. Joe Lowrance, Psy.D., a psychologist who specializes in money issues, adds that money is like a blank screen for many of us. "We can project any dream, wish, or need onto it," he says. "Money is often used in attempts to feel a sense of power, security, or self-worth." Of course, that feeling is only temporary. We have to keep spending to maintain that momentum.

You don't need years of therapy to make progress on fixing your bad money behaviors. Instead, vow to track them closely to find the triggers that set them off, Klontz says. If you're an overspender, he recommends writing down every purchase for at least a month. If you're a bad investor, wait 24 hours before every trade. If you're a workaholic, think about what's happening at 5 p.m. each day when you should be going home. Ask yourself these questions: *What's my mindset right now? What am I thinking? Am I happy doing this, or under stress from it? Do these thoughts sync up with my money scripts?*

Then act on those harder realities, not the imaginary ones you're inclined to follow. Put down that new jacket at the mall. Check out of the office and deal with that "crisis" tomorrow, Klontz says.

BAD MONEY HABIT #5
You're not thinking logically.

Your next step is to formalize your more constructive worldview about money and use that to fend off trouble. Tweak your scripts so they more closely reflect your own values rather than a belief you may have inherited. Example: Your hippie parents taught you that "money isn't important." As a result, you never ask for a raise, and you ignore your finances. That strategy isn't working for your wife and kids, who depend on you. So try this: "Money isn't important, but my family is." Remind yourself of this when you ask your boss for that raise or dive into researching college savings plans. The realization will calm you and help you make smarter decisions, Klontz says.

Changing your behavior is not about distracting yourself; it's about focusing on your most uncomfortable money-related feelings in order to overcome them. George Kinder, a certified financial planner and founder of the life-planning movement, says that accepting these painful feelings will help you separate them from the destructive or obsessive thoughts that attach to them.

BAD MONEY HABIT #6

You're using money to buy stuff, not a better life.

Kinder has a theory about why no investment guide or financial calculator can help us make peace with our cash. When we're children, he says, we're innocent—blissfully ignorant of money or blindly accepting of what we're told about it. Then we experience pain when we realize that we're all enslaved to money in one way or another. As we grow up, we understand money's power and some nuts-and-bolts facts about how it works, and then we use our knowledge to overcome destructive money beliefs that stem from innocence or pain.

You don't have to be a Zen master to understand yourself. Consider this: When guys make mistakes with money, it's usually because they don't really know how they should be spending it, Kinder says. They're bored, lazy, tired, angry, or frenetic—anything but truly purposeful—and their spending reflects that. Purpose is derived from meaning, so what really matters to you?

If you suddenly acquired all the money you needed, what would you do with your life? If you had 5 or 10 years left to live, how would your priorities shift? If you had 24 hours left to live, what would you regret? The answers should give you some idea of how to spend your time—and your money.

Money Talk

No matter how awkward and uncomfortable, these are six conversations you can't afford to blow.

Money. It's a taboo topic in polite company and rarely even broached among friends. At home, conversations about the green stuff can torpedo family harmony. In fact, a recent T. Rowe Price survey discovered that parents find it easier to talk to their kids about drugs and alcohol than about the family finances. Why are we so touchy that way? Confrontations about financial success or failure, or even stray comments about spending habits, can put people on the defensive and make them feel judged.

"In our culture, money and work are closely tied to our identities," says Dalton Conley, Ph.D., dean of social sciences at New York University. "Money conversations have a distinct moral tinge to them, which makes people uncomfortable."

Handled properly, though, financial chats can be liberating, enlightening, and valuable. So we consulted psychologists and financial pros to uncover the ways you can talk about any money matter with confidence—and maybe improve your bottom line along the way.

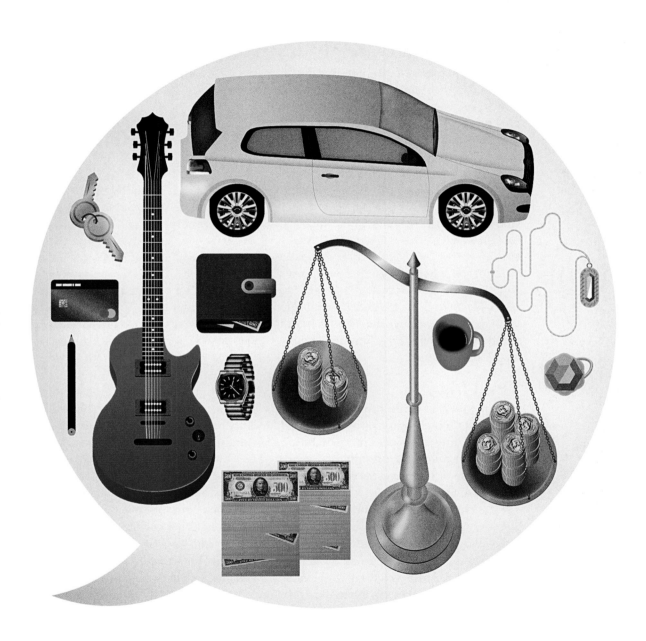

Are your parents financially fit?

There are plenty of legitimate reasons to ask your parents about their finances. Maybe you want to ensure that they have enough to retire comfortably—and to find out how your own money situation could change if they don't. You also want to make sure they don't fall prey to scam artists who target older folks.

But often, in all but the most functional of families, such questions are interpreted as either "What can I expect to inherit?" or "Am I going to have to take care of you when you're in need?" says Jane Isay, the author of *Walking on Eggshells: Navigating the Delicate Relationship between Adult Children and Parents*. It's no wonder those conversations frequently end in stony silence.

Try This

If Mom and Dad think you're angling for control of their resources, you might find yourself facing roadblocks immediately.

"It's very hard for parents to give up their sense of independence," Isay says. "They often lie."

Mention people you know who were glad they could help their parents financially when the need arose. If you think you have reason to worry, ask them how the market has affected their retirement savings. Be wary if they insist they're fine when you suspect they're not or if they make excuses about neglecting certain home or car repairs. Tell them you and your siblings are all doing okay and that you want them to know you're there to help. If your own finances are limited, suggest a certified financial planner (find one at cfp.net), but the most important thing to do is indicate your emotional support, Isay says.

Okay, so how much will you inherit?

This is the mack daddy of all awkward money talks. Just be warned: Unless you've received explicit promises of inheritance, you should not think of your parents' money as your own, says Conley.

"There's a reason a will is read after death," Conley says. "There can be a huge cost to opening the dialogue." Assume from the outset that you'll inherit nothing.

Try This

If you have reason to believe money is coming your way, approach the topic tactfully but clearly, says financial therapist Amanda Clayman, M.S.W., who founded the blog The Good, the Bad, and the Money.

Say to your folks, "Look, I know this is a bit awkward, but over the years you've mentioned that various assets will be left to us. You know I've been putting my financial house in order, and I was hoping you might share some of your intentions."

If this is really about your needing money, ask your parents outright for a loan or gift, Clayman advises. "It's better just to ask than to try to manipulate the inheritance," she says.

Why doesn't your girlfriend chip in on dates?

Even if you're doing fine financially, covering the tab for every date can be irksome. But whatever you do, don't let it reach the point of confrontation.

"This will shut her down and cause an immediate rift in a budding romance," says therapist Sharon O'Neill, Ed.S., author of *A Short Guide to a Happy Marriage*.

Try This

Now's your chance to learn more about what makes her tick. A discussion about who pays and how each person's income and expenses play into the equation can reveal a lot about each other's moral code and ability to negotiate.

BET ON THE HOUSE

With a little work on your part, real estate can still be a great investment. Here's how to renovate your mindset.

Cashing in on houses used to be easy. "When we started investing in 1996 and 1997, we could pick up a property, do very little to it, and make $20,000," says Drew Scott, who with twin brother Jonathan renovates older homes on the HGTV show *Property Brothers*. Flipping homes is tougher in the current economy, but you can make a bundle improving an existing property. When buying a fixer-upper, start by recognizing variables you can't easily change, such as location and major structural elements. Then . . .

Start in the kitchen. "No room is used more than the kitchen is," Jonathan Scott says. "This is why most potential buyers consider the kitchen a make-or-break factor in their decision."

What to invest in: "Instead of laminate countertops for $500, spend about $1,800 and go with granite or quartz," Jonathan says. "It's okay to pair higher-end countertops with store-bought kitchen cabinets."

Use the savings from the cabinets for a commercial-grade stainless-steel range hood with glass accents (about $800), dual wall ovens ($1,500), or a wine fridge ($250). Those little extras can pay off big when it's time to sell. Jonathan recently spent $400 on a wet bar, and that was the feature the buyers said put them over the top. "We've done several new kitchens that cost around $25,000 and increased market value by $35,000," Drew says.

Move on to the basement. Look for high ceilings. Say you can save $20K if you pick a home with low basement ceilings over a similar one with the standard 8-footers. "Go for the more expensive home," Jonathan says. Low ceilings will prevent future buyers from appreciating even a full renovation.

What to invest in: For about $5,000, you can add a media room to a finished basement. The brothers recently mounted a 60" LCD TV ($900) with surround sound ($400), and built cabinets and shelves ($500) to house the electronics. Then they added six leather theater-style seats for $2,600 and a bar for $800. "We've seen buyers pay up to $10,000 extra for a theater room that cost us only half that."

Then renovate the bathrooms. You want a master bath with space for two sinks.

What to invest in: Premade bathroom units with porcelain sinks and a granite top can cost less than $1,000. And, "if space allows," says Jonathan, "consider a separate shower and tub. A shower-whirlpool combo with a glass divider (less than $3,000) can really give the space a spa feel." The Scotts say that a new $15,000 bathroom can easily add $20,000 in home value.

Confrontations about financial success—or failure—can put people on the defensive and make them feel judged.

"These situations can teach you about your girlfriend's values and expectations," O'Neill says.

So point out that while you really enjoy treating her, you both make a good living, so it's only fair to start bouncing the bills back and forth a bit. If she seems uncertain about how to respond, throw out a plan for a future date. You pick up dinner and she springs for the concert tickets, for example.

"If she still balks, don't just assume she's a selfish gold digger," Clayman says. "Sometimes people are brought up with certain financial and gender roles but have never really questioned them. She may need to consciously work through some of her own beliefs before she can meet you halfway."

MONEY CHAT #4
How much money does your wife want to make?

Maybe you're sensing an imbalance: You spend a lot of time focusing on your career,

FUZZY MONEY

Unclear thinking can impact your bottom line. Beware of these four self-delusional money traps.

Don't count on future success. Overestimating your ability to accumulate money in the short term—to pay off that $1,000 stereo in the next few months, say—can lead you deep into trouble, says Kathleen Gurney, Ph.D., the author of *Your Money Personality.* Think in the present. "If you can afford it today, buy it," Gurney says. "If you can't, wait until you have the cash at hand."

Keep collateral costs at the fore. We tend to forget how much those big purchases really cost. That $600-a-month car payment doesn't cover gas, maintenance, or insurance costs. The data plan for that iPhone isn't cheap, either. In fact, it's safe to assume that costs will be 50 to 100 percent higher than projected for many items we spend big on, says Frank Murtha, Ph.D., coauthor of *MarketPsych.*

Check that ego. Don't save weeds and cut flowers: Holding on to a stock that's down 15 percent and hoping it'll bounce back, and then selling profitable winners to supplement that loss, just leaves you with a sinking portfolio, says Murtha. Put rules in place: If a stock drops 10 percent, you're out. "You think, 'If I loved it at 50, I'll love it at 40, and I'll love it at 20,' and so on. By the time you stop loving it, it's too late."

Stop confusing luck with skill. A rising stock in a booming market doesn't make you a talented investor. If you bought the stocks without understanding the numbers, you're reinforcing a habit that will eventually bring down your entire portfolio. Use television shows like *Mad Money* to explore stocks, but don't ever buy on impulse, says Murtha.

but she doesn't. Or the opposite: She's the hard charger while you're more blasé. In either case, bringing up the topic of perceived motivational disparities can put people on the defensive. "Never start a discussion from a negative stance," says O'Neill.

Try This

Flip the conversation around to make it about her goals, talents, and aspirations.

"Make it safe for her to explore why she may not be professionally ambitious," Clayman says. "Is she afraid of failure? Does she feel she's doing too much at home to have the bandwidth to take on more professionally?"

Or if she seems too focused on her career, ask what she wants her life to be like over the long haul—how she wants to enjoy herself and the relationship. Say, "I don't want your goals to become lost. They are just as important as mine. And if you really are fine with where your career is, let's talk about a way to make it work for both of us." Shifting the focus from your careers to your lives together can help both of you approach the problem from a different perspective.

Can your buddy really afford that new car?

Short answer: It's none of your business. That said, friends look out for each other, and seeing a buddy potentially overextend himself financially can be worrisome.

"Men can be very protective of their male friends and usually want to see them succeed, especially when it comes to material gain," says Geoffrey Greif, D.S.W., a professor of social work at the University of Maryland and the author of *Buddy System: Understanding Male Friendships*. But bringing up the subject of financial wherewithal can hurt your pal's ego.

"Men often see their income as a measure of their self-worth," Greif explains. "A guy who's overspending may be uncomfortable with some aspect of himself and need reassurance, so he may be looking for material ways to build himself up."

Try This

First, keep in mind that you never know where people find their money, Greif says. Maybe your friend's parents helped take a bite out of his bill for that new car or vacation in Cancun. Or maybe he just acts as if he's stretched thin most of the time when in reality he's a big saver.

Use the purchase as an opportunity to broach the subject discreetly. Start by suggesting that you might benefit from his savvy: "Wow. Nice ride. Did you work any magic on the sales guy? I'd love to get some of this action."

Let him lead the conversation from there. He might level with you about the financial hit he's taking, and you could offer up a similar story of your own—about how, for example, a financial planner helped you deal smartly with a splurge and keep all your other bills paid at the same time. If he clams up, back off—fast—and just enjoy the ride.

Does your kid really need that pricey prom dress or electric guitar?

No, she doesn't—and being this blunt is actually the correct strategy here.

"We tend not to be direct about economic matters with teenagers, even though they're old enough to understand," says Jean Twenge, Ph.D., a professor of psychology at San Diego State University and the author of *Generation Me*.

Try This

While you manage to still remain true to your financial reality and money values, you can spin the problem quite differently. Tell your daughter that since the expensive item is out of your reach, she now has the tremendous opportunity to be creative and stand out from the crowd.

"Teenagers today have been raised with a very strong emphasis on being special and not caring what others think of them. This is language that's familiar and a message that might resonate," Twenge explains.

So suggest that your daughter shop around for a cool vintage prom dress or a funky, unique six-string.

If your teenager digs in her heels, Twenge recommends, give her the long view. Say that if you spend money on this now, there won't be enough for college later. Then tell her to go out and find a job!

DO IT YOURSELF?

Some projects don't always need a contractor. Jonathan Scott suggests one you can tackle on your own—and one you shouldn't.

HARDWOOD/LAMINATE FLOORING

Do it yourself, and consider a single-board laminate product. Some new varieties of sturdy single-board laminate are indistinguishable from engineered hardwood and are a breeze to install.

Cost: Laminate sells for $1.50 to $2.50 a square foot. In a 1,000-square-foot space, that translates to a total savings of about $3,000 over professionally installed hardwood floors.

Payoff: A $2,000 investment adds $5,000 in home value.

CARPETING

Hire help! Carpet is quick and cheap for pros to install, and they'll make it look right. You'd have to buy special tools, and I guarantee you don't know how much the carpet stretches—the carpet would either bind or come up short at the far end of a long room.

Cost: Decent-quality carpet is $2 to $2.50 a square foot, and most big-box stores offer whole-house installation deals for $250 or less.

Payoff: You'll recoup your costs, and the place will sell faster without the gross old carpet.

MONEY TIPS FROM THOSE WHO KNOW

We asked three fiscal wizards to tell us the best financial advice they ever received. Now their mentors are yours, too.

"The best finance advice I ever received came from the cable and telecom executive Bruno Claude, with whom I worked in Europe and the United States. His advice to me, at age 22: Have passion for what you do, save much of your salary, ignore your potential bonus, and diversify your portfolio—except in the areas you know better than most others and which you can directly control."

—Christopher Winfrey,
EVP and CPO, Charter Communications

"My grandfather always kept a piece of graph paper in his pocket with the daily closing prices of about 50 stocks he owned. He'd pull out that paper, show it to me, and have me choose a company to analyze. We'd then look at the company's numbers. I learned two things from this. First, there is no substitute for rigorous analysis. Second, never invest in a business you don't understand. Good advice from a good man."

—Spencer Rascoff,
CEO, Zillow

"When I was 14, I had a friend who lived with his grandfather, a very successful man named Louis Tepfer. He'd started 17 different companies, from chicken farms to software development. I once asked him what his secret was. He said, 'You need a willingness to fail and a willingness to keep trying and keep learning.' Like him, I've had a lot of failures, but if it weren't for them, I would not have achieved the success I have."

—Chris Friedland,
CEO, Build.com

The Financial Crisis Survival Plan

You can build wealth in troubled times. Here, the smartest and bravest minds in finance tell us how to weather the unpredictable.

If this roller-coaster economy has you feeling stressed and confused, you're not alone. Mixed messages are coming from every corner. The government has been trying to encourage us to spend and borrow by keeping interest rates low. The finance industry keeps urging those of us with still-decent credit to buy houses, apply for new credit cards, and try out hot new investments. But we've been burned before. Why should we put money on the line when jobs are still insecure and markets are about as stable as the Washington Monument in a 5.8 temblor?

When the financial deck seems stacked against the common guy, it's hard to know who to trust. So we turned to some of the few people who saw the financial crisis of 2008 coming. This elite cadre of traders, economists, and money managers had the courage to speak out about the building storm, earning the derision of their peers and clients—until history proved them right. We asked this crew how to survive and thrive through the next crisis. They argued the importance of saving heavily, keeping debt low, and investing in your own career—but beyond those basics, their

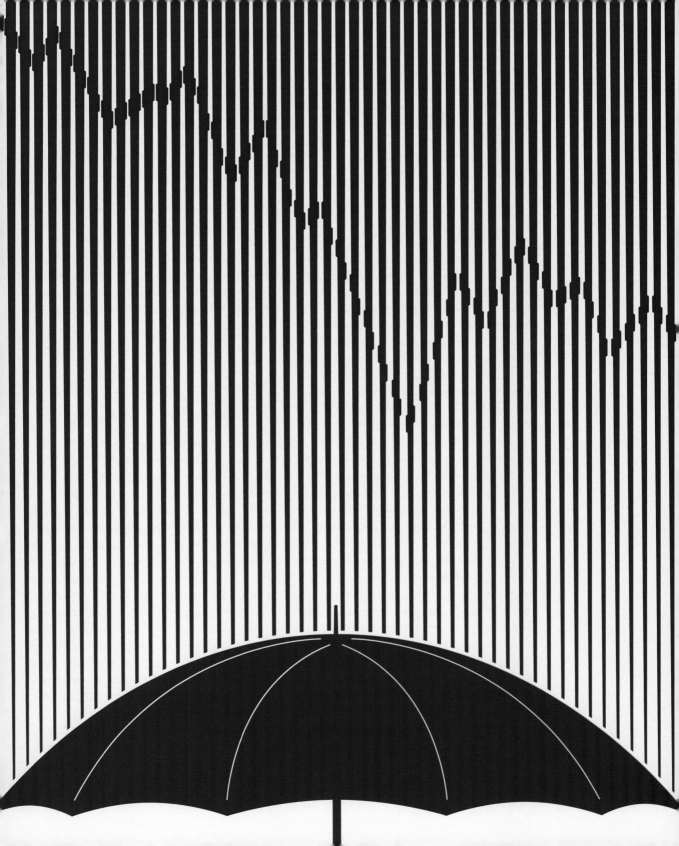

views diverged radically and often contradicted. Some of their prescriptions are unorthodox and unproved, and just because these experts were right once doesn't mean they know what's right for you. On the other hand, whose advice are you taking now?

Don't Lose Hope

It's only natural to believe that the future will look a lot like the past. Just as many of us had assumed that the most recent boom would last forever, we might also assume that today's bust will persist as well. Finance professor Frank Partnoy, of the University of San Diego school of law, who called out Wall Street excess, wants to avoid that mistake. Partnoy, the author of *F.I.A.S.C.O.: Blood in the Water on Wall Street,* was a successful Wall Street trader who turned his back on his former colleagues to warn that their excesses would lead to catastrophe. He doesn't think Washington's reforms have done enough to rein in those excesses, but he has enough faith in America's economy to believe it can ride out the busts.

Take the long view. Partnoy recommends a long-term strategy for retirement. Pick out about a dozen companies that sell products you know and understand and research them. You'll still be taking risks, but at least you'll understand those risks. Buy the stocks and then forget about them. Research shows that investors tend to buy stocks when the prices are high and sell them when they're low. That's the fastest way to lose money in the market.

"You need to resist the short-term temptation to buy and sell based on what's hot and what's not," Partnoy says.

Have some faith. Unlike other advisors, Partnoy thinks stocks are a good buy for the long run. He arrived at that perspective by studying history—particularly the Great Depression, when dire predictions about the future were rampant.

"Over the long run, our economy grows," Partnoy says. "People become better off, and technology improves our lives. If you come out of the blogs and news feeds and look at the arc of history, it's a story of human beings getting better over time. So stay optimistic."

Stay in Crisis Mode—Permanently

In 2006, while the U.S. economy was still a raging bull, money manager Robert Wiedemer and his brother David, an economist, predicted the housing crash, the stock crash, the credit crunch, and the recession. Today Wiedemer believes that the measly "recovery" of the past couple of years is just a bump on the way down to the dollar's collapse and high inflation caused by government debt. Wiedemer, coauthor of *Aftershock: Protect Yourself and Profit in the Next Global Financial Meltdown,* says the government's money policies will prop up the economy for a year or two. After that, and unlike Partnoy, he recommends getting out—not only from stocks but from bonds as well.

Go for gold. Wiedemer likes gold and historically stable currencies like the

Swiss franc, the Canadian dollar, and the Japanese yen. It's easy today for the average investor to buy all these through exchange-traded funds, or ETFs. Most financial planners consider both gold and currency to be very high-risk investments, but Wiedemer is unapologetic: "The days of comfortable investing are over," he says. "You're trying to make money in a crisis."

Be protective. If your focus is on protecting what you have, then you might want to keep most of your money in cash and eventually move into Treasury Inflation-Protected Securities (TIPS). Wiedemer also believes we're stuck in a long-term recession that will endanger many industries. Luxury goods will suffer as the rich finally get poorer, and a slowing economy will cripple companies that make autos and other big-ticket items. So he suggests aiming your career at businesses that produce basic necessities, like medical care, food, repair and maintenance, education, and utilities.

Focus on Your Cash Flow

Janet Briaud, president of Briaud Financial Advisors, is one of the small coterie of investment experts who had the foresight to move their clients' money out of stocks in time to avoid both the dotcom crash and the financial crisis. While most financial planners advise against "timing the market," she suggests a simple rule: Wait until prices are so low that your friends say they'd never consider buying stocks again, and then buy heavily.

Strive for balance. If you're just starting out in your career, don't try too hard to make money in the markets, Briaud says. Instead, focus on earning more, saving heavily—as much as 20 percent of what you earn—and paying off debt. Are you carrying a credit-card balance at 16 percent? Paying it down is like getting a 16 percent risk-free return on your money.

"If I could make 16 percent, I'd do it in a New York minute," Briaud says. If you have "emergency" cash reserves in your bank account but also a credit-card balance, Briaud even suggests draining the cash from your reserve account to pay it off. After all, if emergency strikes, you can still use your cards. (Just be aware that you can't pay for everything with a credit card.)

Be Ready for Disaster

A statistical wizard and distinguished professor of risk engineering at the Polytechnic Institute of New York University, Nassim Nicholas Taleb, Ph.D., predicted the Black Monday stock market crash of 1987. Then came his mega-selling *The Black Swan: The Impact of the Highly Improbable* in 2007. Taleb says our complex financial system is vulnerable to earthshaking yet unpredictable events—his Black Swans. He argues that we can't predict anything but unpredictability. The wise man can only "invest in preparedness."

Stay out of the middle of the road. Taleb suggests putting virtually all your nest egg in safe investments that will stay just ahead of inflation—like TIPS or CDs.

Then put up to 20 percent of your savings into high-risk, high-reward investments, such as venture capital firms or start-ups in risky areas such as biotech or clean energy. The low-risk side protects most of your money from Black Swans. The high-risk side exposes you to those that might pay off.

Be ready for a storm. Have cash in the bank—"a lot more than you think you need," Taleb says. Also maintain high deductibles on your insurance, and be wary of debt. "The more debt you have, the more precise you have to be about your future income," Taleb says.

Make Yourself Valuable

In 2005, Raghuram Rajan, an economist at the University of Chicago Booth School of Business, presented a paper that predicted the exact course of the financial crisis we're dealing with now. Luminaries in the field protested angrily, but time proved him right. Then his book *Fault Lines: How Hidden Fractures Still Threaten the World Economy* gave an unexpected reason for the calamity long before protestors began camping out on Wall Street: He identified our key problem as the growing gap between the haves and the have-nots.

The quest for the American dream initially played out in the housing market— the finance industry encouraged homeowners to take out dicey home loans—and now it's happening with education. People who are out of work or desperate for advancement are being lured into for-profit career schools by recruiters promising the moon. Students at these schools take on 45 to 80 percent more debt than students at public or nonprofit private schools. Their graduation rates are only a third as high, and they're four times more likely to default on their student loans. Your income is your most valuable asset, so your financial planning should revolve around your career and your ability to keep working no matter what happens to your investments. Here are three key imperatives in that vein.

Stay vigilant. Keep your antenna up about which skills will be in demand 5 or 10 years down the road. "It doesn't mean you have to go to college," Rajan says. "Just look for assignments that can move you into areas where you'd have a future." Find people who seem successful and secure doing what you'd like to do, and find out how they got there. They'll be flattered you asked, and you'll have an honest answer about whether school is the best route.

Stay mobile. The labor market is much stronger in some parts of the country than in others. Finding the best jobs might require moving around. Home prices may seem appealing these days, but beware: The economics of home ownership can lock you in place for years.

Stay humble. Don't let pride stand in the way of your financial future. Does tech still seem geeky to you? Nursing too girlie? Well, nothing wilts manhood like chronic joblessness, and nothing revives it like being the financial rock of your family.

"Nursing may not seem like a macho job, but compared with an autoworker, a nurse has many more years of well-paid employment, especially one who develops specialties," Rajan says. "The trick is to develop skills that are in demand but be able to switch if your skills become oversupplied."

Steer Your Money Away from Big Banks

While he was chief economist at the International Monetary Fund, Simon Johnson saw the recession coming early. His book, *13 Bankers: The Wall Street Takeover and the Next Financial Meltdown*, describes exactly how a cabal of big banks gambled with our money, wrecked the economy, and then accepted huge taxpayer bailouts, all the while paying out gigantic bonuses and fighting financial reform. Johnson, a professor of entrepreneurship at the MIT Sloan School of Management, thinks the economy will be at risk as long as the megabanks are in charge. In the meantime, he has a suggestion: Take your money out of those banks.

Go small. Johnson advocates pulling your loot out if it's in one of the six biggest banks: Bank of America, JPMorgan Chase & Co., Citigroup, Wells Fargo, Goldman Sachs, and Morgan Stanley. Smaller banks and credit unions consistently garner better customer satisfaction ratings, and they care for their customers when it counts; they've proven much more likely than the big banks to negotiate with homeowners at risk of foreclosure. Take an especially good look at credit unions: Independent research confirms that these member-owned not-for-profit organizations offer lower fees as well as consistently lower interest rates on loans.

BE CREATIVE

We want you to think outside the box—and in this case, the box is a coffin. Creative men live longer, according to a study from Purdue University. For every $1\frac{1}{2}$-point increase in a man's score on a 9-point creativity scale, his chance of dying in the next 18 years fell by 12 percent. Creative men might be better able to cope with stress and its harmful effects, the researchers say.

UPGRADE YOUR MEMORY

Stretch your body and your brain: Practicing yoga might improve your memory, a study from Brazil found. Men who added twice-weekly yoga sessions to their workouts for 6 months did better on memory tests than men assigned to other forms of exercise. Yoga might reduce levels of cortisol, a stress hormone that can impair memory when elevated, says study author Regina Silva, Ph.D. Visit MensHealth.com/yoga to find a class.

HAVE A POWER LUNCH

Lunch at your desk might not be the best career move. New research from Sweden reveals that exercising during office hours can increase your productivity. Employees who exercised $2\frac{1}{2}$ hours a week during work hours reported accomplishing more at the office than those who didn't exercise on the job. One theory: Exercise

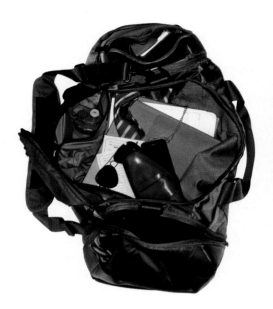

boosts oxygen consumption, which may help improve concentration and problem-solving ability. Can't make it to a gym? Take a walk during lunch or schedule walking meetings.

Plus, employees who exercised at work also required fewer sick days.

DECOMPRESS

Even if you're chained to a desk, you can still shift your mindset. Fifteen minutes of chair-based yoga can curb work stress, according to an Australian study. When people performed a series of seated yoga poses, their stress levels fell. The slow, steady breathing in yoga can cut tension by reducing sympathetic nervous system activity, says study author Bobby Cheema, Ph.D. Clasp your hands, lift your arms above your head, and slowly bend to each side for 30 seconds.

EAT SMARTER

Can smart eating make you wise? Choline might improve your mental performance, research in the *American Journal of Clinical Nutrition* reveals. People in the study who ate more of this nutrient did better on cognitive tests than those who took in less. Dietary choline may aid production of the essential neurotransmitter acetylcholine. The Institute of Medicine recommends 550 milligrams of choline a day for men.

This brain-benefiting nutrient is found in high amounts in beef liver and poultry giblets—but see the chart below for some more-appetizing options, according to the USDA.

AVOID FAT HEAT

The closer science looks at trans fats, the worse they seem to be. Researchers at Oregon Health & Science University found that people with higher blood levels of trans fats had more problems with memory and cognition. Trans fats might displace healthy fatty acids in the brain's neurons. Nix products that contain partially hydrogenated vegetable oils and eat more vegetables, fish, nuts, beans, and citrus fruit, all of which foster brainpower.

LEAK BUT DON'T TOUCH

Public restrooms can be nauseating—literally. Scientists at the University of Colorado found that a typical lavatory harbors 19 phyla of bacteria. While many are harmless, each family has potentially bad bugs, says study author Gilberto Flores, Ph.D. So wash your hands and use a hand sanitizer.

Here are some particularly bad bugs.

- *Propionibacterium acnes,* which causes acne and eye infections

- *Streptococcus pyogenes,* the culprit behind strep throat

- *Staphylococcus aureus,* which can leave you with a skin infection

- *Clostridium tetani,* responsible for tetanus

FOOD	CHOLINE CONTENT (MILLIGRAMS)
½ fillet sockeye salmon (5½ ounces)	175
1 large hard-boiled egg	147
3 oz braised veal (top round)	120
½ fillet halibut (5 ounces)	119
1 cup roast turkey (5 ounces)	116
3 oz braised beef bottom round	111
1 cup canned blue crabmeat	109

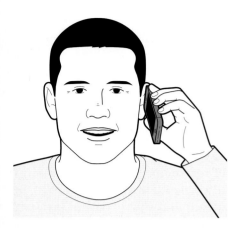 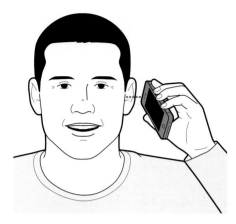

Q How can I make my smartphone safer?

A: Smart call to ask. Although the research is still divided over the cancer risk posed by cellphones, you're better off assuming that there's some danger.

In 20 years we might view cellphones much as we currently view asbestos, says Devra Davis, Ph.D., M.P.H., the author of *Disconnect: The Truth about Cell Phone Radiation*. Use these tips to protect your brain—and the rest of your body—from these wireless worst-case scenarios.

THREAT TO YOUR BRAIN AND SALIVARY GLANDS: cancer
The solution: Use a headset or speakerphone, or at least hold the phone farther than 2 inches from your ear (and your brain). Be especially careful in your car: Each time your phone's signal jumps from one cell antenna to another it goes to max power, says Davis.

THREATS TO YOUR EYES: Eyestrain, headache
The solution: "Hold the phone 16 inches or farther from your eyes," says Mark Rosenfield, O.D., Ph.D., a professor of optometry at SUNY. Take a break and look away for a few seconds every 2 to 3 minutes.

THREATS TO YOUR SWIMMERS: lowered sperm count, DNA damage
The solution: Keep your cellphone out of your pants pocket, where radiation can easily reach your testicles, says Davis.

THREAT TO YOUR SLEEP: disturbed sleep
The solution: "Unplug 2 hours before bedtime to reduce the stress that comes from always being 'on,' " says Sara Thomee, Ph.D., a researcher who studies cellphones and sleep.

Q **After I kept getting spam texts on my phone, I called my provider. The rep said they couldn't do anything about it. Who can?**

A: You can. In 2003, Congress passed a law to curb spam. Assuming the incoming texts are "commercial messages" trying to sell you something, you can file a complaint with the Federal Communications Commission to try to shut the sender down. This would not necessarily include follow-ups on products you bought or with companies you've had contact with. But if it's "cold spamming," then do us all a favor and freeze them out.

Q **Who has a right to know my Social Security number?**

A: The SSN has come to be a crucial piece of personal I.D., though it was never intended for that. You can refuse to provide it, but you risk having a business, landlord, or bank turn you away. Expect to be asked for it for financial transactions, tax returns, background checks, government benefits, and license applications, to name a few. Sure, withhold it if you can—but you might have little choice.

Q **I wake up in the middle of the night worrying about work, which makes me tired the next day. Help!**

A: Warning: This is going to sound like psychotherapy. You need to establish a "worry window" during the day, says Todd Farchione, Ph.D., director of the intensive treatment program at Boston University's center for anxiety and related disorders. "To stay calm throughout the day, which can make you less likely to wake up in a panic at night, schedule 15 minutes in the afternoon or early evening (just not right before bed) to be your worry window. Whenever a worry pops up throughout the day, promise yourself that you'll deal with it, but only during this preassigned time. This can keep you focused through the day."

When it's time to look at your worries, Farchione recommends running through each worry with these questions: How likely is it that this fill-in-the-blank catastrophe will happen? (You can use only facts, not your feelings, as evidence.) What would you do if it did happen? By applying a dose of objective reality to both the perceived danger and the possible consequences, you'll find the calm and perspective you need for a good night's rest, says Farchione. If you do wake up during the night, jot down your worries on a piece of paper so you won't forget what you need to address the next day.

Q **My boss demanded that I postpone my back surgery until I finish a big project. Can an employer make a request like this?**

A: If your company employs 50 or more people and you have worked there for at least a year, then it must provide you with up to 12 weeks of medical leave or family leave a year without the threat of losing your job. The company can demand a doctor's note to let you go and even to have you return, but it can't just refuse your request. If you want to work there again, however, be as accommodating as possible while making it clear you need the time off.

Q **I'm Facebook friends with some colleagues. Am I protected from being fired for anything they might write there about our boss?**

A: Probably not. Most employees can be fired for any reason unrelated to age, race, gender, and so forth. Fireable offenses include trashing your boss (or even colleagues) on Facebook. But recent rulings from the National Labor Relations Board suggest that complaining in social media forums about workplace conditions or union activities is probably protected speech. So if you must vent, focus on general office conditions, not your boss.

Q **What's a reasonable weekly allowance for my 10-year-old son? I'd like him to learn a lesson with the money I give him.**

A: Maybe 5 or 6 bucks. That assumes you started at $1 a week in kindergarten and increased a buck a year from there. But it also depends on what the money is for. My philosophy on allowances is simple (and time-tested by my two teenagers): You give them enough to pay for a few things that you have explained, up front, that you will no longer be paying for. Maybe that list includes the school store, iTunes downloads, bake sales. When they spend it all, you don't bail them out. That's how they learn to budget.

Q **I'm traveling to Europe. How can I limit the exchange-rate hit?**

A: Exchange at your local bank to avoid pricey airport kiosks. Once overseas, exchange at an ATM (preferably from your bank, to minimize transaction fees). The goal: Make fewer exchanges for larger amounts, but take only what you need. Credit cards are often better bets abroad. Some (including all Capital One cards) don't charge a foreign transaction fee.

Q My bank charges a fee anytime I use a debit card. Is that even legal?

A: Unfortunately, yes. The Federal Reserve recently tried to limit the fees that banks can charge merchants each time a customer uses a debit card for a purchase. Now the banks want to recoup those dollars in the form of higher fees on checking accounts that use debit cards. So while retailers might be charging less, you may be paying more.

Q What's the best strategy for letting go of anger?

A: Stop brooding: Australian researchers found that angry people reported being able to chill out when they positively reappraised the event that set them off instead of dwelling on the negative aspects.

"When you're angry, think about what you can learn from the episode," says study author Michelle Moulds, Ph.D.

Q What quality will make me a better supervisor at work?

A: Humility.

Humble bosses rule. They're more effective and better liked, according to new research in the *Academy of Management Journal*. Study author Bradley Owens, Ph.D., cites these keys to leading with humility: Admit your mistakes, spotlight your employees' strengths, and model teachability—in other words, show how you're continuing to learn and grow.

PART 6

Live Longer, Live Better

Your Stress—Smashed

It's no secret that stress beats up your body. But is the way you deal helping you—or hurting you?

You know you should take a few deep breaths when you feel stressed. Instead you inhale a doughnut (or five). Strange? Not at all. Your strained brain craves instant gratification, often in the form of a quick fix like food or alcohol, says James Herman, Ph.D., a neuroscientist at the University of Cincinnati. "These things activate reward pathways while quieting the amygdala—the emotional, over-wrought area of your brain."

The trouble with the Krispy Kreme cure—besides the inevitable risk of obesity and the powdered sugar on your neckties—is that it's really just a stress Band-Aid. In the long term, you might feel more mentally steamrolled than ever.

And when your psyche suffers, so does your body. In fact, in a new Oregon State University study, researchers found that chronically stressed middle-aged men were almost 50 percent more likely to die during an 18-year period than other men who experienced fewer stressful events. Which of these guys do you want to be?

Good choice. Now follow this plan for replacing your current so-called coping strategies with techniques that'll feel like a shiatsu massage for your mind.

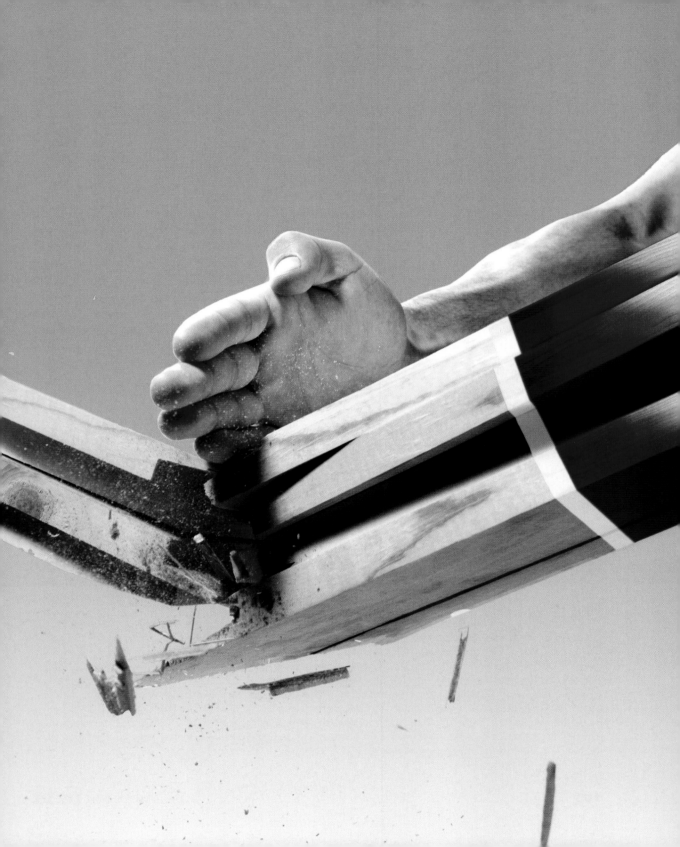

COPING STRATEGY #1
Down a Dessert.

There's a reason you equate sugar with serenity. When you consume the sweet stuff, your prefrontal cortex, a part of your brain that helps control emotions, is activated, says Herman. The danger of a sugar binge: Men with higher anxiety are also more likely to have elevated glucose levels, according to scientists in Japan. In fact, the American Diabetes Association warns that long-term stress might push your blood-sugar levels into the diabetic range if they're already higher than normal.

DO THIS INSTEAD
Savor a small portion of ice cream.

The stress-busting benefits of dessert are due more to the flavor than the fat and calories, says Herman. "High-calorie foods often taste better, but calories aren't necessary for food's effects on stress." Buy a single-serve treat and take half an hour to eat it. Savoring the flavor can extend the calming effect.

COPING STRATEGY #2
Pour a Drink.

After a few shots of Jack, the office jackass is the last person on your mind. When alcohol enters your bloodstream, it seems to activate reward pathways for temporary relief. Ultimately, though, it may intensify your depression, says William Pollack, Ph.D., a *Men's Health* mental health advisor. In a University of Chicago study, stressed-out men injected with alcohol felt anxious longer than guys in a placebo group. Booze might disrupt your body's calming process, prolonging the mental misery.

DO THIS INSTEAD
Self-medicate with music.

A study in the journal *Nature Neuroscience* found that listening to favorite tunes or anticipating a certain point in a song

CAN STRESS SABOTAGE YOUR WORKOUT?

It's tough to lift if you're carrying a mental load. From now on, do a stress check before you hit the weight room. A 2011 study published in the *European Journal of Applied Physiology* found that people who lifted weights while mentally stressed became fatigued more quickly and experienced greater strength declines than they did when they were worry-free.

"When you're stressed, your muscles are at a higher level of arousal and your heart rate is elevated," explains study author Ranjana Mehta, Ph.D. That means your body is already on its way to wearing out before you've even completed your first set. The fix? Work out in the morning, when you're naturally less stressed. Or if you rely on evening lifting to decompress, extend your warmup. Low-intensity exercise can help switch off the fight-or-flight response that saps your strength, says Mehta.

can cause a pleasurable flood of dopamine. Listen to a few songs in a row several times a day.

"These doses of dopamine can lower your stress, removing the trigger that causes you to seek alcohol," says Edward Roth, MT-BC, a professor of music therapy at Western Michigan University.

DEBUG YOUR BRAIN

Technology can fry your mind. Here's how to stay connected without powering down your productivity.

Adults spend about 8½ hours a day on the Internet, watching video, or using mobile gadgets, according to estimates from eMarketer. "The problem is that we get glued to our devices and forget we have a life offline," says Gary Small, M.D., a professor of psychiatry and biobehavioral sciences at UCLA. Don't let technology rule your life. Here's how to know if it's gone too far.

The Problem:
CHRONIC MULTITASKING

You multitask to accomplish more in less time, right? Yet an experiment at Stanford University revealed that heavy media multitaskers were less efficient than people who multitasked less often. They also had difficulty ignoring irrelevant information.

"We become faster but also sloppier," Dr. Small says. Research also suggests that chronic stress from multitasking can make your brain's memory center more vulnerable to damage.

The solution: Live now.

Don't snap a photo of every meal, or tweet about that concert while it's happening.

"Consider enjoying a seminal experience fully before posting about it," says Daniel Sieberg, author of *The Digital Diet*. "There's always time to update your social network, but life is worth living in the moment first." Dr. Small suggests designating e-mail time in the morning so you don't sweat it all day.

The Problem:
DIMINISHED SOCIAL SKILLS

The tech-addled brain "drifts away from fundamental social skills, such as reading facial expressions during conversation or grasping the emotional context of a subtle gesture," Dr. Small writes in his book *iBrain*.

The solution: Find quiet.

In *iBrain*, Dr. Small advises creating a quiet environment, even if it's only temporary, to ease anxiety. That might mean silencing gadgets, disabling alerts and alarms, or instituting a no-phone zone. "No charging the smartphone in the bedroom," Sieberg says. "Keep the room a sanctuary and you might even aid intimacy."

The Problem:
"TECHNO-BRAIN BURNOUT"

People who work online for several hours nonstop report feeling spaced-out, fatigued, irritable, and distracted. Dr. Small calls this digital fog "techno-brain burnout." It causes your brain to alert your adrenal glands to secrete the stress hormones cortisol and adrenaline. Over time, this process can impair cognition and alter the neural circuitry in brain regions that control thought and mood.

The solution: Fall asleep.

In an experiment at Harvard, Sara Mednick, Ph.D., and her colleagues were able to reduce the negative impact of techno-brain burnout in volunteers by adding variety to mental tasks and by introducing strategic power naps—a reminder that "sleep mode" has advantages for human beings, too.

COPING STRATEGY #3
Play *Call of Duty* All Night.

The lure of a record-breaking kill/death ratio isn't the only thing keeping you up till 3 a.m. Stanford researchers found that playing video games stimulates the brain's mesocorticolimbic system, a key reward region. And the more you win, the more the area lights up.

The downside: Most video games are sedentary and mimic the competitiveness of a stressful job, which might negate any brain benefits, says Michael Addis, Ph.D., a psychology professor at Clark University.

DO THIS INSTEAD
Build a fence.

Learn to braise meat. Practice the ukulele. Activities that give you a sense of mastery can also activate the mesocorticolimbic system, deploying a rush of dopamine. Plus, as you practice your new skill, you enter a healthy psychological state known as flow.

"You lose track of time and are completely immersed in what you're doing," says Addis. "It's incredibly relaxing to the mind."

COPING STRATEGY #4
Drive too Fast.

Why do guys love Vegas? Or consider cliff jumping a worthy pastime? The same reason they speed: Risk taking produces a surge of endorphins, which numb pain, says Cleveland Clinic psychologist Michael McKee, Ph.D. But if you chase those thrills while you're stressed, they could kill you. Your judgment tends to become clouded,

ARE YOU TECH-ADDICTED?

Find out with this self-assessment from *iBrain*, by Gary Small, M.D., and Gigi Vorgan. Answer each question and give yourself a score from 1 to 7 based on this scale. Then add up your answers.

1-2: Usually   **3-5**: Sometimes   **6-7**: Rarely

Do you snap at people when they interrupt you while you're online or using a mobile device?

Do you use technology to escape uncomfortable feelings or situations in your life?

Does the time you spend engaged in tech-related activities interfere with your work or social life?

Are you defensive or secretive about your computer gaming or other tech-based activities?

Do people complain about the time you spend on the Internet or using other technology?

SCORING

Above 25: You are not a tech addict.

15 to 25: You show addictive tendencies.

Below 15: You just might be hooked.

so it's harder to take calculated risks, explains Addis. "You're more likely to put yourself in unnecessary danger."

Hightail it to the gym.

But don't default to your regular workout. If you're bored with your routine, you might not experience the normal post-gym endorphin rush, making exercise less effective as a stress fighter than it could be, says Addis. So try something new: Sign up for a martial arts class, check out an indoor rock-climbing center, or go mountain biking. These activities combine physical exertion with a bit of benign risk taking.

COPING STRATEGY #5
Bury Yourself in Work.

It's tempting to battle the stress of a massive workload by immersing yourself until it's done. Don't do it. "Concentration and productivity suffer when your brain doesn't have a chance to unwind, relax, and reset," says McKee. And your work performance may not be the only thing to suffer. In a new British study, people who worked 11 or more hours a day were nearly 70 percent more likely to develop heart disease over a 12-year period than those who worked 7- to 8-hour days.

DO THIS INSTEAD
Take a 60-second vacation.

Each hour, spend a minute perusing a funny blog. (We like passiveaggressivenotes.com.) Periodic breaks help you process and absorb new information, increasing your efficiency, says McKee. During your hiatus, take 10-second breaths—inhale 4 seconds, exhale 6—to bolster your heart's ability to recover from stress.

COPING STRATEGY #6
Hibernate in Your Cave.

If stress makes you want to retreat and hole up at home, here's why: Research shows that men generally favor the fight-or-flight stress response, whereas women are more likely to "tend and befriend" when they feel stressed. Which way is better? A 2009 British study linked social isolation with a more prolonged spike in heart-straining systolic blood pressure after a stressful event, and higher stress-hormone output throughout the day.

DO THIS INSTEAD
Watch the game with your buddies.

And don't spend halftime bitching about your boss. Venting can actually be counterproductive; with men, it often turns into a stress-inducing "who has it worse" showdown, says Addis. Besides, the social aspect alone is enough to activate your brain's GABA receptors, which control fear and anxiety, in turn triggering feelings of calm and satisfaction, says Pollack.

Health Saboteurs

You're doing it wrong! Here are 11 ways you might be sabotaging your health—when you think you're saving it.

Some tasks in life are so mind-numbingly simple that you don't even think twice about them. You're essentially on autopilot, feet up in the cockpit, content in the knowledge that you'd have to try to screw these things up.

Or would you? What if you've actually been botching things you thought you had mastered long ago? Take flossing: Couldn't be easier, right? You're probably doing it wrong. And if you aren't, well, then we'll bet you don't know how to dry your hands.

Or apply sunscreen. Or slip on a condom. Yes, we mean stuff that simple.

The point is not to make you feel stupid but to help you do something smart. In other words, we want to help you take hold of the controls before you crash.

"Making small corrections to the things you're already doing can have a major impact on your overall health," explains Ted Epperly, M.D., the *Men's Health* family medicine advisor. Now about that condom . . .

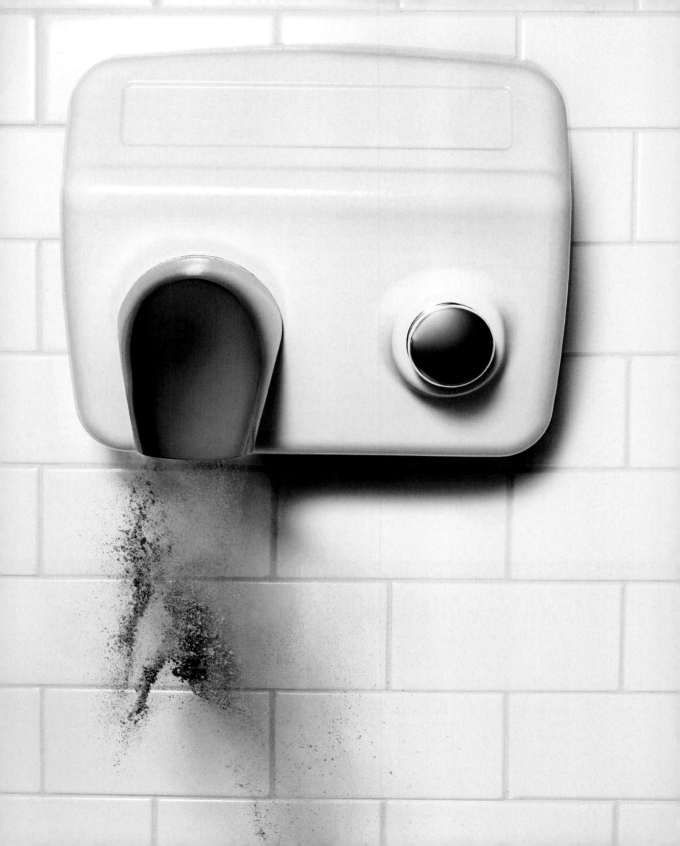

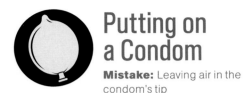

Putting on a Condom

Mistake: Leaving air in the condom's tip

The banana-condom demos clearly aren't cutting it. According to a 2012 Kinsey Institute review, men tend to make one of two condom mistakes: They either forget to leave space for their semen to collect at the condom's tip, or if they do leave a little room in their rubber, they fail to squeeze out the air. Both of these boners can increase your risk of breakage. So what's the proper technique for gloving up?

"To leave space and remove the air, use your thumb and forefinger to squeeze the tip as you're rolling the condom down all the way to the base of your penis," says study author Robin Milhausen, Ph.D.

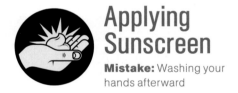

Applying Sunscreen

Mistake: Washing your hands afterward

This is one time you don't want to wash your hands. If you suds up after slathering on sunscreen, you leave a crucial surface exposed to harmful UV rays.

"I frequently see accelerated aging on the hands because people forget to apply sunscreen there," says Northwestern University dermatologist Amy Derick, M.D. Apply about as much sunscreen to your hands as you would if you were moisturizing with lotion—and don't forget your nails. Yes, they're dead cells, but the tissue underneath is active and susceptible to melanoma and other skin cancers, the Skin Cancer Foundation warns.

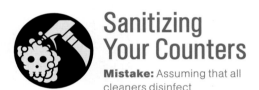

Sanitizing Your Counters

Mistake: Assuming that all cleaners disinfect

That blue stuff you spray on your windows might be great on glass, but it's a dud as a disinfectant. Scan the label before you buy: Only cleaners labeled with an EPA registration number, such as Clorox Any-

MISTAKE MANAGEMENT

Don't let a blunder kill your confidence.

You've just made a stupid mistake at work, but it might not be your boss's wrath you need to worry about.

"People engage in harsh self-criticism thinking it will help them avoid the same error in the future," says Jeff Szymanski, Ph.D., author of *The Perfectionist's Handbook: Take Risks, Invite Criticism, and Make the Most of Your Mistakes*. "The problem is, beating yourself up doesn't tell you what to do instead."

It's okay to mentally evaluate your blunders—as long as you're solution oriented. For example, instead of telling yourself, I'm a total idiot for screwing up those reports, make this your mantra: I screwed up because I took on too many projects. Next time I'll delegate to Dan. How to tell if you've truly moved on? You'll be able to talk about the mistake with others, and the thought of a repeat mishap won't freak you out, says Szymanski.

where, are true germ killers.

"If you use a cleaner that's not a disinfectant, you run the risk of not killing bacteria, spreading microbes, and contaminating more surfaces," says University of Arizona microbiologist Charles Gerba, Ph.D. Once you start cleaning, step away after you spray. "It takes 30 to 90 seconds for a disinfectant to kill germs, so let it sit before wiping it off," Gerba says.

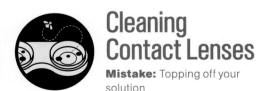

Taking a Shower

Mistake: Taking a shower every day

Unless you punch the clock in a sewer pipe, you're probably overdoing it.

"The outermost layer of skin is essential for locking in moisture," says Dr. Derick. Frequent showers with serious scrubbing can remove the layer's oils and lipids, which help fend off dryness. Shower every day if you need to—just keep the water lukewarm and your time to 10 minutes or less, Dr. Derick says. Afterward, skip the vigorous towel-dry routine, which can also dry your skin. Instead, gently blot your body with a soft towel and smear on CeraVe, a moisturizing cream that contains skin-fortifying fatty acids, says Dr. Derick.

Cleaning Contact Lenses

Mistake: Topping off your solution

If you never changed your car's oil and only topped it off, do you know what you'd

> You love the idea of having sex like clockwork. But for your wife, having to hook up anytime she's ovulating, can make her wish your Big Ben would break.

end up with? An engine full of dirty oil. Well, you're practicing the same poor maintenance with your contacts. In a University of Texas study, 90 percent of people thought using fresh solution meant simply adding a few drops to what was already in the lens case. The harm? Leftover solution is sapped of its disinfecting power, which the FDA says can raise your risk of vision-damaging infections. Your move: Clean, rinse, and air-dry the case each time you remove your lenses from it. Then refill it with fresh solution.

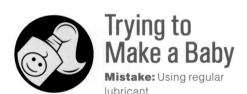

Trying to Make a Baby

Mistake: Using regular lubricant

You love the idea of having sex like clockwork. But for your wife, having to hook up whenever she's ovulating—horny or not—can make her wish your Big Ben would break.

"Three out of four women report increased vaginal dryness when they're trying to conceive," says Ashok Agarwal, Ph.D., director of research at the Cleveland

> "Most dryers draw in air from the bathroom and then can expel any contaminants onto your hands."

strained less than when they sat normally on a toilet.

Clinic's center for reproductive medicine. Unfortunately, a lube might alter the pH of her vagina and act like a spermicide, he warns. Stick to those that say "safe for use when trying to conceive," such as Pre-Seed Personal Lubricant. This means the FDA has deemed it sperm-safe.

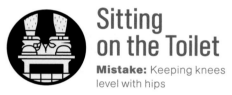

Sitting on the Toilet

Mistake: Keeping knees level with hips

Even if you're a fan of fiber, you can still find yourself straining on the toilet. Most commodes are now "comfort height," which means your knees are level with your hips. This puts a crook in your rectal canal, interfering with the smooth transit of your turds.

"In the natural squatting posture, with your butt below your knees, the rectal angle is straighter, minimizing straining," explains Dov Sikirov, M.D., the author of an Israeli study on the topic. To help straighten your canal, try placing a 4-inch footstool under your feet. In Dr. Sikirov's study, people who did this

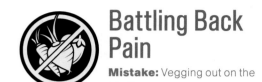

Battling Back Pain

Mistake: Vegging out on the couch

Lounging in front of the TV for all eight seasons of *House* won't cure a bad back.

"Lying down for a prolonged period of time is one of the worst things you can do for low-back pain," says Carmen Pichard-Encina, M.D., an assistant professor of orthopedics at Johns Hopkins Medicine in Baltimore. "It increases stiffness in the muscles of your back. Over time, inactivity can also cause those muscles to weaken, making them even more prone to injury and pain."

This doesn't mean you should exercise as normal, though. Opt for low-impact activities, such as walking or swimming, which target muscle stiffness without jolting your joints, suggests Dr. Pichard-Encina. That said, if even these activities are unbearable or if the pain doesn't let up in 5 to 7 days, schedule a doctor's appointment.

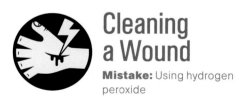

Cleaning a Wound

Mistake: Using hydrogen peroxide

Bleach is a powerful disinfectant, but you don't pour the stuff on a cut, right? And yet many of us reach for a bleach called hydrogen peroxide, not realizing that while it's murder on germs, our skin also suffers.

"It reduces the number of fibroblasts, a type of cell that's crucial for cleaning and repairing damaged tissue," says David Bar-Or, M.D., director of trauma research at the Swedish Medical Center in Colorado and the author of a study on the perils of peroxide.

Instead, just clean the wound with soap and water and apply a petrolatum-based cream (such as Aquaphor). Then cover it with an adhesive bandage. The petrolatum creates a moist environment, which promotes the healing of minor wounds, according to researchers in Germany.

Flossing Your Teeth

Mistake: Flossing before and not after brushing

In your mind's eye you can picture the floss dislodging food particles, which brushing can then sweep away. Except for one thing: The benefits of flossing have less to do with freeing the lettuce wedged between your teeth than clearing the debris you can't see—in your mind's eye or the mirror.

"Flossing is better able to remove the microscopic debris between your teeth after you've brushed off larger particles that were in the way," says Manhattan dentist Jennifer Jablow, D.D.S. After brushing, spit out the excess toothpaste, but hold off on your final rinse until you've finished flossing. Doing this can help transfer the toothpaste's fluoride into the crevices between your teeth, maximizing its germ-fighting action, says *Men's Health* dentistry advisor Kenneth Young, D.D.S.

Drying Your Hands

Mistake: Skipping the paper towels

Anyone who says electric hand dryers are more sanitary than paper towels is full of hot air. Rubbing your mitts under a traditional dryer can boost the number of bacteria on the surface of your skin by up to 45 percent, a recent study in the *Journal of Applied Microbiology* found.

"Most dryers draw in air from the bathroom and then can expel any airborne contaminants directly onto your hands," says University of Westminster microbiologist Keith Redway, M.Sc. Another problem: Rubbing your hands together can stir up bacteria in your pores so they rise to the surface of your skin. Your best bet is still the paper route, which reduces microbe levels on your palms by nearly 60 percent. Don't worry about paper waste: Many facilities now use biodegradable towels made from recycled paper.

Your Heart, Stopped Cold

Winter weather might trigger an avalanche of arterial trouble. Don't let it bury you.

A lift ticket might not be the only tag you wear in the winter. If you tangle with Old Man Winter, you could end up in the morgue with a toe tag. Cause of death? Heart attack. The incidence of chest-clutching catastrophes spikes 40 percent during the colder months compared with summertime, Japanese researchers say.

"Snow shoveling is probably the winter heart threat that's most familiar to men," says John Elefteriades, M.D., a *Men's Health* cardiology advisor and director of the Aortic Institute at Yale–New Haven Hospital. "But there are lesser-known seasonal factors that can place your heart at risk."

Fortunately, sidestepping the most chilling heart threats is simple—if you know what to do. Read on to find out how you can downgrade the danger to bunny-slope level.

WINTER HEALTH HAZARD #1
Frigid Air

Cold weather strains your heart as much as your heating budget. The average person's heart attack risk climbs 2 percent with every 1.8°F drop in temperature, British scientists report.

"Inhaling very cold air through your mouth chills your coronary arteries, which then constrict," says NYU cardiologist Howard Weintraub, M.D. This can dangerously reduce the volume of blood being pumped to your heart, especially if your arteries are clogged. "If you have a mild to moderate blockage—say, 20 to 40 percent—an hour of exposure to cold air can amplify that to upwards of 80 percent," says Dr. Weintraub. This can lead to chest pain during low-intensity outdoor activity, such as walking uphill. If you have a more severe blockage, it could even trigger a heart attack.

Protect Yourself

Wrap a scarf loosely around your nose and mouth so the icy air is warmed before it hits your lungs, says Dr. Weintraub. But watch out: As your moist breath makes the scarf clammy, its warming properties diminish. So if you brave the cold for longer than an hour (especially during exercise), wear a face mask lined with a moisture-wicking material.

Pay extra attention to your hands and feet. Freezing temperatures constrict blood vessels in your fingers and toes, forcing your heart to work harder to pump blood to your extremities.

All bundled up but still feel chest pain or pressure? Call 911 immediately.

WINTER HEALTH HAZARD #2
Short, Dim Days

In the winter, your body's supply of vitamin D drops right along with your tolerance for Christmas music. That's bad news for your heart: According to a 2010 study conducted at Utah's Intermountain Medical Center, people with the lowest levels of vitamin D are 45 percent more likely to develop coronary heart disease or have a heart attack than those with normal levels. The reason isn't entirely clear, but study author J. Brent Muhlestein, M.D., points to

CAUTION: ROADS ARE SLICK (AND YOU'RE NOT)

We asked Ted Plank, road supervisor for Colorado's Boulder County department of transportation, how to avoid the winter driving mistakes men make most often.

Driving too fast.
You should stay 10 to 20 miles per hour below the speed limit, especially if the air temp is between 25° and 40°F. When snow is slushy, it doesn't cling to your tires, so you're more likely to slide.

Racing with semis.
Truckers sit three times higher than you do; at your level there's more visual interference. For better visibility, buy winter wiper blades. Their rubber jackets keep ice out of the moving parts.

Ignoring your tires.
Check your all-weather tread: If it's less than half its original height, invest in winter tires. Inflate winter rubber 3 to 5 psi higher than all-season tires to boost the stability of the softer compound.

Driving back roads.
"These are the guys we find stuck in snowdrifts," says Plank. Stick to main roads and keep your gas tank at least half full. The extra weight provides traction for freeing your vehicle if you do get stuck.

research showing that vitamin D keeps a lid on your kidneys' levels of renin, an enzyme that can elevate blood pressure.

Protect Yourself

Reach for fatty fish, which are packed with vitamin D. Salmon, tuna, and mackerel are good choices, as are eggs and D-fortified milk. Although the Institute of Medicine recommends 600 IU of D a day, request a 25-hydroxy vitamin D blood test so your doctor can customize your dosage, says Dr. Muhlestein.

If you do require an extra dose of D, opt for a D3 supplement and take it with your largest meal of the day. Doing this might increase your absorption of the vitamin by 50 percent, say Cleveland Clinic scientists.

WINTER HEALTH HAZARD #3
Forgotten flu shot

Which would you prefer: a little jab in your arm, or a crushing pain in your chest? A Texas Heart Institute study found that people's likelihood of death due to heart attack spiked 30 percent when influenza rates peaked. The viral infection causes inflammation, which can disturb arterial plaque and cause clots to form, explains study author Mohammad Madjid, M.D. He estimates that if all eligible Americans were vaccinated every year, heart-related deaths would drop by 90,000 annually.

Protect Yourself

Roll up your sleeve. Even after the holidays, it's not too late for a flu shot, because the virus could stay active until March. And make sure your family follows suit, says Dr. Madjid.

"The flu vaccine isn't 100 percent effective, so if someone brings the virus into your home, your chance of becoming infected increases—even if you've been vaccinated." If you do get sick, don't fight the chills with a dunk in the tub. A hot bath on a cold day could raise your heart-attack risk. How? The rapid increase in body temp can lead to a heart-stressing drop in blood pressure, a Japanese study found. Instead, sponge off with lukewarm (about 70°F) water.

HARD TRUTH

53

The percentage of men who underestimate their heart disease risk, according to the journal Gender Medicine.

WINTER HEALTH HAZARD #4
An Overzealous Workout

Don't try to make up for a whole season of sloth and gluttony with a few days of sweat and grunting. A recent Tufts University analysis found that a person's risk of having a heart attack more than triples 1 to 2 hours after exercise. If you're fit you shouldn't worry, since your baseline risk of a heart attack is probably low. But if your most recent workout involved the lever on your La-Z-Boy, strenuous exercise could spell trouble.

"Your body's response to exercise—a rise in heart rate and blood pressure—may be exaggerated when you're deconditioned," says Gordon Tomaselli, M.D., chief of cardiology at Johns Hopkins University. "If you have undetected heart disease, this could result in heart attack and death."

Protect Yourself

This isn't a doctor's note to skip the gym. Simply monitor your heart rate to keep your intensity at a safe level. For the first 2 weeks, aim for 60 percent of your heart rate max (subtract your age from 220, then multiply the result by 0.6), and maintain that intensity for 20 minutes.

"You'll improve your fitness without creating undue cardiac risks," says *Men's Health* fitness advisor Alex Koch, Ph.D. Gradually increase your target heart rate by 5 percent every 2 weeks.

WINTER HEALTH HAZARD #5
Too Much Holiday Cheer

Tossing back the yuletide libations too quickly can have a sobering effect on your heart. It's what doctors call "holiday heart syndrome," a disruption of your heart's normal rhythm caused by overconsumption of alcohol.

One night of binge drinking could be enough to trigger an abnormal heartbeat.

"One night of binge drinking may be enough to overstimulate the nerve pathways that regulate your heart's rhythm," warns Laurence Sperling, M.D., director of preventive cardiology at Emory University. This usually has no lasting impact in otherwise healthy folks; if you have an underlying arterial blockage, however, the abnormal heartbeat caused by the condition could provoke a heart attack, says Dr. Sperling.

Protect Yourself

Limit yourself to two or three servings of alcohol per occasion. In a 2010 Canadian review, men who downed about five drinks' worth of alcohol had a greater risk of abnormal heartbeat than nondrinkers did. To pace yourself, hold your drink in your nondominant hand; you won't raise your glass to your lips as automatically, says Dr. Sperling.

Then rethink your buffet binge: Salty foods can spike BP, while fatty foods can cause arteries to spasm. Overindulging in either (or both) can conspire with alcohol to increase your risk of holiday heart.

Allergies Amok

Clearing the air on allergies, we separate fact from fiction to stop your sniffling, sneezing, and wheezing for good.

You don't need WebMD to decode allergies. The reason for your sniffling is simple: Your immune system encounters a foreign substance (pollen, say), registers it as a threat (it's not), and launches a counterattack. Cue the runny nose and itchy eyes. Straightforward, right?

In fact, that might be the only thing about allergies that is straightforward.

"Many people suffer quietly with allergies for decades," says William Reisacher, M.D., an assistant professor of otorhinolaryngology at Weill Cornell Medical College. "They don't tell their doctors because of the false belief that allergies are a trivial problem with no solution." Breathe a sigh of relief: We've uncovered the truth about allergies—and the best ways to keep airborne enemies at bay.

Fact or Fiction?

Allergies are on the rise because we've sanitized our lives.

Probably true: But Purell isn't entirely to blame. One leading theory is that the uptick in allergies began with our shift away from farm life and has accelerated because of our obsession with antibiotics and cleanliness, says Estelle Levetin, Ph.D., head of biological science at the University of Tulsa.

As a result, we're exposed to fewer infectious agents than ever before—with a very unexpected side effect. In the absence of its usual targets, your immune system might become overly sensitive and attack harmless particles, says Levetin.

Your Move

There's no need to play FarmVille in your backyard. But the next time your doctor prescribes an antibiotic, ask if it's absolutely necessary. When your immune system is forced to focus on invaders that matter, it might eventually start to ignore allergens, say researchers in France.

Here's another strategy: Eat more fermented foods, such as sauerkraut and kefir. They're full of good bacteria that might boost your immune system and, say scientists in Pakistan, further help prevent it from reacting to allergens.

Fact or Fiction?

Special pillowcases and mattress covers will banish dust mites from your bedroom.

False: You won't win this pillow fight. Simply covering your bedding with mite-proof covers isn't enough to reduce your symptoms, a 2011 Cochrane review concluded.

"Covers will work as part of a plan that includes other dust-mite control measures," says Thomas Platts-Mills, M.D., Ph.D., director of the University of Virginia's asthma and allergic disease center.

Your Move

The first step in your mite-control mission: choosing the right pillow and mattress covers. Skip the cheapie versions. Their weave isn't tight enough to block the little buggers, says Dr. Platts-Mills. Instead, invest in Mission: Allergy Premium Microfiber Allergen-Proof Shams and Mattress Encasings ($28 to $170, missionallergy.com).

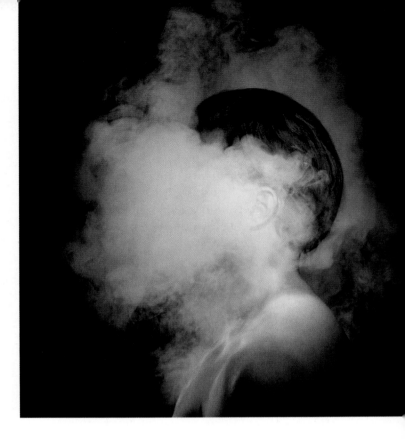

Also, regularly wash your sheets and pillowcases in hot water and clean your floors with a HEPA vacuum, such as the Hoover WindTunnel Self-Propelled Bagless Upright ($250, hoover.com). In a Rutgers study, HEPA filtration reduced dust-mite allergens by 81 percent. The key: After vacuuming, the scientists waited 2 hours to let any agitated particles settle, and then they vacuumed again.

Fact or Fiction?

You might have allergies and not even realize it

True. You've pegged your runny nose as a cold symptom, but could it be allergies?

"Many people misdiagnose allergies as a cold or the flu, so they never receive appropriate care," says Stanley Naides, M.D., medical director for immunology at Quest Diagnostics.

This could prime your body for more misery: Untreated allergies can predispose you to sinusitis (a sinus infection due to fluid buildup), middle ear infections (inflammation/fluid buildup in your ear), or even asthma.

Your Move

Take this test from the American College of Allergy, Asthma, and Immunology.

1. How did your symptoms start? Cold symptoms evolve, but allergy symptoms often strike all at once.
2. How long have you been miserable? Colds typically clear up within a week or two, whereas allergies may drag on.
3. Achy and feverish? Probably a cold or the flu.
4. Itchy eyes? Allergies, most likely.
5. Sore throat or coughing? Generally a cold.

Bottom line: Don't let symptoms linger. After 2 weeks of suffering, visit your doctor, who can spot subtle signs of allergies, such as pale nasal mucous membranes, says Jeffrey Demain, M.D., director of the Allergy, Asthma, and Immunology Center of Alaska.

Fact or Fiction?

Hypoallergenic pets won't stir up your symptoms.

False. Don't expect a hypoallergenic pet to sneezeproof your pad. In a recent Henry Ford Health System study, allergen levels in homes with "hypoallergenic" dogs were found to be no lower than in homes with other breeds. The reason: The particles sloughed off the dog's tongue and saliva—not its fur—are what trigger your reaction, says study author Christine Cole Johnson,

FOOD ALLERGY OR FALSE ALARM?

Here's why you might no longer need to be afraid of your plate.

While a child's peanut allergy is nothing to sneeze at, many adults may not need to skip the Skippy after all. A recent study review in the *Journal of the American Dietetic Association* found that even though one in five people alter their diets because they fear adverse reactions, fewer than one in 10 truly have a food allergy. The tests used for diagnosis are partly to blame: So-called positive results can be wrong nearly half the time, indicating a food allergy where none exists, says allergy researcher Michelle Conroy, M.D., an assistant professor of medicine at the University of Massachusetts medical school.

"Some of the issue related to the insane increase in food allergies is potentially in part related to overdiagnosis," she says. If the results of your skin-prick or blood test are unclear or inconclusive, your doctor can confirm the diagnosis with a food challenge, during which you eat increasing amounts of a food at regular intervals under carefully controlled conditions.

Ph.D. Plus, pets are often covered in other allergens, such as pollen, dust, and mold.

Your Move

The Obamas were smart to adopt Bo, but not because of his so-called allergy-free coat. A dog can be an allergic person's best choice because cat dander is "stickier" and thus tougher to eliminate, says Dr. Reisacher. Shampoo your pooch regularly, and blow-dry its fur on low heat to fight "wet dog" smell, which is caused by mold. Finally, use bleach or a color-safe alternative to destroy any dander clinging to your clothes.

Fact or Fiction?

Nasal sprays are a safe steroid treatment.

True. You might associate steroids with meat-heads, but what they use are anabolic steroids, which mimic male hormones. The corticosteroids in nasal sprays, on the other hand, are inflammation-fighting hormones.

"They have fewer side effects than antihistamines because they go directly into your nasal tissue instead of throughout your body," says Timothy Mainardi, M.D., an allergist at Columbia University. Studies also show that corticosteroid sprays reduce nasal blockage and discharge more effectively than antihistamines do.

Your Move

Start spraying a couple of weeks before your allergy season typically begins, suggests Dr. Mainardi. Red, itchy eyes? Opt for Veramyst, a new corticosteroid spray

Untreated allergies can predispose you to sinusitus, middle ear infections, or asthma.

that controls nasal and eye symptoms. Or pair Nasonex or Flonase with a second-generation antihistamine, such as Claritin or Zyrtec.

Fact or Fiction?

Skin testing is a waste of time. You'll react to everything.

False. If your test results say "allergic to the world," find a new allergist. Skin reactions need to be at least 3 millimeters across to indicate an allergy that can cause symptoms, says Dr. Demain. Another key to avoiding false positives: Share your medical history before testing. If you now eat eggs without problems despite a childhood egg allergy, your allergist can skip that test.

Your Move

This is one exam you don't want to cheat on. Avoid antihistamines 3 days prior, because they might dampen your allergic response and skew your results, say Mayo Clinic scientists. And at your appointment, provide the full rundown: timing of your symptoms, family history, suspected triggers, and previously diagnosed allergies. Your allergist will then decide which allergens to test for.

The Drugstore War

Addicts are infiltrating our pharmacies, placing themselves and everyone else in danger.
Is it time for the man in the white coat to don the white hat?

Ryan Donnelly had it down cold. Three years ago he was a 25-year-old Navy vet who had been booted from the service for a failed drug test, cycled through cocaine to alcohol, and finally landed on a 560-milligrams-a-day oxycodone addiction. To maintain his habit, Donnelly stole prescription pads. When those ran out, he dipped legitimate scrips in nail polish remover to strip away the physicians' scribblings. He then took his forgeries to more than 20 pharmacies in and around his hometown of Toms River, New Jersey.

Today when the clean and sober Donnelly looks back on those years, he knows there were obvious signs of his addiction that anyone, especially an experienced pharmacist, could have picked up on.

"When you're withdrawing, your upper lip and your forehead sweat; you look like you have the flu," says Donnelly, who now runs FreeFromHell.com, a social support website for recovering addicts. He says sometimes he'd even put on a suit in an effort to look normal. "You try to pull it together, but you end up looking like a hoodlum."

If the red flags were there for all behind the counter to see, why didn't anyone turn Donnelly away—or better yet, turn him in? Fortunately, a family intervention finally

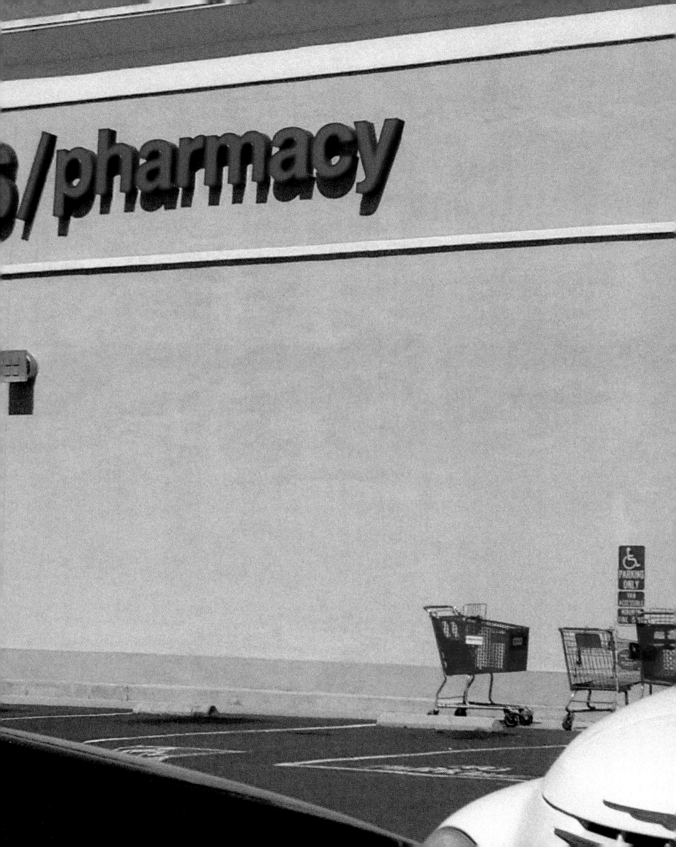

pushed the pillhead to rehab before he could hurt himself or anyone else.

Things ended more tragically in the case of David Laffer. In June 2011, Laffer walked into a Long Island pharmacy and shot the pharmacist, a 17-year-old employee, and two customers while stealing hydrocodone, a semisynthetic opioid derived from codeine. In the 12 days before the killings, he had filled six prescriptions from five different doctors for a total of more than 400 pills, according to one Long Island newspaper.

"We sometimes lose sight of the fact that pharmacists are trained to spot drug-seeking behavior," says Luis Bauza, director of investigations at RxPatrol, an alliance formed between local law enforcement and the drug company Purdue Pharma, which makes OxyContin, to track pharmacy fraud and thefts across the country. "I see pharmacists as our last line of defense."

Armed and Dangerous

Opium from Afghanistan's poppy fields helps fund the Taliban, but you could

THE RX FOR AVOIDING ADDICTION

Here's how to find pain relief without becoming hooked on the feeling.

Make it the med of last resort. "OxyContin is at the far end of the spectrum of pain medication and should be reserved for the most extreme circumstances," says Adam Carinci, M.D., a pain management physician at Massachusetts General Hospital. First step: Try taking an over-the-counter anti-inflammatory, such as ibuprofen. If that doesn't help, ask your doctor for a prescription muscle relaxant or a lower-grade, short-acting opioid, such as tramadol, says Dr. Carinci.

Go under the microscope. Your doctor should monitor your symptoms closely, adjust your dosage as needed, and watch for signs that you're abusing the drug (taking extra pills and/or crushing and snorting them). "Monthly follow-ups might not be enough, and you might need to go in every 2 weeks," Dr. Carinci says. If you want to play it especially safe, you can even ask your doctor to randomly test your urine for elevated opioid levels.

Own up to your demons. If you have a track record of doing drugs, bingeing on booze, or overeating, avoid opioids. "People are more likely to abuse these medications if they have a history of abusing something else," says Michael Weaver, M.D., an associate professor of internal medicine at Virginia Commonwealth University. Family history of drug abuse? You may be genetically predisposed to addiction, says Dr. Weaver.

Check your motives. Are you depressed? Anxious? You have a higher risk of developing psychological dependence on opioids, which can lead to addiction, says Dr. Weaver. "Some people take painkillers to help them with things that are emotionally uncomfortable, to sleep at night, or to unwind after a hard day." Even if you have no history of psychological problems, if you reach for the pill bottle for any of these reasons, tell your doctor.

Don't play doctor. Take meds exactly as prescribed. "A common myth is that people should take only the lowest dose and take it as infrequently as possible—and just grit their teeth and bear the pain to avoid taking too much," says Dr. Weaver. "That can lead to more problems." If you can manage your pain with your prescribed dose, then you'll be less likely to take extra pills or crush or snort pills for faster absorption, which can accelerate you into an addiction.

argue that it's the synthetic stuff that poses the most immediate threat to U.S. national security. In 2008 alone, 14,800 people died after taking opioid painkillers such as oxycodone, according to the CDC. More recently, a 2010 survey by the Substance Abuse and Mental Health Services Administration found that an estimated 1.9 million people had abused or been dependent on prescription painkillers in the past year. And increasingly, the addicts who don't kill themselves are becoming desperate enough to endanger others. The U.S. Drug Enforcement Administration reports that 686 armed pharmacy robberies took place in 2010, an 81 percent increase from just 4 years earlier.

Pharmacist Mike Donohue has witnessed the change firsthand. In 2009, a man walked into Donohue's Seattle pharmacy and slipped the technician on duty a piece of paper that read, "Give me your OxyContin. I have a gun." Luckily for the people in the store that afternoon, Donohue noticed what was going on, pulled out his own gun, a Glock 19 loaded with hollow-point bullets, and chased the would-be robber out the door.

Donohue has been working behind a drugstore counter for more than two decades. He remembers a time not so long ago when a holster wasn't part of his uniform. In fact, in the late 1990s, medical boards across the nation were chiding doctors for often under-treating patients' pain and recommended the increased use of opioids for difficult-to-manage cases. According to Donohue, pharmacy boards encouraged reluctant pharmacists to dispense narcotics in such situations, in amounts that were significantly larger

> "I had a guy come in with a falsified scrip. I called the doctor, turned the guy away. He came in again; I called the cops."

than what the pharmacists were used to doling out.

"They said people were suffering needlessly," he recalls. "We were told that with proper documentation and a legitimate prescription, dispensing these narcotics was appropriate. The word out then was 'Pharmacists are not police officers!'"

They're not physicians either, but if pharmacists don't intervene when suspicious customers proffer scrips, they expose themselves to as much liability as doctors do when they prescribe drugs inappropriately. Under the Controlled Substances Act, a clause commonly known as "corresponding responsibility" stipulates that a pharmacist who fills a prescription when there's reason to doubt its intent for legitimate medical use can lose his or her license and even be prosecuted for a felony.

Yet even at the risk of possible legal ramifications, many pharmacists don't step in early on. This is despite the fact that in a 2005 report from the National Center on Addiction and Substance Abuse at Columbia University, 52 percent of pharmacists said the patients—not physicians or drug companies—were mostly to blame for the problem of unlawful prescription drug use.

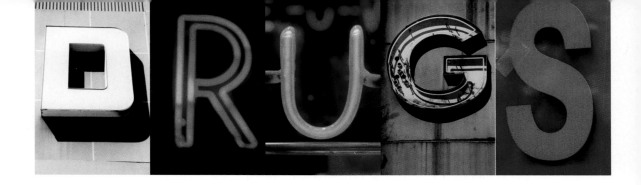

One reason for their reticence is that pharmacists don't feel adequately prepared to spot patients with problems. A study of Florida pharmacists found that less than a third of those surveyed had more than 2 hours of addiction and substance-abuse training in school. Worse, nearly 30 percent said they'd received no training at all.

"It's not something you can really teach in a classroom," says Lauren Schlesselman, Pharm.D., an assistant clinical professor at the University of Connecticut's school of pharmacy. She estimates that less than 1 percent of the UConn curriculum is dedicated to spotting signs of addiction in customers. That course work includes students viewing mock patient profiles, looking for signs of doctor shopping (trying to fill multiple scrips from different physicians) and pharmacy hopping (trying to fill the same scrip at different places), and noting the numbers of attempts at early refills. But the best lesson—witnessing the physical signs of a customer who's slipping into addiction—isn't found in a textbook. That's why Dr. Schlesselman believes pharmacists should be honing their observational skills on the job during their internships.

That said, she also admits that pharmacists and pharmacy techs would be able to spend more time evaluating the legitimacy of a prescription held by, say, the fifth customer in a 10-person line if they weren't stretched so thin already. With much of the population aging into a medication-reliant culture, pharmacists are in high demand. Adding to their work stress is the fact that they now often provide immunizations, and Medicare is requiring them to become more involved in counseling patients. And while enrollment in pharmacy schools is up, most stores can't afford to hire enough pharmacists, says Dr. Schlesselman. She also points out that just about every transaction—even the basic ones handled by technicians, such as counting pills—must be overseen and approved by the pharmacist.

"With chain stores, frankly, they are trying to move you through the line as fast as possible," she says. "And the small shops are also trying to fill as many scrips as fast as they can so they can afford to stay in business."

Virtual Training

A possible compromise between classroom education and hands-on prescribing would be to train pharmacists in the virtual world. When researchers from the Philadelphia College of Pharmacy tested a Web-based learning program on second-year pharmacy students, the results were encouraging. The study, published in the *American Journal of Pharmaceutical Education* in 2010, found that after answering a series of questions on addiction and then sitting through a Web-based tutorial, students' scores on the questions improved by 30 percentage points.

Of course, it isn't enough simply to spot an addict. The hard part is stopping one.

"Pharmacists have only a few options," says Dr. Schlesselman. "They can approach the prescriber with their suspicions in an effort to obtain confirmation, they can confront the patient, they can warn other pharmacists in the area, or they can call the police."

Ryan Donnelly doesn't know how many of the pharmacists who filled his scrips suspected he was hooked, but he believes they all acted appropriately by not challenging him.

"I don't think it's worth it for them to get involved," he says. "The longer you use and the more desperate you get, eventually you'll end up doing something stupid."

"Pharmacists are positioned at a critical intervention point," says Sherry Green, CEO of the National Alliance for Model State Drug Laws. "But we can't expect them to be the sole gatekeepers, to take all this on themselves. That burden has to be shared."

To that end, Green's organization has been pushing state governments to institute prescription drug monitoring programs (PDMPs), computer databases that are set up to track and share information on prescriptions as those scrips flow from doctor to patient to pharmacy. With access to such data, a pharmacist can run the details of a prescription through the system and look for suspicious activity. The

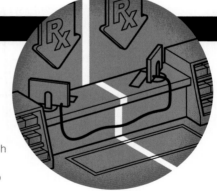

NO MORE STATE SECRETS

Here's how improving communication among drugstores can help stop border-hopping addicts.

One of the most powerful weapons in any pharmacist's arsenal is a state prescription drug monitoring program (PDMP). This computer database connects drugstores around the state, making it easier to catch suspicious customer activity. The problem with PDMPs, however, is that they're weapons with a limited range—few reach beyond their borders to share information with neighboring states.

"Improving communication across states is essential," says Jermaine Jones, Ph.D., an assistant professor of clinical neuroscience at Columbia University who studies opioid abuse. "We know that many people do what we call 'doctor shopping,' going to multiple doctors to obtain quantities of opioid meds, and that can cut across state lines."

In March of 2012, Ohio senator Rob Portman and Kentucky congressman Hal Rogers introduced the Interstate Drug Monitoring Efficiency and Data Sharing Act of 2012, which will create a system that allows states to share information from their PDMPs. Ask your legislators to support the bill (senate.gov, house. gov).

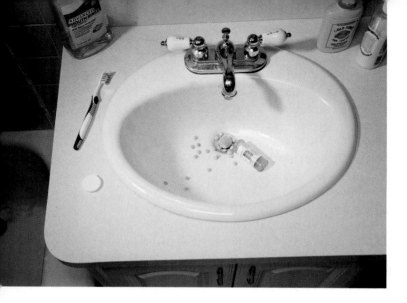

24 states have begun sharing data with the PDMPs of other states.

Another issue, Green says, is that the laws surrounding each state's system differ. In some states, pharmacists can only enter information; they aren't allowed to access it.

Mike Donohue, for one, is willing to give this technology a chance. He has recently installed new software in his Seattle pharmacy that will pipe him into Washington State's PDMP, which allows full access to pharmacists. But while he appreciates the convenience of the new system, he feels it's no replacement for a pharmacist's intuition.

"We do this all day," Donohue says. "We know when we should say no to a customer and when we should say yes. If you use common sense and good judgment, you'll be okay."

On the Front Lines

As a banker on Wall Street, Michael Altman dealt with risk all the time. So it didn't surprise anyone when 9 years ago, at the age of 36, he left the stress of the Street to take a chance on starting his own business: a pharmacy in the small village of Hastings-on-Hudson, less than 20 miles from Manhattan.

The gamble paid off, at least financially. But as the decade passed, an unexpected problem emerged. Altman began to notice unfamiliar faces infiltrating his closely knit core of local customers. People came bearing prescriptions from doctors in the Bronx or Brooklyn. Many of the scrips being presented were on photocopied

database can then reveal whether a patient is doctor shopping or pharmacy hopping, for example, or whether specific physicians are prescribing inordinate amounts of painkillers to many different patients.

Forty-one states have already installed and launched PDMPs, and all other states except Missouri and New Hampshire have enacted legislation to do so. Reluctance in the two holdout states, Green says, is due to privacy concerns about the government maintaining a database of personal prescription information. Nevertheless, she believes that the benefits of the monitoring program will outweigh any negatives. "With early detection, the appropriate professionals can intervene early and help resolve potential problems."

So far the implementation of these systems has been problematic. Because each state decides how to set up its database, each system is different. That means communication among state databases is difficult if not impossible, resulting in loopholes that border-hopping pill poppers can exploit. As of February 2012, only

paper, some obviously altered with an extra digit penned in to change, say, 20 pills to 120. Some of these customers insisted on paying cash. And all of the prescriptions were for painkillers—usually oxycodone.

"I had a guy come in with a falsified scrip on a stolen prescription pad," says Altman in a thick New York accent. "I called the doctor, turned the guy away. He came in again; I called the cops. He was arrested right outside the store, right in front of his friend, who was waiting in the car."

Then Altman delivers the punch line: "The next week, the friend comes in with the same pad. It's a game to them."

If there's a lesson in Altman's experience, it's that now it's more critical than ever for pharmacists to stay connected to the communities they serve.

"The pharmacist needs to know the patients who come into the pharmacy," says Bauza from RxPatrol, "and he or she should also have relationships with the doctors in the area." When these connections are made, the pharmacist not only comes to trust the prescription, adds Bauza, but also becomes familiar with the circumstances surrounding treatment and can possibly even provide the customer with useful advice.

"I want my pharmacist to call my doctor if any questions arise about a medication I'm supposed to be taking," says Bauza. "It's like getting a second opinion."

John Burke, president of the National Association of Drug Diversion Investigators, recommends that a pharmacist extend that same familiarity to local law enforcement.

"Don't wait until there's a robbery to meet the cop on the beat," he says.

If the pills don't go down the drain, the addict's life almost certainly will.

Whether it's the nationwide adoption of PDMPs, a renewed focus on adequately educating pharmacists to spot addiction, or a conscious move toward building stronger and more personal customer relationships, no single prescription can cure the problem of painkiller abuse everywhere. Each individual pharmacy needs to figure out a combination of strategies that works best for the particular community it serves.

There is, however, one last-resort measure that no pharmacist wants to implement. Altman eventually saw it as his only option for protecting himself, his staff members, and his customers. He printed up signs and then taped them to the windows of his pharmacy. They read: WE ARE NO LONGER CARRYING OXYCODONE.

"It's worked," he says. "The calls for the drug have largely stopped."

Altman doesn't relish the idea of denying people with real medical needs—his neighbors—access to pain relief, nor does he look forward to the inevitable hit to his bottom line. But he also knew he had to do something.

"Everybody should take the situation into their own hands as part of our civic responsibility," says Altman. "If we allow these people to become junkies just so we can make a profit, we're no better than the people selling on the street."

Time Delay

Discover science's newest secrets for never growing old.

It's not just women who define aging by what they see in the mirror. LeBron James has lamented his receding hairline on Twitter. Simon Cowell admits to being a regular guest in the Botox chair. And Donald Trump's comb-over is a daily source of media derision. But really, it's what's on the inside—your heart, your lungs, your brain—that matters, at least when it comes to dominating on the basketball court, belting it out like an *X Factor* winner, or ruling the business world.

Unfortunately, while we're living longer than ever, our "health span"—the stretch of time when we're healthy enough to actually enjoy life, not just hang onto it—isn't gaining much ground.

"Much of the decline that we experience as we age is not a necessary function of aging. It's a result of our expectations and mindset," says Ellen Langer, Ph.D., a professor of social psychology at Harvard, who studies aging. "We expect to fall apart, so we allow ourselves to fall apart."

But what if you decided to stay 35 forever? New science suggests that you can turn back the clock on the ravages of time. Read on for our tips. They're like Botox for your brain and hair dye for your DNA.

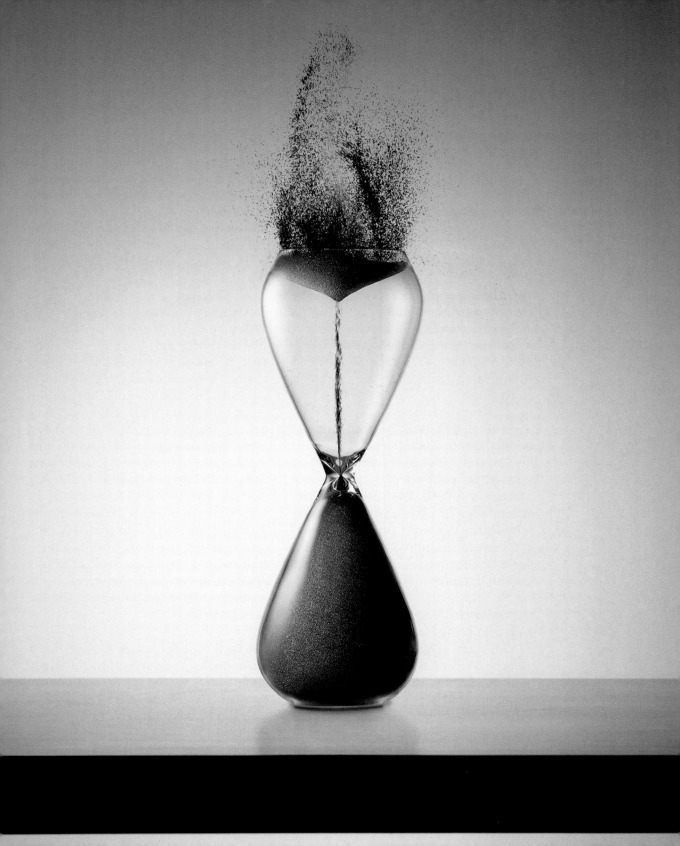

Only your fittest brain cells survive into your 20s— and the Jell-O shots and Jagermeister aren't entirely to blame.

Your Brain

The damage: Only your fittest brain cells survive your 20s—and the Jell-O shots and Jagermeister aren't entirely to blame. A 2011 study published in the *Proceedings of the National Academy of Sciences* noted that around age 25, the human brain starts to slowly decrease in size.

And your mental capacity might be shrinking right along with it. As your brain starts to shrivel, its white matter becomes less efficient at nerve signaling, says Deborah Little, Ph.D., a professor of psychiatry at Texas A&M University. The effect: Your working memory—your short-term ability to reason, comprehend, and retain information—might gradually begin to slip. Hmmm . . . now where did I leave that Jell-O?

HIT REWIND: Playing with balls might help your brain bounce back. In a 2009 British study, people who practiced juggling for 6 weeks strengthened the structural integrity of their white matter. It didn't even matter if they dropped the balls; the benefit was linked to time spent training, not proficiency.

The reason? Practicing a new skill might encourage the formation of myelin, the white matter that helps conduct nerve impulses, the scientists say. Start with the three-ball cascade—this was the basic juggling skill the study participants practiced. (Watch "Learn How to Juggle 3 Balls," by master juggler Jason Garfield, on YouTube.) Work on it at least 30 minutes a day, 5 days a week. Or try another pursuit that combines learning with physical activity, such as archery, surfing, or bowling, says study author Jan Scholz, D.Phil.

Your Lungs

The damage: Even if you've never touched a cigarette and you always avoid secondhand smoke, your lung function might have declined by the time you blow out the candles on your 40th birthday. Although your lungs hit their peak around age 25, it's not until your mid-30s that aging kicks into high gear. Your alveoli—the tiny air sacs in your lungs that allow oxygen to cross into your bloodstream and carbon dioxide to exit—begin to lose surface area, say scientists at Georgetown University. This makes your lungs less efficient at transporting oxygen. The result: You might find it harder to breathe during exercise.

HIT REWIND: Don't wipe away that milk mustache; it's a sign of youth. A 2010 study published in the *Journal of the American College of Nutrition* found that people who consistently downed two daily servings of low-fat dairy, such as reduced-fat milk, yogurt, and cottage cheese, showed fewer signs of disease-related lung damage. Credit the vitamin D in fortified dairy products: This nutrient may help improve lung function, the scientists say.

In addition, milk is loaded with vitamin A, which is thought to switch on genes involved in the production of new lung tissue, says Matthew Hind, M.D., Ph.D., a researcher and physician at London's Royal Brompton Hospital, who has studied the effects of vitamin A in animals. Aim to eat two or three servings of fortified dairy a day, and you'll be taking in up to 10 micrograms of vitamin D and up to 455 micrograms of vitamin A.

Your DNA

The damage: Remember W's "axis of evil"? Well, never mind Iran, Iraq, and North Korea—the "axis of aging" in your cells poses a clear and present danger, says Ronald DePinho, M.D., who heads the University of Texas's MD Anderson Cancer Center. The axis starts with special strands of DNA called telomeres that cap off each of your chromosomes, protecting them from mutation when your cells divide.

The problem is that your telomeres begin to shorten and fray as you grow older; once they a drop below a critical length, your cells are no longer able to divide, so they start deteriorating. At the same time, your mitochondria, the energy powerhouses of your cells, start losing steam.

HIT REWIND: Think of this as *Extreme Makeover: Telomere Edition*. In a recent

As your heart shrinks in your 40s, your risk of a chest clutcher might climb.

study, Dr. DePinho and his team managed to shift the aging process of rodents into reverse by restoring their truncated telomeres. The little guys suddenly had fewer signs of DNA damage, more-efficient mitochondria, and healthier organs! And while more study is needed, humans might reap the same benefits, says Dr. DePinho.

Luckily, you might be able to revitalize your own telomeres. In a recent University of California study, people who regularly meditated over a 3-month period had more active telomerase, an enzyme that helps preserve telomeres. Start with a 10-minute session before breakfast, says Alfred W. Kaszniak, Ph.D., a professor of psychology, neurology, and psychiatry at the University of Arizona.

"Find a comfortable seated position in which you can stay upright, relaxed, and alert," he says. "Then, focusing on either the sensation of your breath at your nostrils or the rising and falling of your abdomen just below your navel, count each exhalation, from 1 to 10, and then start at 1 again."

Your Heart

The damage: The clock may be ticking on your ticker. Starting around age 40,

Why slow the sands of time when you can stop them?

elastin, a flexible protein in your heart's aorta, is gradually replaced with collagen, a stiffer, more fibrous protein. As a result, your heart no longer pumps blood as efficiently, says Joao Lima, M.D., director of cardiovascular imaging at Johns Hopkins Hospital.

"In your 40s, your body also begins to replace myocytes—muscle cells—with scar tissue, so your heart becomes smaller," says Dr. Lima. This forces it to work harder, potentially raising your risk of a chest clutcher.

HIT REWIND: Every minute you log on the treadmill helps turn back time. By keeping your heart muscles and arteries flexible and by slowing your resting heart rate, exercise interrupts the cardiovascu-

lar aging process, Dr. Lima says. Interval training is ideal for fitness gains, but a steady pace may be best for heart health.

In a recent study in the *International Journal of Cardiology*, men who hit the treadmill 3 days a week for a solid 30 minutes per session showed renewed arterial flexibility, improved bloodflow, and increased levels of progenitor cells, a type of bone marrow cell that repairs artery walls. Running intervals, on the other hand, boosts arterial flexibility but won't impact progenitor cell circulation, a new British study reports.

Your Bones

The damage: Your skin might be smooth with youth, but inside your body your bones are already wasting away. A recent Mayo Clinic study found that the thickness of the trabeculae—the spongy, supportive material inside bones—shrank in men by almost 30 percent from age 24 to 48.

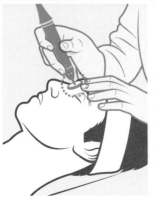

THE NEW AGE ERASER

Before you Botox, consider zapping away the years.

To bluff your way through the aging game, you need to avoid two tells that can tip your hand: wrinkles and sagging. So how do you perfect your poker face? Radiofrequency skin tightening, a nonsurgical procedure that applies heat to jumpstart collagen production. In a Johns Hopkins study, it reduced sagging and wrinkles in 80 percent of patients.

"Bipolar" radiofrequency tightening uses two electrodes for better heat control, and it might be paired with a laser or light pulses to improve results. Unlike with Botox, the effects of a single session ($1,000 and up) can last for years. Make sure your dermatologist has performed the procedure daily for at least a year, says *Men's Health* dermatology advisor Adnan Nasir, M.D.

Then, around age 65, your bones begin shedding more of the mineral building blocks that make them strong, a process that causes even faster degeneration, says Bahram Arjmandi, Ph.D., R.D., chairman of the department of nutrition, food, and exercise sciences at Florida State University.

HIT REWIND: The go-to fruit of grandparents may be the secret to younger bones.

"Prunes are one of the most effective fruits for reversing bone loss and preserving bone mass," says Arjmandi. His research has shown that men who add prunes to their diet can boost their bone density by 11 percent. "Prunes have unique polyphenols with antioxidant properties that help fight osteoporosis. Plus, prunes

Your skin might be smooth with youth, but inside your body your bones are already wasting away.

may increase the magnesium content in bone," he says. And higher magnesium translates to stronger, denser bones. Shoot for three prunes a day, with a glass of water to keep the fiber and sugar alcohol from dehydrating you. (Try adding diced prunes to trail mix or oatmeal.) For extra insurance, eat two medium apples or 2 ounces of fresh blueberries. Both promote bone growth by reducing the amount of calcium lost in your urine, says Arjmandi.

PUT THAT BOTTLE BACK

Don't go the herbal route to treat prostate problems: Saw palmetto extract does not relieve the symptoms of prostate enlargement (a.k.a. BPH), according to a study in the *Journal of the American Medical Association*. We also recently reported that finasteride, an Rx for BPH, can cause lasting sexual side effects. Luckily, the FDA recently approved the erectile dysfunction drug Cialis to treat BPH. Talk to your doctor about its pros and cons.

HARD TRUTH
60
The percentage decrease in your odds of developing BPH if you take cholesterol-lowering statin meds, according to the British Journal of Urology International.

SEE THE SIGNS

Adult acne can be an eyesore, but it's what you can't see in the mirror that should scare you: Pimples might signal insulin resistance, a precursor to type 2 diabetes. In a study published in the journal *Endocrine*, men with acne had fasting insulin levels that were nearly double those of guys with clear skin. One theory:

Excess insulin spurs overproduction of male hormones, triggering oil secretion and zits, says study author Antongiulio Faggiano, M.D., Ph.D. If you're breaking out, ask your doctor for an oral glucose tolerance test.

CHECK THE ERECTION RESULTS

Straining in the bathroom might leave you limp in the bedroom. Hemorrhoids might signal an increased risk of erectile dysfunction, a study in the *International Journal of Andrology* reveals. Men with ED were nearly twice as likely as those without the condition to have hemorrhoids. (ED sufferers under age 30 had an even higher hemorrhoid risk.) Swollen veins in your rectum might irritate nerves around your prostate, the researchers say. Cut your toilet time—and maybe lift your love life—by eating 20 to 35 grams of fiber a day.

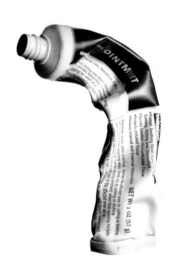

FLOSS TO FIGHT CANCER

Dental floss is definite MacGyver material. This is unusual use #46: Floss can help you escape stomach cancer. New York University researchers found that people with precancerous gastric lesions were nearly three times as likely to report that they flossed infrequently as people who didn't have the lesions. Study author Yu Chen, Ph.D., M.P.H., explains that if you don't maintain good oral hygiene, bacteria may build up in your mouth and eventually migrate to your stomach, where they can trigger cancer-causing inflammation. Here's a tip for the forgetful: Jot down a plan of when, where, and how you'll floss each day and you'll be more likely to actually do it, a German study found.

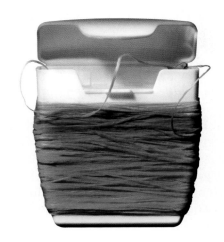

ACHY JOINTS? SNACK ON CHOCOLATE

Call it the chocolate touch: Cocoa powder may help reduce inflammation associated with arthritis, says a Spanish study. Scientists fed rats with achy joints a high-cocoa diet and saw signs of inflammation decrease. Cocoa might bolster immune responses in the body by regulating disease-fighting T cells.

EAT MORE BUGS

Sometimes you need a bug to beat a bug. Consuming "good" bacteria might help you fend off colds, according to a study review by the Cochrane Collaboration. When people took probiotic supplements or ate yogurt, 42 percent fewer caught colds or other upper-respiratory infections than people who took placebos. Two of the probiotics studied can be found in Culturelle capsules and DanActive yogurt.

Why? Experts think that probiotic capsules may condition your white blood cells to more effectively fight viral invaders.

BANISH BACK PAIN

If you're plagued with back trouble, kettlebell swings might be your answer, say researchers in Canada. The reason: "Kettlebell swings require you to move your hips while your core works to prevent motion of your spine. This may help prevent back injury," says study author Stuart McGill, Ph.D. Watch the perfect swing at MensHealth.com, keywords "kettlebell swing." (Don't do it if your back hurts when you swing heavy loads.)

PREVENT A PAIN IN THE APP

As amazing as iPads are (have you read *Men's Health* on one?), they have a downside: Tablet computers can cause neck pain Harvard researchers found that people who rested a tablet on their lap or any flat surface tended to tilt their neck at an awkward angle in order to see the screen better. Over time, craning like this can cause neck and shoulder pain, says study author Jack Dennerlein, Ph.D. When you're tired of holding your tablet, set it on a table and use the case to adjust the screen to a 45-degree angle.

COMMUTE WITH CARE

Danger: False sense of security ahead. German researchers suggest that car accidents may be more likely to happen at uncrowded intersections. Using a driving simulator, study participants who made right turns at unsignaled intersections were more likely to have collisions when few cars and no crossing pedestrians were present. The reason for the recklessness? If the coast seems clear, drivers accelerate too quickly and don't watch their right side.

PICK UP STICKS

Freshen your breath and your attitude at the same time. Chewing gum can improve your mood and help you focus, say Japanese researchers. People who popped a piece of gum twice a day for 2 weeks lowered their scores on tests of depression and mental fatigue by as much as 47 percent—while those who sucked on a mint instead saw almost no change.

The act of chewing might keep you happy—and alert!—by increasing bloodflow to your brain and reducing your levels of stress hormones, says study author Chifumi Sato, M.D. Note: You need to keep chewing for at least 5 minutes to experience any benefit.

SPEND LESS, LIVE LONGER

You're not just burying your abs when you eat junk food. An unhealthy diet might cost more than a healthy one, according to USDA economics researchers. They studied about 4,400 foods through three cost-analysis measures (price per calorie, price per edible gram, and price per portion), and they discovered that healthy foods are cheaper than unhealthy ones and contain more nutrients for your buck.

TAKE THE DEATH TEST

Your doc might soon be able to peer deeper into the coronary crystal ball. Researchers in Sweden recently found that people with the highest levels of an inflammatory protein were 62 percent more likely to die of heart disease in the next 8 years than those with the lowest levels. The next step is to see how the predictive power of the protein, called cathepsin S, stacks up against cholesterol and triglycerides.

BEAT NICOTINE WITH A NECTARINE

Scientists from the University at Buffalo report that eating fruits and vegetables can help you quit smoking. In the 14-month study, people who consumed at least four daily servings of produce were three times as likely to stub the cigs for good as those who ate less than two servings. Study author Jeffrey Haibach, M.P.H., says smokers often mistake hunger for tobacco cravings, so the satiating effect of fiber-rich produce might keep them from lighting up. Another benefit: Fruits and vegetables worsen the flavor of that Marlboro, making it taste as disgusting to you as it smells to everyone else.

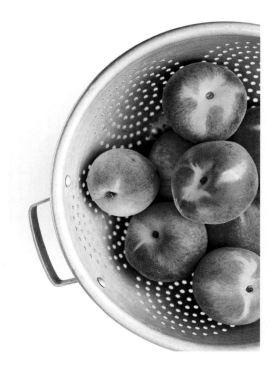

Q The different cholesterol numbers confuse me. Which ones matter?

A: Even we have trouble wrapping our heads around the heart math. So we asked *Men's Health* advisor Prediman K. Shah, M.D., the director of cardiology at Cedars-Sinai Medical Center in Los Angeles, to help us make the numbers less fuzzy.

"The single best predictor of cardiovascular disease is your non-HDL cholesterol, which is your total cholesterol minus HDL," says Dr. Shah. That's because this calculation results in a figure representing your LDL and more esoteric artery-clogging particles, such as VLDL and Lp(a). In a study recently presented at the American Heart Association conference, Dr. Shah and his colleagues found that non-HDL beat every other cholesterol calculation in predicting who would develop heart disease over an 11-year follow-up period. To stay in the safe zone, aim for a non-HDL level of 130 or less.

Q Is the DASH diet legit or just hype?

A: In case you're scratching your head right now, the acronym stands for Dietary Approaches to Stop Hypertension. The plan was developed by the National Heart, Lung, and Blood Institute and involves maintaining your total calorie consumption at 55 percent carbs, 27 percent fat, and 18 percent protein while keeping your sodium intake under 2,300 milligrams a day. A typical DASH menu focuses on fruits and vegetables, whole grains, and protein from poultry, fish, beans, and nuts while minimizing added sugars and salt.

So yes, as a way to fight high blood pressure with food, the DASH diet is completely legit. In fact, a study in the *Archives of Internal Medicine* found that it can lower systolic blood pressure by up to 16 points in 4 months in people with high BP.

But even if your pressure is perfect, you still might want to give it a shot: Research shows that the diet can also lower your LDL cholesterol as well as your risk of diabetes and colon cancer. Need more incentive? Try this: A University of Rhode Island study suggests that a reduced-calorie DASH diet paired with resistance training 3 days a week can help you lose 7 pounds in 10 weeks, gain muscle, and decrease body-fat mass by 11 percent. Visit nhlbi.nih.gov/health/public/heart to download a free guide.

Q Is it possible to have a stroke and not know it?

A: You're thinking of a silent stroke, a brain attack that happens just as a regular stroke does—when a blocked or leaking blood vessel disrupts circulation, damaging surrounding tissue.

Where the two differ is in the symptoms: With a silent stroke, you don't notice an immediate change in cognitive or physical function, says Adam M. Brickman, Ph.D., an assistant professor of neuropsychology at Columbia University. "It could be that the stroke didn't affect a large enough area of the brain, or it could be in a region that doesn't control some major function."

Still, the event is far from harmless. In a new study, Brickman found that silent-stroke sufferers had poorer memory and a smaller hippocampus (a part of the brain that governs memory) than people who'd never had silent strokes. These brain changes could lead to a full-on stroke and may set you up for dementia.

Reduce your risk of silent stroke by keeping your blood pressure below 120/80 and your LDL cholesterol under 100. Exercising at moderate to heavy intensity might also help protect your brain: A study published in the journal *Neurology* shows that people who regularly ran, bicycled, or swam were 40 percent less likely to suffer silent strokes than other people who stayed put.

Hard Truth

55

The percentage increase in your stroke risk if you have hypertension— high blood pressure of 120 to 139 systolic or 80 to 89 diastolic, according to Neurology.

How can I avoid going for a colonoscopy?

A: You could opt for the less invasive fecal occult blood test. This screening simply involves providing a stool sample.

But while having this test is better than doing nothing, you are taking a risk: It catches only 20 percent to 32 percent of advanced cancerous growths, versus 100 percent for a colonoscopy, according to a German study. A colonoscopy gives your doctor a better shot at detecting suspicious growths, and it also reveals problem polyps that can be removed immediately, says Robert Sedlack, M.D., a gastroenterologist at the Mayo Clinic. "Depending on risk factors, it's recommended that men have them every 5 to 10 years starting at age 50."

In fact, a study in the *New England Journal of Medicine* shows that the removal of precancerous polyps during colonoscopy reduces your risk of dying of colon cancer by 53 percent. What's more, the 20-minute procedure itself is actually painless because you're sedated. And now there's even a slightly less onerous option for the standard bowel-cleansing prep of chugging a gallon of polyethylene glycol. Ask your doctor about split-dosing it, says Dr. Sedlack. It's equally effective but causes less discomfort.

Q Should I pay extra for "pharmaceutical grade" omega-3 and CoQ10 supplements?

A: Don't blow your dough. "Pharmaceutical grade" is marketing talk, says Tod Cooperman, M.D., president of ConsumerLab.com, a company that tests health products. "There's no FDA definition of the phrase for any supplements."

Instead, scan the label for words worth something: NSF International Certified or U.S. Pharmacopeial Convention (USP) Verified. Both certifications ensure that the supplement contains the type and amount of ingredients listed. If you'd rather not squint at fine print, buy USP-verified Nature Made supplements: The 1,200-milligram fish oil capsules have 180 milligrams of EPA and 120 of DHA, and cost 8 cents apiece; the 100-milligram CoQ10 soft gels contain oil to improve your body's uptake of the antioxidant, and cost 53 cents a pop.

Q Could sitting in heavy traffic every day damage my lungs?

A: You might be giving new meaning to the phrase "killer commute." Because you're surrounded by idling cars, you're basically sitting inside a cloud of exhaust fumes.

"The danger comes from high concentrations of toxins, such as particulate matter, that can accumulate in the air circulating inside your car," says Jeff Gearhart, M.S., research director at the Ecology Center, a Michigan environmental organization. These unseen enemies can cause lung trouble (including an elevated risk of cancer), and they can also raise your risk of a heart attack.

So what's a road warrior to do? Start with the obvious: If you're entering bumper-to-bumper hell, roll up your windows and set the ventilation to recirculate. Doing this reduces your exposure to particle pollution by at least 70 percent, say researchers at the University of Southern California. For extra insurance, Gearhart recommends replacing your car's dust and pollen filter (a.k.a. cabin filter) with one containing activated carbon (or charcoal), such as the Fram Fresh Breeze (available at Advance Auto Parts). Unlike standard paper filters, those with activated carbon also trap particulates and chemicals in vapor form, significantly improving the quality of the air.

Q What's the germiest thing in my home?

A: Your kitchen sponge. When scientists from NSF International tabulated the germ count on 30 household items in 22 homes, they found kitchen sponges and dishrags to be the top germ hot spots.

"We found a variety of bacteria, yeast, and mold that can cause foodborne illness," says study author Robert Donofrio, Ph.D. His advice: Sanitize sponges daily by rinsing them in water and then microwaving for 2 minutes; and replace them often, at least every 2 weeks. Change dishrags every other day, and disinfect them in your washing machine's hot water cycle with bleach.

Q When I have a hangover, what's really happening to my brain cells?

A: Those same chemicals in alcohol that tickle your cerebral cortex in the moment also hammer nails into it in the a.m. Here's the chain of intoxicating events: Your body metabolizes booze into acetaldehyde (similar to formaldehyde), which is turned into acetate (similar to vinegar), which is then processed into a neurochemical called adenosine, says Robert Swift, M.D., Ph.D., a professor of psychiatry and human behavior at Brown University. "Acetaldehyde is toxic to brain cells, and adenosine dilates blood vessels in your brain. The effect is a pounding headache."

But it doesn't stop there: Alcohol can lead to a drop in blood sugar, which creates a power shortage for your mental machinery.

"When your blood sugar is low, your brain cells can't produce enough energy and can't work properly, which slows your thinking," says Dr. Swift.

Your best bet to expedite recovery: Eat high-fiber carbs, such as oatmeal, to slowly raise your blood sugar; drink lots of water to combat dehydration; and sip caffeinated coffee to thwart the effects of adenosine metabolism, says Dr. Swift.

Q Is video chat just as good as meeting a psychologist in person?

A: There isn't enough clinical evidence to say, but one thing's certain: It's a hundred times better than doing nothing, says William S. Pollack, Ph.D., an associate professor of psychiatry at Harvard medical school. "Men who might be reluctant to slink into a shrink's office may feel more comfortable receiving treatment through video chat; plus, they're using a familiar technology, and that can help them open up."

It's also convenient for people who travel. And while Pollack prefers to meet a new patient in person first to make a connection, he has done initial consults through video chat. Before you bare your soul over Skype, make sure the psychologist has a doctorate (Ph.D. or Psy.D.) and a state license.

Also check your insurance coverage. There is a billing code for long-distance treatment, but not all providers reimburse it. Finally, ask the psychologist how many other people are being counseled remotely. "You want a therapist who's tech savvy and has had success treating people this way," says Pollack.

Q Do I really need to drink water all day to stay hydrated?

A: No, you can eat your H2O too. "Produce contains high percentages of water as well as antioxidants and essential minerals," says Leslie Bonci, M.P.H., R.D., director of sports nutrition at the University of Pittsburgh's center for sports medicine. You probably consume 20 percent of your fluids from food, and you can boost that percentage with highly saturated snacks. Of course, every time you eat a meal you should also drink: Sip 16 ounces of water or another low-cal beverage.

Hydration helpers: (Percentages indicate water content by weight.)

- **Cucumbers:** 97 percent
- **Raw radishes:** 95 percent
- **Celery:** 95 percent
- **Watermelon:** 91 percent
- **Raw broccoli:** 89 percent
- **Peaches:** 89 percent
- **Yogurt:** 88 percent
- **Raw carrots:** 88 percent
- **Plums:** 87 percent
- **Apples:** 86 percent

Q How worried should I be about BPA?

A: It's smart to be vigilant, but you don't need to be fitted for a hazmat suit. CDC research shows that as an average American, you carry a certain amount of BPA and other potentially toxic chemicals in your blood and fat. This is known as your "body burden," and it can be measured through a series of blood, breath, urine, and hair tests. The downside is that these tests are expensive and raise more questions than answers. "Body-burden testing isn't something I would routinely recommend," says Leonardo Trasande, M.D., an associate professor of environmental medicine and health policy at New York University. "However, if you can recall exposure to specific chemicals and are suffering from vague, chronic symptoms that have stumped doctors, it's worth consulting an environmental health expert." (Find one at aoec.org/directory.htm.) In the meantime, here's how to minimize the amount of new chemicals creeping in.

BPA (Bisphenol A)
The threat: Linked to hypertension, diabetes, and reduced sperm quality.
Where it lurks: Bisphenol A has been found in plastic water bottles, plastic food containers, and canned foods. To limit your exposure, buy cans labeled "BPA-free," says Ted Schettler, M.D., M.P.H., science director of the Science & Environmental Health Network. Never heat any plastic in the microwave; that promotes chemical leaching of BPA.

PBDEs (Polybrominated Diphenylethers)
The threat: These chemical flame retardants may disrupt thyroid function.
Where they lurk: Flame-resistant upholstered furniture, computers, and electronics can harbor PBDEs. Since you can't tell for sure if your sofa has flame retardants, eliminate what you can by keeping the dust in your home

under control. "Dust becomes a repository for the flame retardants that have migrated out of products," says Dr. Schettler.

PFOA (Perfluorooctanoic Acid)

The threat: Linked to high cholesterol and disruption of thyroid function.

Where it lurks: PFOA may be in nonstick cookware and some food packaging, such as popcorn bags and pizza boxes. Make popcorn in an air popper or on the stovetop, and tell the pizza delivery guy you don't want a nonstick box. If you get one anyway, remove your pizza promptly, Dr. Schettler says. You may be able to reduce your exposure by limiting contact time.

Phthalates

The threat: Researchers have found that phthalates can interfere with testosterone production and may be linked to weight gain and insulin resistance.

Where they lurk: Shower curtains made with polyvinyl chloride (PVC), plastic food containers, personal-care products, and fragrances can all have phthalates. If a plastic container's recycling symbol shows the number 3, then it's PVC. Choose grooming products that are phthalate-free; check the ingredient list. Fragrances and any products that list "fragrance" as an ingredient could also have phthalates. Go scentless.

Q Can I train myself to have lucid dreams?

A: You'll have to master the dark but illuminating art of realizing when you're dreaming. "We call it 'dream control,'" says W. Christopher Winter, M.D., medical director at Martha Jefferson Hospital sleep medicine center and *Men's Health* sleep medicine advisor. "It can have many psychological benefits, such as relieving stress, as well as making your dream life more exciting." Your apprenticeship starts by learning these reality checks.

1. Study your hands. "Dream hands" tend to be a different color or have a missing or extra digit because you rarely focus on your hands, says Dr. Winter. Study your hands a few times each day, picturing how they look. Each time, say this mantra to yourself: "I'm awake; I'm not dreaming."

2. Push on your palm with your finger. If you do this in a dream, your finger will probably go right through the middle of your hand, says Dr. Winter. That's because your brain has a hard time replicating a physical sensation during a dream. At various times throughout the day, press your index finger into the center of your palm. When you feel the pressure, repeat the mantra.

3. Flip on a light switch. It's difficult for your brain to simulate light changes in a dream, says Dr. Winter. Anytime you flip a light switch, take note of the contrast in bright and dark, and then say the mantra.

Once these reality checks become part of your daily routine, they will emerge in your dreams, says Dr. Winter. When they appear, you'll realize you're dreaming and have the ability to dictate which scenarios you want to play out.

PART 7

Improve Your Game

The *Men's Health* Guide to Running Faster

What is the best way to do this simple sport? New science reveals surprising strategies to sprint faster, sidestep injury, burn more fat, and strengthen your brain and heart. Don't get left behind!

Left foot, right foot, repeat a gazillion times—how hard could running be? Turns out there are plenty of ways to do it better. Here, we talk about preparation, fine points, diagnostics, and even inspiration to help you run faster.

Preparation

With the rise barefoot-style running and the five-fingered minimalist shoe, the science of stride mechanics—once the arcane province of running geeks—has entered the mainstream. Has running, the most elemental of sports, really become so complex? Does the average guy hoping to go out for a pain-free run really have to fret about all this?

Men's Health joined forces with *Runner's World* magazine to bring you the best answers to these questions. You'll find out how to clean up your stride, strengthen your legs, blast belly fat, prevent injuries, train for a half marathon without losing muscle, and approach that cute speedster in hip-huggers and a sports bra. Here's to happy running!

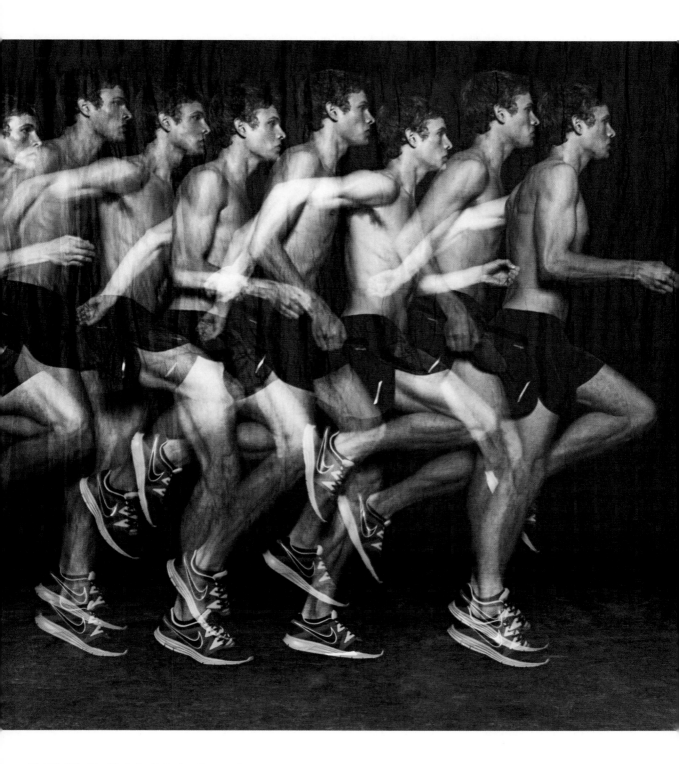

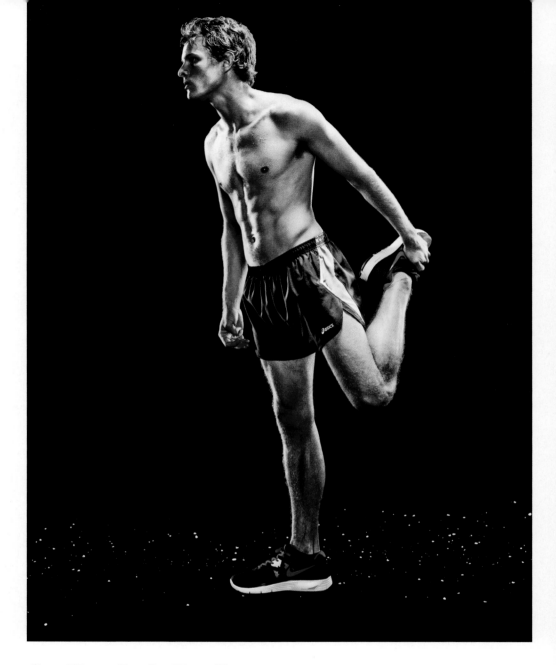

Can Your Body Handle Running?

With each stride, up to five times your weight slams through your feet, ankles, knees, hips, and spine. If your muscles are weak, you risk injury, says Bill Hartman, P.T., of Indianapolis Fitness and Sports Training.

Do this drill 3 days a week to strengthen your weakest areas.

Ankle Mobilizer

Helps with: ankle flexibility

From a staggered stance, palms on a wall, bend your knees and shift forward until you feel your forward ankle stretch. (Try not to raise your heels.) Bring your front knee close to the wall. Hold for 3 seconds. That's 1 rep. Do 20 reps, switch legs, and repeat.

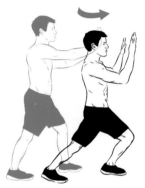

Reverse Lunge and Rotation

Helps with: hip mobility

Step back with your left foot and lower your body into a lunge as you rotate your upper body to the right. Return to the starting position. That's 1 rep. Do 3 sets of 12 and then repeat, this time stepping back with your right leg while rotating to the left.

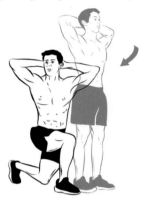

Single-Leg Straight-Leg Deadlift

Helps with: hip stability

Hold a dumbbell in your left hand. Lift your right foot as you slowly bend and lower the dumbbell. Once it reaches mid-shin, return to upright. Complete 12 reps on one leg, and then switch sides and repeat. Do 3 sets.

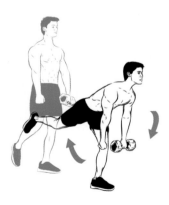

Wall-Press Abs

Helps with: core strength

Lie down. Now brace your core and push against a wall as you lower your bent right leg and touch your heel to the floor. Reverse the move and repeat with your left leg. Keep alternating for 60 seconds, and then rest for 1 minute. Do 2 or 3 sets.

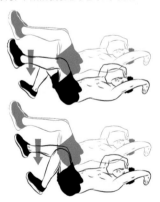

The Fast Lane

What's the secret to faster gains? Doing intervals—alternating hard efforts and recovery periods—yields performance gains similar to steady-state training, but in a fraction of the time. As a bonus, you benefit from greater fat loss and better blood-sugar management. But ease into it. Your first workout should be half the time or distance and half as many reps as your ultimate goal, says exercise physiologist Janet Hamilton, C.S.C.S. Then gradually increase the number of repeats. Use this guide to match your goal to the right workout.

Turbo-Charge Your Fitness

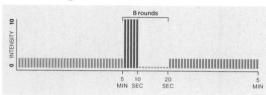

Total time: 14 minutes

"These ultra-intense intervals not only burn fat and reduce insulin resistance but also increase aerobic and anaerobic conditioning, making you a better athlete," says Nathan Trenteseaux, the owner of Underground Fitness Revolution in Alachua, Florida. Do them 3 days a week; after 4 weeks, switch to 20 seconds on and 10 seconds off.

Blast Your Belly

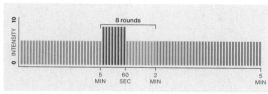

Total time: 34 minutes

In a 2011 Canadian study, people running intervals lost 12.4 percent of their body fat after 6 weeks. The reason: The intensity makes you burn extra calories even after the run is over. Other research shows that this kind of interval can boost Levels of HDL (good) cholesterol by 25 percent and improve blood glucose control. Do these 3 days a week.

Boost Your Speed

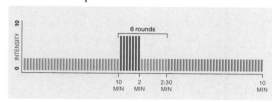

Total time: 47 minutes

This kind of interval boosts your aerobic capacity, says Hamilton. The more oxygen you can take in and utilize, the faster you can run. A 2011 University of Western Ontario study found that runners who did three weekly interval sessions for 6 weeks improved their time on a 2,000-meter run by 4.6 percent. Work up to 8 rounds.

Extend Your Stamina

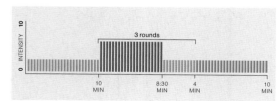

Total time: 57:30 minutes

Most people start a long run too quickly and then slow down. This plan teaches you pace discipline—sticking to a steady speed that you can sustain over the long haul. It also trains your muscles to be more efficient at faster speeds, says Hamilton. Do these once a week, building to 6 rounds. Note: Instead of timed intervals, you can run 1 mile.

Fine Points

"There has to be one best way of running," Alberto Salazar once said. "It's got to be like a law of physics." The iconic American marathoner is pursuing that theory with his elite coaching program, the Nike Oregon Project. His new book is out now, *14 Minutes: A Running Legend's Life and Death and Life.*

Fix Your Form

You can run with fewer injuries, greater efficiency, and ultimately more pleasure, if you follow the four simple rules from Salazar that follow and do regular sprint drills. (See "Speed School" on page 310.)

Lean forward. Aim for a slight forward tilt—about two or three degrees, says Salazar. You don't want to lean too far forward or too far back. Too far forward, and you shove your full body weight into the ground with each stride. Too far back, and you jam your heels.

To promote a properly tilted and aligned neck and torso, allow your eyes to guide you. Instead of looking down at the ground, let your gaze settle on the horizon. Keep your chin tucked in instead of letting it jut out.

Take a hand. "The typical runner never thinks about his hands, but in fact they're crucial," Salazar says. "Your arms should swing back and forward, not across your body." With each stride, bring your hand to the vertical midpoint of your torso, but don't let your hand cross that midline. If it does, your body will rock from side to side.

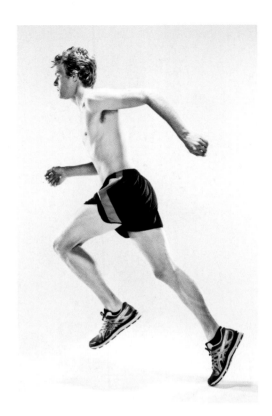

To release tension in your hands and arms, run with your hands forming a loose fist; imagine that each hand is carrying a pretzel that you don't want to break.

Be on the ball. "If you land on your heel, you're almost certainly overstriding," says Salazar. "You're pounding your leg into the ground with each stride and increasing your risk of injury. When you land on the balls of your feet, you flow with your forward energy." A recent study of Harvard runners supports Salazar's theory; it found that forefoot strikers have fewer injuries than heel strikers.

Flick back your heel quickly after contact; visualize pawing the ground with the balls of your feet.

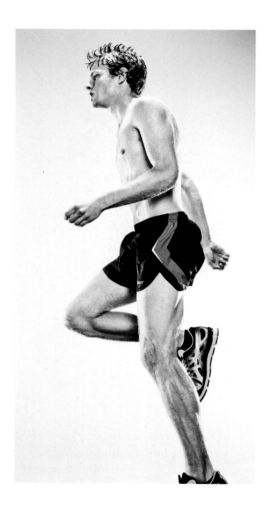

Speed School

Jog 5 minutes, and then do each of these drills for 30 seconds. They help you run on the balls of your feet.

Arm Circles with Skip

As you skip, swing your arms in a forward circular motion as wide and as high as you can. After 30 seconds, swing backward.

Cross-Body Toe Touch

Every three steps, lift your leg as high as you can and swing your opposite arm to touch your elevated toes. Alternate sides each rep.

"A" Skip with Knee to Chest

Skip, but every three steps lift your knee toward your chest. Alternate sides. This pushes you onto the balls of your feet.

"B" Skip

Follow the "A" skip pattern, but kick your leg out in a quick burst once your leg reaches its apex. Try to do it as fast as possible.

Fast-Leg High-Knees

Do a single high-knee as fast as you can, and then jog a few steps and switch knees.

Fast-Leg Butt Kicks

Your hamstrings and quads have opposing functions. Butt kicks warm up both. Do a butt kick as quickly as you can, jog a few steps, and switch the kicking leg.

Use your arms. The fourth key to a successful stride, Salazar says, is arm carriage. "Your shoulders need to be relaxed and sloping down, and your elbows should be slightly bent," he says. "If you tighten your shoulders and let them point up instead, your arms start to flail and you lose that circular, forward-flowing drive."

As fatigue sets in, your shoulders tend to lift and tighten. When this happens, briefly drop your hands and shake out your arms to relax your muscles.

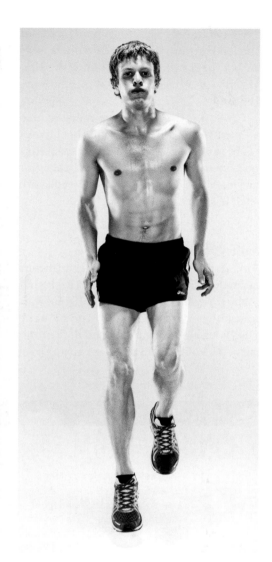

Find a partner. If you spy an interesting runner, compliment her stride or her shoes, says Olympian Kara Goucher. Or join a club (rrca.org). You'll meet educated, fun, and fast women!

Create a mantra. Think brief, positive, and instructive. For instance, says *Runner's World* editor-in-chief David Willey, to fight fatigue when powering up a hill, think, claw the ground.

Strike like a ninja. Listen to your stride: ninja good, elephant bad. "Lean forward slightly," suggests Scott Berlinger, coach at Full Throttle Endurance. It will help you touch down on your forefoot.

Zoom up hills. "Increase your arm swing, as if you were pulling yourself quickly up a rope," says Larry Indiviglia, a coach based in San Diego. "And lift your knees higher."

Ignite your stride. If you're tiring during a race or while doing intervals and need a mental boost, imagine you're on hot coals, Galloway says. Hot damn, you'll speed up your stride!

Run for a cause. "It boosts your incentive. With social media you can now gain support from friends and family non-invasively," says *Runner's World* chief running officer Bart Yasso.

Outfox negativity. "If you hit a bad patch, try counting your steps," says Goucher. "When you hit 100, start over at 1. It can help take your mind off your troubles and put you back on track."

Join treadmill U. "The rhythms of treadmill running boost learning," says coach Matt Barbosa. You can use an easy run to rehearse a presentation or listen to an educational podcast.

Boredom Busters

Running can be a head game. Use the following motivational tips to come out on top.

Shift to walk speed. Going long? Break up the tedium by running 4 minutes and then walking 30 seconds, coach Jeff Galloway says. "You'll recover faster and can finish quicker."

Diagnostics

With running, like so many things, it's going great—until it's not. Here's how to figure out why your run is in a rut, or worse.

Where Does It Hurt?

First, let's dispel two myths. New research reveals that running isn't bad for your knees and won't give you a heart attack. Use this guide to diagnose regular injuries and run pain-free.

Achilles Tendinitis

The problem: Your Achilles tendons tense and extend with each stride. Weak calves strain them.

The big risk: Running uphill increases the load on your calves and Achilles, says Bryan Heiderscheit, P.T., Ph.D., of the University of Wisconsin sports medicine center.

The fix: Do calf raises: Balance on a step on your right foot so your heel hangs off it; raise your left foot behind you. Rise onto your toes; then lower your heel as far as you can. Do 2 sets of 10 to 15 reps with each leg twice a week.

Iliotibial Band Syndrome

The problem: The IT band is a fibrous tissue on the outside of your thigh that stabilizes your knees and hips. If your hips and knees twist too much, the IT band rubs your lateral femoral condyle, a prominent part of your thigh bone, causing pain

---

WHAT YOU CAN LEARN ABOUT RUNNING FROM . . .

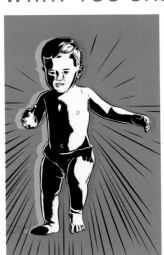

Toddlers: They tend to land on the balls of their feet. Try running barefoot for 2 minutes after your regular run, says biomechanics researcher Peter Larson, Ph.D. You'll adapt to the lack of cushioning by landing closer to your body.

The Road Runner: There's a running method to the madness of the bird's whirring legs. An efficient running economy is about 90 steps a minute per foot, says exercise physiologist Jack Daniels, Ph.D. Count your steps for a minute, and if your number is under 90, shorten your stride.

Forrest Gump: He went for a little run and ended up across the country. *Runner's World* editor at large Amby Burfoot offers two takeaways: (1) Aim to go a bit farther or a bit faster each week; and (2) use races to explore places in America. To find the best races, visit runnersworld.com/racefinder.

Bison: Strong tendons help these burly beasts hurdle 6-foot fences and outrun horses in endurance races. To gain more spring, says decathlete Bryan Clay, do this plyometric circuit once or twice a week: box jump, single-leg hop, lateral jump (3 sets of 10 reps each).

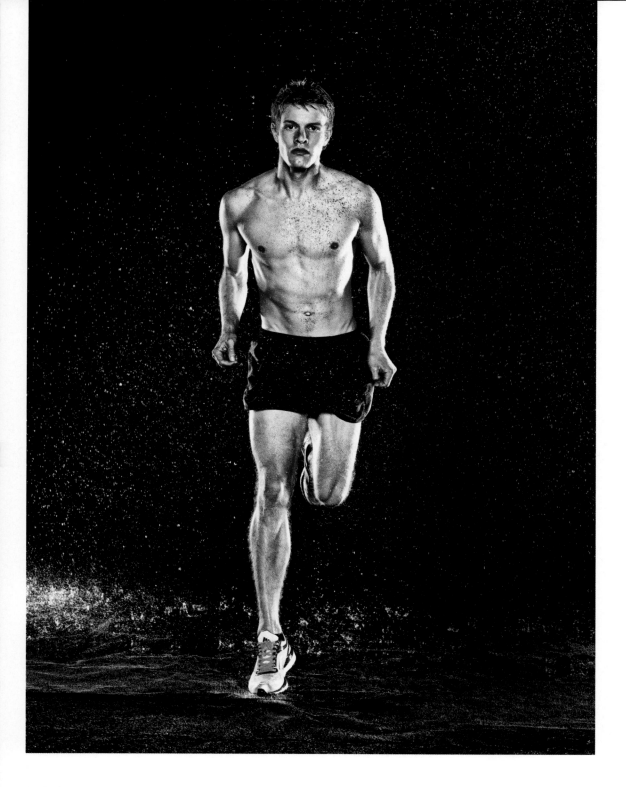

on the outside of your knee.

The big risk: A long stride increases force on your knees and IT bands.

The fix: To shorten your stride, boost your step rate by 5 to 10 percent, Heiderscheit says. Try to avoid landing hard on your heel, and keep your knee flexed about 20 degrees. Have a friend take video of you so you can check your form.

Shinsplints

The problem: You feel pain and soreness because your tibialis posterior muscle is pulling away from your shin bone. This muscle works with a larger calf muscle, your soleus, says Reed Ferber, Ph.D., director of the running injury clinic at the University of Calgary. "Your tibialis posterior is overworked and has to pull more of its weight," Ferber says.

The big risk: Weak muscles can expose you if you're new to running or returning after a hiatus.

The fix: Strengthen your tibialis posterior and soleus muscles with calf raises. Also try seated ankle invertors: Sit with your leg straight and loop a resistance band around your foot. Making sure your leg doesn't rotate, pull the top of your foot inward for 2 seconds, and release for 2 seconds. That's 1 rep. Do 1 set of 10 reps a day, working up to 3 sets a day.

Plantar Fascitis

The problem: The tight, thick plantar fascia supports the arch and works with a network of muscles across the bottom and sides of your foot. You might feel a sharp pain on the bottom of your heel, especially in the morning. (The tissue shortens at night.)

The big risk: Weak foot muscles strain the plantar fascia.

The fix: Do towel crunches: Put a towel on the floor, your heels on the ground, and your toes on the towel. "Make fists with your toes and scrunch the towel up," Ferber says. Do this every day for 15 minutes.

Runner's Knee

The problem: Your thigh bone rotates too far inward, pressuring your kneecap. You feel dull pain under your kneecap, especially when you sit a long time or take stairs.

The big risk: Running on steep or uneven terrain could cause runner's knee.

The fix: Strengthen your hip muscles, which control your thigh bones. Try these two moves, doing 1 set of 10 reps and working up to 3 sets a day. The standing hip abductor: Stand with one foot in the loop of a resistance band and the other foot on top of the band (adjust the length to control the resistance). Move the banded leg 2 seconds out, 2 seconds in. Then work your hip gluteus medius: Loop the band around and face a chair; move the banded leg back to 45 degrees, 2 seconds out, 2 seconds in.

Which Shoe for You?

No doubt about it, your shoe choice is critical to your running success. So much so that recently, *Runner's World* scrapped the system it had used for three decades to rate shoes. Too rigid, the editors said. Now *RW* emphasizes how much shoe a runner needs, noting the shoe's weight and the drop in height from heel to toe. *RW* also factors in body type, stride, and mileage. (For details, visit runnersworld.com/shoeadvisor.)

To identify your ideal pair, listen to your feet. We recently tested more than a dozen shoes with support features that spanned the spectrum from minimal to maximal. A good running shop will let you do the same on a treadmill.

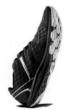

New Balance Minimus Zero
Price: $110
Weight: 6.4 OZ
Heel height: 12 MM
Forefoot height: 12 MM

Having these on is like wearing nothing, which makes any workout suck a little less. That feeling of wearing nothing can be a negative on longer runs.

Asics Gel-DS Racer 9
Price: $100
Weight: 7.7 OZ
Heel height 23 MM
Forefoot height: 14 MM

These feel more stable than the NB Minimus pair, but they're still light and nimble. Consider them for a 10-K race. The mesh sides and vented soles are floodgates in wet conditions.

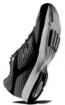

Newton Neutral Performance Trainer
Price: $175
Weight: 9.1 OZ
Heel height 31 MM
Forefoot height: 28 MM

These shoes can change your stride. Four ridges under your metatarsals encourage a midfoot strike. Almost felt like training wheels; pricey, too.

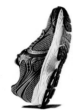

Saucony Powergrid Triumph 9
Price: $130
Weight: 10.9 OZ
Heel height 34 MM
Forefoot height: 26 MM

Wearing these was like running on a cloud. We loved the tongue pocket. They're a bit clunky for speed work.

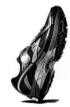

Brooks Ravenna 3
Price: $100
Weight: 10.9 OZ
Heel height 24 MM
Forefoot height: 14 MM

This new model is just as stable and supportive. We prefer the old model; find endangered shoes at roadrunnersports .com.

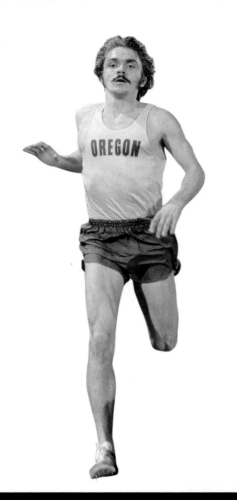

Inspiration

The great ones motivate us to push our limits, whether in a road race or the rat race.

Steve Prefontaine set U.S. records at every distance from 2 miles to 10,000 meters, and narrowly missed a medal at the '72 Olympics. Three years later he was gone—killed in a car crash at 24, like James Dean. To emulate Pre's cool, you could grow a 'stache, lace up a pair of Nike Classic Cortez shoes ($65, nike.com), and slip on his high school #13 singlet ($30, prefontainerun.com).

But to truly be like Pre, you must embrace his attitude: the go-for-broke swagger, the life-is-short tenacity, and the winner's mentality. "To give anything less than your best is to sacrifice the gift," he said. Pre inspires people to run that way, and to live that way, too.

Usain Bolt is a 21st-century version of

FAST ABS

A strong core ensures that any runner is stable at top speeds. Use these moves.

Hip Raise

Lie on your back with your heels on a 30" box; raise your hips so your body forms a line. Hold 15 seconds, then rest 15 seconds. Do 2 sets of 8.

Single-Leg Plank

Hold for 2 minutes; rest 1 minute. Repeat 2 times.

Bicycle Crunch

Do 4 sets of 45 seconds, with 1 minute of rest in between. Stop if you feel back pain.

the young Muhammad Ali. So secure is his sense of destiny and mastery of his craft that he can play the jester. Bolt possesses an uncanny ability to read situations—to pivot from dance to reflection and give whatever the moment demanded. What else is the 100-meter dash but a single, searing moment? He lives gloriously in the moment, even if it's a slow and tedious one, and he reminds us to do the same. In the London Olympics, he won three gold medals and declared himself "the greatest athlete."

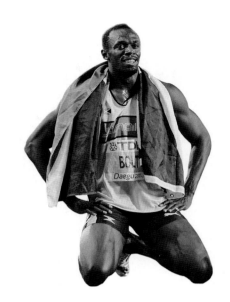

RUNNING MAKES YOU SMARTER!

Sharper memory, better mood, new brain cells—the research is in. Running blows your mind! Here's real-world proof.

The atomic physicist: "I run six times a week first thing in the morning, usually for an hour. Afterward I'm energized: I'm more spontaneous, and in a positive sense I'm more aggressive at getting work done. Running gives me a fresh mind and makes me more focused and efficient."—Wolfgang Ketterle, Ph.D., Massachusetts Institute of Technology, Nobel Laureate in physics

The inventor: "Running focuses my mind and allows me to think around a subject. I still need a workshop to make discoveries, but on a run I might think of a new avenue to explore. Another thing I learned from running is that the time to push hard is when you're hurting like crazy. The moment you should

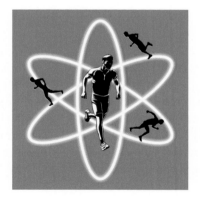

accelerate is the moment you're the most tired. I found that to be so in life as well."—Sir James Dyson, founder and chief engineer of Dyson, manufacturer of vacuums and fans

The tech whiz: "I really started running for meditative purposes. I would pick some problem to have in my head while running—not for the purpose of solving it, but for the purpose of having it bounce around in there. Like when you say you're going to sleep on it; I say I'm going to run on it. Then at some point later on, a solution falls out." —Biz Stone, cofounder of Twitter

The novelist: "I try not to think about anything special while I'm running. As a matter of fact, I usually run with my mind empty. However, when I run empty-minded, something naturally and abruptly crawls in sometimes. That might become an idea that can help me with my writing."—Haruki Murakami, author of *1Q84*

The Flab Assassin

Frank Matrisciano is the most secretive sports trainer in the world. Many also call him the toughest. But survive his training, and you'll emerge a new (fitter, stronger) man. Just ask writer Andrew W. Heffernan. In his own words . . .

Hell's Trainer has no website, no newsletter, and no Facebook page. You can't just drop in on a class to sample a workout. If you do manage to track him down, he'll communicate only by phone. He's 6 feet tall and 230 pounds, with 7 percent body fat. In photographs, he wears a mask. It makes him look like a ninja linebacker.

Yet despite the man's best efforts, the word is out: "Frank Matrisciano [Hell's Trainer's real name] is the best in the world at what he does," says Josh Pastner, head basketball coach for the University of Memphis Tigers. And what he does is an extremely intense brand of strength and cardiovascular conditioning that eschews the sweaty comforts of most gyms for real-world (usually outdoor) workouts that push the limits of human strength, power, and endurance—and inspire seemingly superhuman results.

How intense are those workouts? Seven out of 10 people don't return for a second session, and many tap out just a few minutes in. But the ones who do stick with the program are often transformed dramatically: After a 6-week stint with Matrisciano in the summer of 2011, NBA All-Star Zach Randolph emerged as an entirely new athlete, helping push the

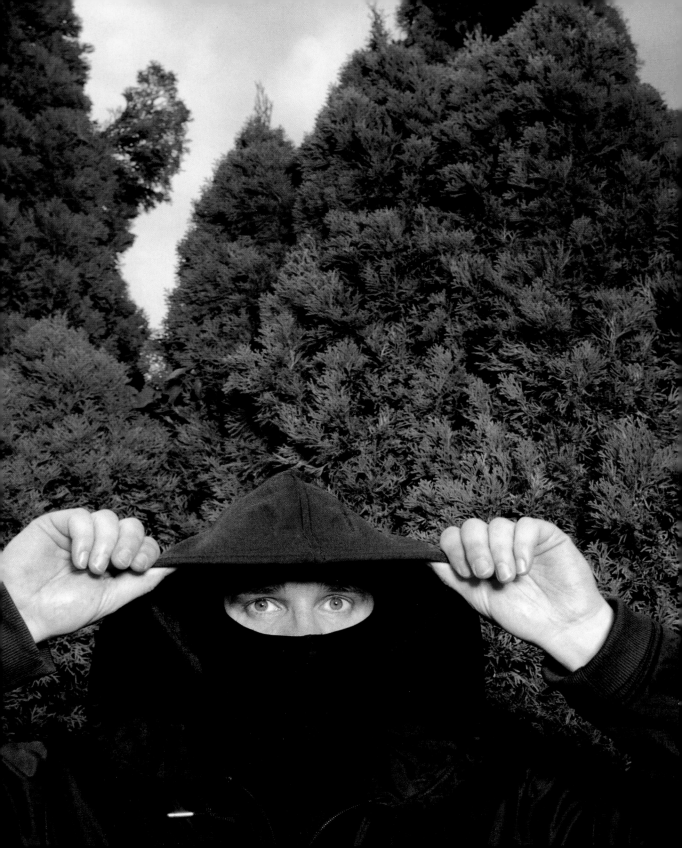

> ## "Compared with the mental challenge of my workouts, everyday stress is nothing."

Memphis Grizzlies to the first round of the playoffs.

As a personal trainer and lifetime fitness obsessive, I'm more than a little skeptical of "gurus," especially those who wear masks. But the buzz around Hell's Trainer was too loud to ignore. Why are so many top athletes seeking out a guy with no apparent credentials, no obvious affiliations, and apparently no face? Has he discovered a new way to push clients past their limits, or are they just enthralled by his Svengali trainer mystique? I decided to find out for myself.

A Meeting

"How ya doing, Sir?" asks Matrisciano, pulling up to my hotel in Memphis. It's 8 a.m., and we're headed to breakfast before joining the Tigers for a workout. It's the first time I've seen his face; his shaved head and New Jersey affect make him look and sound like Travis Bickle's less disturbed older brother.

For a mask-wearing mediaphobe, he turns out to be surprisingly voluble, so I ask him about his disguise. "I don't want to be bothered," he says simply.

When word of Matrisciano's effect on NBA stars like Randolph and Blake Griffin began to spread, sports agents descended on him in droves, looking for the next superstar to emerge from his program. But the trainer wanted no part of that. So now when the cameras come out, the mask goes on. That way, he says, agents can't pick him out of a crowd.

Of course, the disappearing act also draws the attention of journalists and curiosity seekers—like me—who might otherwise leave him alone. But the irony doesn't seem to compute with him. Free of the queries of agents, he can focus on his mission: "We all have a voice in our heads that tells us we can't go on," he says. "My job is to get people to silence it."

Decades of exercise and sports training have helped Matrisciano amass a host of exercises that make the voice kick in quickly. Outdoor activities are among his favorites: running hills; climbing stairs, poles, and ropes; doing drills on playground equipment; running long distances with heavy loads.

Though Matrisciano isn't averse to traditional gym training, he believes that exercising outdoors presents novel challenges—uneven running surfaces, natural obstacles, shifting weather conditions—that force you to pay closer attention to what you're doing and to work harder than you would indoors.

"You have to adapt continually to your environment," says Matrisciano. "My cousin Michael started calling it 'chameleon training,' and I think that describes it pretty well."

CrossFit, P90X, and hard-core military training all share similarities with his approach.

"But those are Chameleon Lite,"

Matrisciano jokes. "One day of Chameleon training is equal to 2 weeks of illusion training," he adds, referring to the cookie-cutter workouts offered by many gyms. "You can do lat pulldowns all day and never be strong enough to climb a rope. But if you can climb a rope, you'll crush the lat pulldown."

Rebuilding bodies, however, is only part of what he does.

"I tell my NBA guys that this training is not just for basketball; it's for their whole life." Same goes for the lawyers, executives, and everyday Joes on his client roster. "Compared with the mental challenge of my workouts, everyday stress is nothing," he says.

Despite Matrisciano's penchant for exercising outdoors, he is sometimes forced to bring his workouts inside. Case in point: the University of Memphis. "There are no hills in Memphis," he notes. "And there aren't many outdoor sites that offer what I need, so I adapted to my environment." Or rather, he created a new one from scratch.

Matrisciano avoids referring to his facility at the university as a gym. It's his Area of Operation (or "A.O."), and it's like nothing I've ever seen. There are no squat racks or benches. No yoga studios or swimming pools. No cute front-desk girls. There's just a large open area covered by black mats; a few carefully selected machines; and a massive, custom-built, two-story steel structure called the "Chameleon."

Matrisciano had it built to mimic the sand hills, playground equipment, and other outdoor features he utilizes in San Francisco, his home base for the past 10 years. On its front is a steep AstroTurf ramp for indoor hill sprints. The back sports an assortment of poles, ropes, and other climbing equipment. It looks like the world's most intimidating jungle gym.

I quickly find that the Chameleon is also booby-trapped with features that make normally tough exercises even tougher. The stairs adjacent to the ramp, for example, are unusually steep. And when I grab a horizontal ladder, the rung spins out of my hand.

As impressive as it is, however, the Chameleon is far from essential; during the 2 months it was being built, all Matrisciano did with the Tigers was body-weight drills. He crushed them.

"It's not about the equipment," he says. "It's about the mindset."

An Hour Later

I'm 3 minutes into the workout alongside four exceptionally fit Memphis Tigers, and I'm getting a very personal taste of the mind games Matrisciano warned me about.

I've had moments of doubt during workouts before, but this is different. The voice is screaming at me: Stop trying to prove yourself! Just sit down and take notes! No one will care.

Puking and passing out feel like very real possibilities, but I swallow hard and continue our circuit of pushups, swims (a dry-land breaststroke), and climbs up an 18-foot fireman's pole using only our arms. We repeat the circuit four times. No rest.

On the next circuit, we switch things up with an exercise called "Save the Kids."

Hanging beneath a pair of 12-foot-high parallel bars, we hand-walk from one end to the other. We're shooting for multiple sets. I hope I'll finish one.

Ahead of me, a 6'9" senior named Wesley Witherspoon hits up Matrisciano for some motivation.

"Who's over there?" Witherspoon asks.

"Your dad!" shouts Matrisciano. "His leg's broken! Go get him!"

One by one, Frank gives each of us a life-or-death scenario to drive us past our fatigue and help us ignore the loud protestations of the voice. When my turn comes, I imagine my 3-year-old son being trapped in a burning building: I'm coming, buddy! I think, and hurl myself across the bars with surprising determination.

And on it goes: three more rounds of pushups and kid saving; two more trips up the pole; more pushups and swims; seemingly endless sandbag drags. Pause for even a second and he's on you.

And then it's over. I've been going for all of 27 minutes, and I'm spent. "Is this a normal workout for you guys?" I ask Witherspoon.

"It's always challenging, physically and mentally," he says. "You want to stop. Your body tells you to stop. But Frank won't let you. It puts you in a mental state you've never been in before."

In the end, it's that ability to help his clients quiet their mental demons that sets Matrisciano apart from other strength coaches. He doesn't keep track of how high his players jump, how fast they sprint, or how much they deadlift. He doesn't know how much they weigh or what their body-fat percentages are. Nor does he care. Empirical markers of progress mean nothing to him.

"If you're doing my workouts and busting your ass, you improve," he says.

Most of us understand intuitively that we're supposed to push ourselves when we

DIY HELLACIOUS WORKOUTS

Here's how to put the science behind Frank Matrisciano's training program to work for you.

TAKE IT OUTSIDE. Gyms are comfortable, convenient, and well lit—and that's exactly why they might be holding you back. Matrisciano prefers to sweat outdoors, where the uneven terrain, unexpected hills, and unpredictable weather force you to constantly adapt, encouraging consistent results.

DIVERSIFY. Instead of following a "routine," Matrisciano regularly incorporates new drills, obstacles, and exercises (or exercise variations) into his workouts. Such nonlinear training can lead to greater gains than less varied routines offer, notes a study in the *Journal of Strength and Conditioning Research*.

FIRE YOURSELF UP. Matrisciano gives some workouts imaginary life-or-death stakes, which help his clients push past physical and mental limits to reach new levels of performance. Chalk it up to fight-or-flight energy. The more you can tap into it, the harder you'll go and the more progress you'll make toward your goals.

BE RELENTLESS. Most trainers schedule strength and cardio sessions on separate days. Matrisciano often combines them into one workout, stringing exercises into total-body circuits with minimal rest. Known as "metabolic resistance training," it's the fastest way to burn fat and increase cardiovascular endurance.

exercise. But when we arrive at the gym, we submit to the siren call of the voice. We tell ourselves that it doesn't have to be so hard. That progress is supposed to be gradual. It's only by silencing the voice—digging in, pushing your limits, and doing the hard stuff, even if it freaks you out—that you'll ever actually run faster, lift more, lose fat, and transform your body. And that's why an increasing number of men are seeking out Matrisciano's help. His true A.O. isn't a basketball gym, the Chameleon, or even the hills of San Francisco. It's the murky, ever-shifting landscape of the mind.

"Train like this for long enough and a weird thing happens," says Matrisciano. "The voice changes; it starts being positive." Instead of holding you back, it spurs you on, helping you build strength and power that translate far beyond the gym. "Whatever you do in life," says Matrisciano, "this type of training makes you better at it."

The Sweat 16

Need more flash in your drives? More lift in your layups? Try these drills from the NCAA's elite strength and conditioning coaches.

Hoops is a game of attrition, a fact that becomes painfully clear every March. The strongest, healthiest, and best-conditioned teams are the last ones standing.

So to help you elevate your game, we recruited 16 of the NCAA's top strength and conditioning coaches, whose teams often play long after everyone else has gone home. Use their favorite training tricks and tips to pick up your performance. But the real reward is this: These routines blast fat and build muscle. Who says your best days on the court—and in front of the mirror—are behind you?

Break Fast

JONAS SAHRATIAN, C.S.C.S.,
University of North Carolina

To make sure his players are the first ones down the court on a fast break, Sahratian has his Tar Heels do resisted sprints: One player runs as hard as he possibly can while a partner stands behind him and slows him down using a special harness. To buy your own, search for "resistance trainers" on the Perform Better website ($45, performbetter.com).

You can achieve a similar workout, though, with an everyday bath towel.

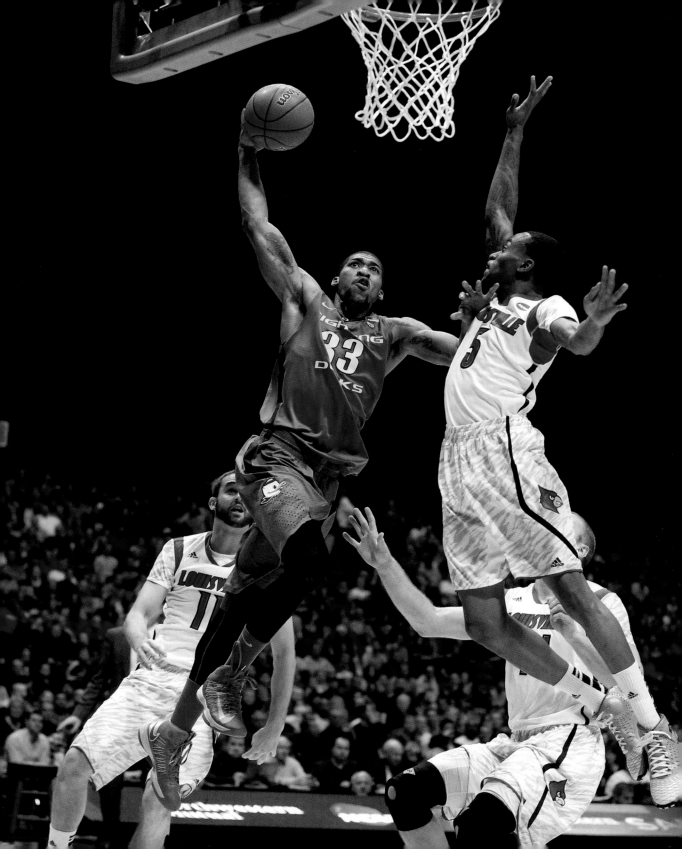

Wrap the towel around your waist and have a workout partner stand behind you and hold its ends. Then run as fast as you possibly can for 10 to 20 yards as he provides resistance. Rest for 30 seconds. Repeat the drill five times, and then try it once without resistance.

To see the total-body conditioning workout that Sahratian uses with the Tar Heels, go to MensHealth.com, keywords "tar heels workout." It's a muscle-building, fat-blasting routine that requires only an 8-pound medicine ball.

Cash the Boards

MIKE MALONE, C.S.C.S.,
University of Kentucky

The Wildcats dominate the boards because of the band overhead squat, a warmup move that adds spring to their steps. Grab a half-inch-wide resistance band, with your hands shoulder-width apart. Stand on the band and spread your feet slightly beyond shoulder width. Press the band overhead and hold it there with your arms straight; this is the starting position. Push your hips back and squat until your thighs are at least parallel to the floor. (Keep your torso upright and your back naturally arched.) Explosively spring back to the starting position. Do 2 or 3 sets of 6 to 10 reps before any game or workout.

Grab and Go

RYAN CABILES, C.S.C.S., Syracuse University
Great basketball requires relentless movement—setting rock-solid screens, boxing out for a big rebound, and playing dogged defense. Cabiles puts his Orange to the test with a drill called around the world: Set an empty container under the hoop. Distribute five cones evenly along the three-point line, or about 20 feet from the container, and place a tennis ball on each cone. Starting at the container, sprint to the ball farthest to your right, grab it, sprint back, and drop it into the receptacle. Spin around, retrieve the next ball, and sprint back. Repeat until you've retrieved all five. Do this drill 8 to 10 times, alternating your starting direction. Rest 30 to 45 seconds between drills.

Stretch Your Boundaries

CHARLIE MELTON, C.S.C.S., S.C.C.C.,
Baylor University

Basketball is a game of length, and the farther you can extend your limbs in every direction without hurting yourself, the more distance you can cover. The Bears boost their range of motion with the spiderman crawl, a lower-body drill that builds mobility. Assume a pushup position. Now take a big step forward with your right foot and place it outside your right hand. Pause for a few seconds, and then lower your head and chest for a deeper stretch in your thigh muscles. Walk your hands out until you're once again in a pushup position, and step forward with your left leg. Do 8 to 10 reps on each side.

Get Tenacious on D

SCOTT HETTENBACH, C.S.C.S.,
University of Wisconsin

To build strength and endurance in the defensive quarter-squat position, the Badgers do the triangle of terror. You'll need an exercise band with handles. Grab the handles and stand on the band, over its center, with your feet shoulder-width apart. Push your hips back, bend your knees, and press your arms straight out from your sides so you're in a D stance. Mimic how you'd move on defense by shuffling 10 steps to the right and then 10 steps to the left. Repeat 5 times. That's 1 set. Do 5, resting 1 minute in between.

Achieve Liftoff

ANDREA HUDY, C.S.C.S., University of Kansas

True power comes from quick, strong movements—similar to what happens when you jump to block a shot. That's why the dumbbell single-arm snatch is a staple of the Jayhawks' workouts. In a hip-width stance, grab a dumbbell in your left hand and hold it, using an overhand grip, at arm's length in front of your hips. Then bend at your hips and knees until the weight hangs just above your knees. Now jump, shrug your left shoulder, pull the dumbbell up, and catch it overhead with your arm straight. Do 4 sets of 3 reps with each arm.

Hunker Down

TIM BELTZ, C.S.C.S., University of Pittsburgh

Squats are tricky for hoops players—long limbs and torsos might make it tougher for them to maintain optimal form. The Zercher squat lowers the center of gravity, so Pitt players stay safe while still squatting heavy. Set the bar in a rack just below chest height. Holding the bar in the crook of your arms, lift it off the supports. Step back, holding it against your abdomen and keeping your feet shoulder-width apart. Squat until your thighs are parallel to the floor. Return to standing. Do 3 sets of 5 reps, resting 2 minutes.

Stick the Landing

BOB ALEJO, C.S.C.S.,
North Carolina State University

The higher you jump, the harder you land, putting you at risk for serious injury. That's why the Wolfpack do eccentric stepups, an exercise that strengthens the muscles that help protect your knees and hips. Holding your arms straight out in front of you, keep your right leg straight and place your left foot on a step or bench that's 18 to 24 inches off the floor. This is the starting position. Without using your right leg, push down through your left heel to lift your body until both feet are on the step or bench. Take 2 seconds to return to the starting position. Complete 12 reps. Switch legs and repeat.

Branch Out

CURTIS TURNER, C.S.C.S., S.C.C.C.,
Vanderbilt University

The Commodores prepare to handle the unexpected with a drill called maps.

Players are given a map of the campus with various highlighted locations, each of which features a fitness challenge. Create your own map drill at a local park. Give yourself five challenges—squats, pullups, squat thrusts, pushups, and agility drills, say—and space them about 100 yards apart. Pick a number of repetitions for each that's difficult yet attainable. Go through the stations as quickly as you can two or three times. Do this once a week.

Think Fast

TRAVIS KNIGHT, C.S.C.S., Gonzaga University

Reaction time can mean the difference between smoking your opponent and being smoked. The Bulldogs use a unique hand-eye drill to build coordination and prepare themselves for intense NCAA game speed and pressure. Find a half dozen or more tennis balls. Mark half of them clearly with an L and the others with an R. Place the balls in a plastic bag. Without looking, reach in, grab a ball, and toss it against a wall. Catch the L balls with your left hand and the R balls with your right. When you miss a total of five, do 10 pushups. Stop the drill when you reach 50 pushups.

Get Warm

MIKE CURTIS, C.S.C.S., University of Virginia

A 2011 study found that a quick dynamic warmup might help players jump higher. So the Cavaliers do the multidirectional lunge: Hold a medicine ball in front of your chest, and stand with your feet hip-width apart; this is the starting posi-

tion. Do 3 lunges with your left leg: Lunge forward, step back. Lunge left, step back. Finally, step across your body with your left leg, turning your hips and shoulders to the right as you lunge. Return to the starting position. Repeat the lunges with your right leg. That's 1 rep. Do 1 or 2 sets of 4 to 6 reps to warm up.

Sweat to the Oldies

JE'NEY JACKSON, C.S.C.S., S.C.C.C., Indiana University

College ballers are magnificently conditioned athletes. Even some team managers could run the average weekend player off the court. The Hoosiers' warmup sequence would be a great cardio workout for anyone, and it works equally well before or after a training session. Stand on one end of the court. Jog to the other end. Backpedal to the start. Now do a high-knee run across the court, and again backpedal to the start. Follow that with a butt-kick run (lifting your heels high enough to kick your glutes on each step), a left-foot-leading side shuffle, a right-foot-leading side shuffle, and a high-kick run (like a drum major's strut) on your next four trips out. Backpedal to the start after each. Do this sequence once for a warmup, or do it 2 to 4 times for a fat-burning finisher.

Drive Hard

CHRIS WEST, C.S.C.S., University of Connecticut

West makes sure his Huskies are as solid as Mack trucks when driving to the basket by training them with the kneeling cable core press, a move that strengthens and stabilizes every muscle from hips to core to shoulders. To do it, attach a D handle to a hip-level pulley on a cable machine, and kneel with your right side next to the weight stack. Hold the handle against your chest. Press your arms straight out, hold for 10 seconds, and return the handle to your chest. Do this 10 times, and then turn around so your left side is next to the weight stack. Repeat the movement. That's 1 set. Do 1 more.

"Jop" Till You Drop
ANDY WEIGEL, C.S.C.S.,
University of Alabama

The next time you watch a game, check out the star players' feet: Sure, the players run and jump, but they also hop, leap, lunge, shuffle, and "jop"—jump off both feet and land on one. It's a lot of impact to absorb with one leg. That's why the Tide train with the multidirectional jop. Stand with your knees slightly bent. Jump forward 12 inches and land on your right foot. Hop backward to the start, landing on both feet. Repeat on your left foot. Next, do the sequence going sideways. Do 2 sets of 4 jops in each direction as a warmup. Or, for a fat-torching workout, hold a medicine ball in front of your chest and perform 4 sets of 4 in each direction.

Catch Air
JIMMY PRICE, C.S.C.S.,
University of Illinois

All else being equal, the guy who can jump highest has a tremendous advantage, so the Fighting Illini do band jumps to add inches to their vertical and improve their overall athleticism. You'll need an exercise band with handles. Grab a very heavy dumbbell and place it on the floor between your feet. Loop the band under the dumbbell and hold one handle in each hand. Curl the handles up to your shoulders, and keep them there throughout the drill. Push your hips back and jump, extending your hips, knees, and ankles as quickly as possible. Jump as high as you can on each rep and take a few seconds to recover in between. Do 3 sets of 5 jumps, resting 30 seconds between sets.

Press Your Luck
FRANK MATRISCIANO,
University of Memphis

We think of basketball as a game of sprints, lunges, and jumps. But it's also a game of nonstop reaches, pushes, pulls, and lifts, which can be hell on your shoulders. For unwavering upper-body stamina, the Tigers do this shoulder drill: Grab an 8-pound medicine ball. Stand with your dominant foot forward, holding the ball chest-high. Press the ball forward as in a chest pass, but don't release the ball. That's 1 rep. Do 30 reps, 6 seconds each. Then slowly press the ball up and slightly forward, as if you're grabbing a rebound. Again, do 30 reps, 6 seconds each. That's 1 set. Rest for 45 seconds, and then do 2 more sets.

Necessary Toughness

In professional football, every down is a man-on-man melee—so some players are gaining an edge by training like brawlers. Welcome to the NFL's new fight club.

The rafters shake as 250 pounds of muscle slam into the floor. The grappler looks dazed for a moment, showering the mat with sweat as he shakes his world back into focus. His opponent seizes the opportunity, straddling the downed man's chest in a debilitating ground-and-pound position. But the advantage is brief; an arm is grabbed, bodies spin, and the tables turn.

Despite a combined weight of nearly 500 pounds, the two giants move with surprising speed and agility, like trained fighters. Still, neither has a single professional bout to his name: Kirk Morrison plays linebacker for the Buffalo Bills, and

his training partner, Akeem Ayers, fills the same position for the Tennessee Titans.

Elsewhere in the gym, defensive star Dashon Goldson is mixing it up with running back Ryan Grant, and Raiders defensive end Lamarr Houston practices a strike-and-evade drill with Atlanta Falcon Brian Banks. Coaching these men through their moves, and occasionally diving into the action themselves, are mixed martial arts (MMA) pros, including eighth-ranked middleweight Brian Stann. And overseeing it all with gleefully profane words of encouragement is a thickly built fire

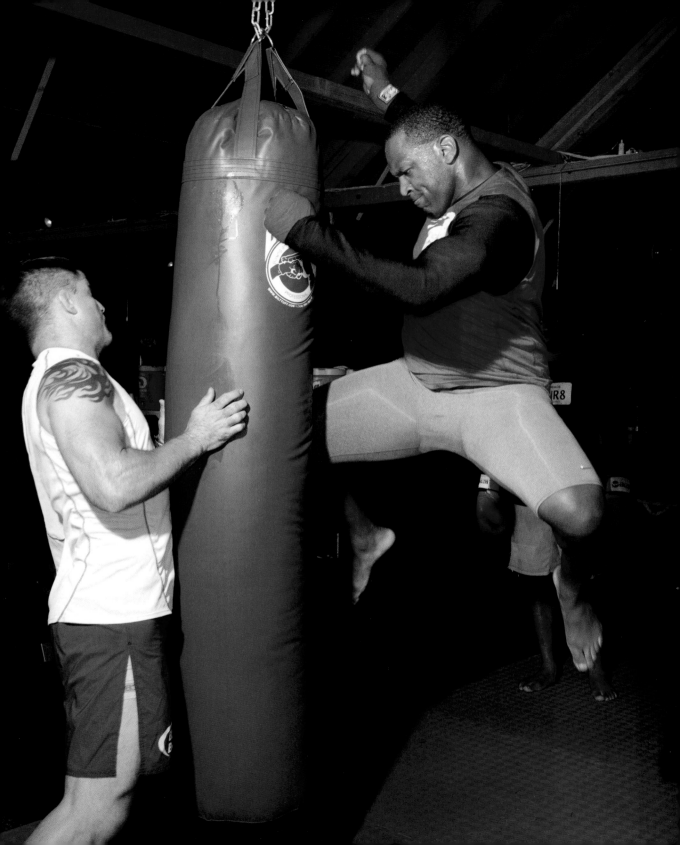

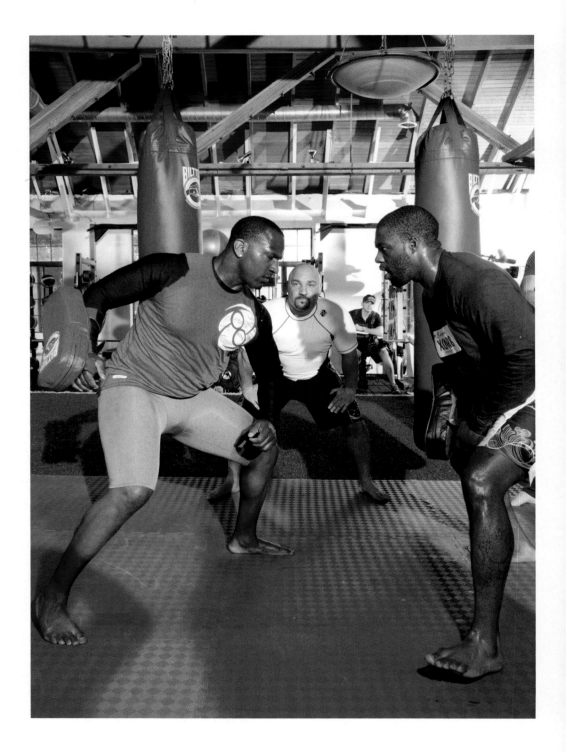

Improve Your Game **MH**

hydrant of a man named Jay Glazer.

"When that game starts, you impose your will out there. YOU OWN YOUR SPACE!" yells Glazer, a journalist for *Fox NFL Sunday* when he's not training the league's top athletes. "The cage is shut, and your goal is to make the guy across from you beg to get out of it."

It's like stepping into the voyeuristic fantasy of some ultraviolent sports fanatic. But this is an everyday sight at MMAthletics, the Los Angeles-based training program that Glazer started in 2008 with UFC legend Randy Couture. Their goal: to train NFL players and other elite athletes to become stronger, faster, and more explosive by using fighting techniques and drills from mixed martial arts. So far it seems to be working.

"Every play on the field is 11 individual battles," says Minnesota Vikings All-Pro defensive end Jared Allen, one of more than 60 players Glazer has trained. "And every snap of the ball is a challenge: How much are you willing to give on this play, this drive, this quarter? Working with Jay has shown me that I always have more, even when I feel like I'm totally tapped out."

Just as important as athletic power and stamina, however, is the warrior mindset that goes hand in hand with such martial conditioning. "The players start to look at their opponents with a fighter's eyes," says Couture. And as today's practice attests, a growing number of them are realizing that such vision can help them improve their game and also dominate the gridiron.

Like many high-end LA establishments, Athletic Gaines, the gym that

"A lot of players use only about 50 percent of their power because their bodies are so locked up."

houses MMAthletics just off Santa Monica Boulevard, is hidden in plain sight. It's set back from the street with no sign on the door, no large windows, and indeed nothing to entice rabid fans. And at 9:30 sharp each morning, the players arrive for what is sure to be the most grueling 90 minutes of their day.

After a brief warmup of jumping rope and slow kicks, Glazer splits the players into pairs. One man lies on his back while the other sits astride him like an opponent ready to strike. The guy on his back grabs his attacker's arms and launches his hips up to throw the attacker off. Soon they find a rhythm—grab left, throw left; grab right, throw right—and continue for an exhausting 60 seconds.

Many trainers would call this drill a core builder, but it's more than that. Sure, it stresses the legion of muscles between the hips and shoulders, but after just 30 seconds of grabbing and throwing, it becomes exhaustingly clear that it hits everything else, too, including the heart and lungs. And working against a fighting opponent is decidedly harder than lifting inanimate weights; as your adversary shifts and resists, each rep becomes different, forcing you to adapt to new forces on the fly.

"You can squat and leg press all day,"

says Jaguars tight end Marcedes Lewis, "but body-on-body work takes place on a whole different level."

Allen agrees. "An opponent helps you translate what you learn into the real world."

Next up are muay Thai kicks—fast-spinning roundhouses requiring exceptional flexibility—and then tackling drills on the heavy bag. After a few sessions at MMAthletics, most of the players can crash through the 135-pound bag like it's a pinata, so the trainers loop an exercise band around each player's waist to hold him back as he charges it. The bands slow the guys down a little, but more important, they provide horizontal resistance—a challenge most standard gyms don't offer.

The players' kicks are similarly thunderous, but Couture points out that drills like these do more than just rattle the floor. "The guys move their hips into positions that they're not used to in football," he says. Like classical musicians dabbling in jazz, they expand their range and transform themselves into more formidable athletes. "It's easier to keep my knees high when I run, making me harder to tackle," says Grant.

Indeed, many of the moves translate directly to the field. The hammer fist is one example: As one player extends a padded arm—like a lineman throwing a block—another whacks it away using the edge of his forearm.

"It's a short, quick move," Glazer tells them. "But it has to be done with violence. Instead of slapping their hands away, I want you to smash their forearms."

Soon they're all throwing hammer fists that could shatter concrete. When Morrison finds his groove, a cannonball-size dent forms on his partner's pad. Glazer seems pleased. "Hit your opponent like that a few times and he'll think twice about putting his hands on you!"

Morning workouts typically end with "30-30-30" drills: six to 20 rounds of 30-second, high-intensity moves performed back-to-back. Because most of the players are conditioned for brief bursts of activity lasting only a few seconds—the duration of an average football play—even 3 minutes can feel like an eternity.

"Plenty of guys come in here saying, 'Yeah, yeah, I've boxed before. I know what I'm doing,'" says Grant. "Very quickly they realize they have a lot to learn."

Today, Glazer ups the ante with seven drills that last a minute each. It leaves the men tired, winded, and soaked with sweat, but far from finished. Glazer gives them a moment's rest before launching into part two of their training: weightlifting.

"It's like a constant sprint," says Allen. "After my first few months of doing MMA, I was able to push myself much, much harder on the field."

Glazer's goal, like that of a dedicated drill sergeant, is to drive his charges past what they think are their breaking points.

"That way, when it's the fourth quarter and the other team's tongues are dragging, they still have plenty left in the tank," he says.

Allen, Goldson, Morrison, and the other players don't sign up just to develop stamina, however, and most of them arrive with plenty of strength. But what they invariably lack after years of heavy lifting is the type of fluidity and effortless

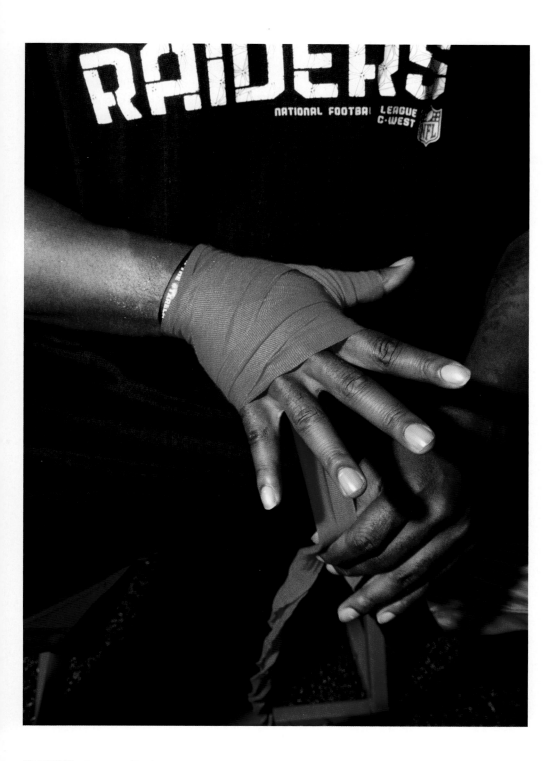

"Good fighters tense up only at the moment of impact. The rest of the time, they're relaxed."

efficiency that can give them a leg up on other gridiron giants.

"A lot of players use only about 50 percent of their power because their bodies are so locked up," says Stann.

Kneeing and kicking drills give them greater mobility. Punching and grappling help them develop leverage, reach, and multidirectional power, making them not only big and strong but also explosive and economical. And hand-to-hand drills give them the quickness and coordination they need to tackle the storm of fists, elbows, and knees that follow every hike.

"Good fighters tense up only at the moment of impact," says Morrison. "The rest of the time, they're relaxed. It's true of great football players as well."

The players also talk about how MMA training instills a killer instinct that helps them hit that much harder, run that much faster, and dig that much deeper than their opponents. Just as important, they say, is its ability to shore up weaknesses and keep them in the game.

"Both MMA fighters and NFL players understand what's at stake," says Couture. "We all know it's possible to lose big—even catastrophically." Players in the NFL—the most punishing of professional team sports—see the evidence every day. Teammates are injured. They lose a step. They spend more time on the sideline. And sometimes they even lose their jobs. Morrison estimates that he's seen a thousand teammates come and go during his 7 years in the NFL, which only underscores the precariousness of their careers.

But that's precisely why this unlikely brotherhood gathers here every day. "When you have this level of conditioning," says Couture, "you can walk onto any field with the confidence that you'll be the last man standing."

ARE YOU OCTAGON FIT?

Upgrade your workouts with these MMA pointers.

Train fast.

Life doesn't happen in slow motion. Neither do sports. So why train that way? Whether you're lifting weights, running intervals, or working the heavy bag, do it fast. "And skew your workouts in favor of explosive movements like cleans, push presses, and anything with kettlebells," says MMAthletics cofounder Randy Couture. All of these target your fast-twitch muscle fibers.

Train with a partner.

By definition, mixed martial arts training requires an opponent. But you don't have to swap punches to benefit from sweating with a partner. A buddy can help motivate you: "I'm smaller than most NFL guys," says Couture. "But when I train with them, they realize they might not be as tough as they think they are, and that knowledge makes them work that much harder."

Train everything.

Forget the "back and bis" and "chest and tris" routines you learned in JV football. "We've come a long way from isolation training," says Couture, who notes that muscles rarely work alone in the real world. Every movement, from swinging a toddler to shoveling snow, is a team effort. If you want to build strength that translates beyond the gym, work your entire body every time.

Train differently.

Workouts are like anything else: Keep doing the same thing every day and your workouts will become stale. Worse, your gains will grind to a halt. "Whether we're talking hand-eye coordination, flexibility and mobility, or even a better understanding of body mechanics, new exercises and activities strengthen weaknesses and fill the gaps in your game," says Couture.

A Smack Upside the Head

NHL and NFL concussions get the ink. But your head is on the line, too.

Matt Mastrantuono remembers a lot about that Sunday last April, but not the crash. One minute he was guarding his man during an Ultimate Frisbee tournament in Walla Walla, Washington, the disc sailing in his direction. The next thing he knew he was splayed on his back, trying to figure out why that strange guy was standing over him. Turns out, that guy was one of his best friends. "I didn't even know why I was on the ground," says Mastrantuono.

The seconds that escape his memory have since come to define his life. Mastrantuono's head had rammed into the shoulder of an opposing team member.

The filmmaker from Portland, who's in his 20s, was knocked cold when his brain rocked from one side of his skull to the other. He sustained a brain injury of the least severe and most common kind: a concussion.

The "Common" Concussion

Most of the concern about traumatic brain injuries, or TBIs, used to focus on the obvious, most severe scenarios: skull fractures,

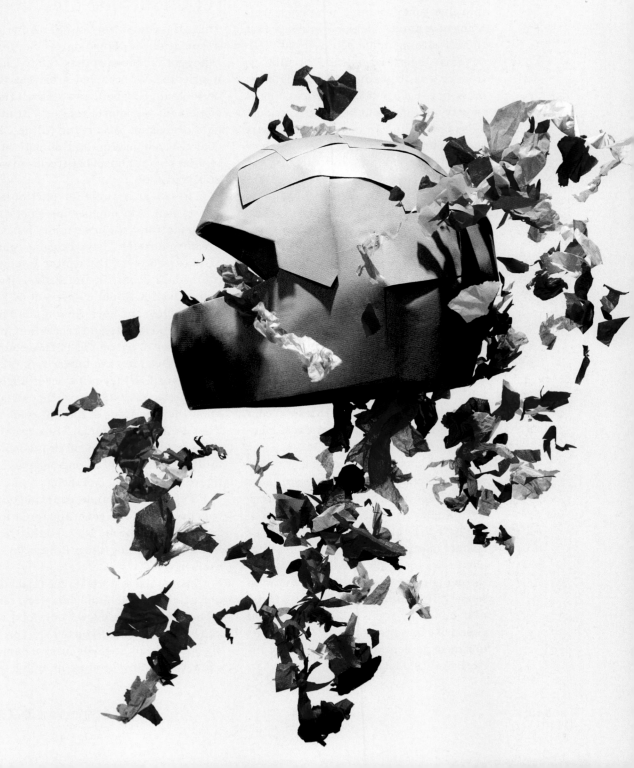

hemorrhages, patients wheeled comatose into emergency rooms. The worry is widening now, amid undeniable evidence that there's nothing mild about a "mild" TBI. Organized sports leagues and the military, from peewee to pro and raw recruit to top brass, have been publicly soul searching as they try to figure out how many concussions one brain can bear, how far apart these injuries can safely happen, and how to improve diagnosis and care for the wounded. Studies suggest that even a single impact to the head might light a fuse to dementia or Alzheimer's disease.

But one fact is often lost as we fret over the brains of veterans, pro athletes, and wannabe pros. The vast majority of concussion victims are ordinary citizens—weekend warriors, aging gym rats. That is, you. For every concussion victim meticulously counted and monitored on youth and pro teams, many more people are sustaining concussions as they go about their daily lives. Perhaps millions are living with the consequences of blows to the head. The science suggests that even concussions that go unnoticed can cause mental impairment.

"You don't have to be tackled by a 350-pound lineman to injure your brain," says Brent Masel, M.D., medical director of the Brain Injury Association of America. You just have to be on a ski slope and lose your balance on an unexpected veneer of ice. Or have a few too many and then let testosterone get the better of your common sense. ("Hey, man, watch this . . .") Or be rear-ended by some texting maniac on your drive to work tomorrow. "It happens to a huge percentage of us in our day-to-day lives," Dr. Masel says.

A Concussion Epidemic?

Think this couldn't be you? The American Association of Neurological Surgeons reports that more sports-related head injuries in 2009 occurred on bicycles than on football, baseball, and softball fields combined, and sports-related TBI numbers are rising. According to the CDC, emergency room visits for traumatic brain injuries rose by almost 15 percent between 2002 and 2006.

This is an issue that particularly affects men. "The number one genetic risk factor for traumatic brain injury is having a Y chromosome," says Douglas Smith, M.D., director of the center for brain injury and repair at the University of Pennsylvania. About 59 percent of TBIs occur in men and boys. Among adult participants in sports and recreation, men account for 70 percent of TBIs, according to the CDC. Men are bigger risk-takers than women, so they suffer accordingly.

But experts acknowledge that we don't know the true scope of the TBI epidemic. The CDC's tally of annual TBIs treated in E.R.s or admitted to hospitals is about 1.7 million, but almost no one believes this figure accounts for all of them.

"There's a vast undercounting of the concussions in the general population," says Julie Gilchrist, M.D., of the CDC's National Center for Injury Prevention and Control.

An organized sports league might document every head bump, but if you crash on your bike tomorrow, the only folks who know will be the ones you tell—i.e., probably nobody. Nor does concussion damage show up on any kind of imaging test.

Concussions are among the few major injuries that are largely invisible, and the sufferers themselves must be relied on to catalog symptoms—some of which may not appear until the collision is old news. And by then, a complete recovery might not be possible.

Dr. Masel describes a recent case in point, a buddy beaned by a soccer ball while playing in a weekend rec league. The friend "had his bell rung" for a few minutes but then caught his breath and finished the game, believing the common myth that if he wasn't knocked unconscious, he couldn't have had a concussion.

"Then a couple of months later he started feeling tired," Dr. Masel says. "It wasn't just, 'I'm a little tired.' He was thinking about selling his business—that's how tired he was."

Only when Dr. Masel asked him about any recent head trauma did the man recall the fateful play. Dr. Masel traced the man's symptoms to a growth hormone deficiency that had been triggered by the trauma to his pituitary gland. Treating the deficiency helped him recover completely, but who knows how many other men are walking around with unexplained fatigue, headaches, or mental fogginess and not connecting their symptoms to an incident that occurred some time ago?

"Most of the nonathlete population just doesn't make it to the doctor," says Summer Ott, Psy.D., director of the concussion program at the Memorial Hermann Ironman Sports Medicine Institute in Houston. These injuries may actually be worse in some aspects than the ones seen among the pros. Athletes risk concussion week after week. But with regular guys, injuries tend to occur when they're not braced for impact. Plus, they don't have the neck muscles of a Hereford bull. (There is a widespread theory that neck strength might lessen the g-forces inside the brain.)

Unlike a pro athlete's head injury, your own concussion isn't likely to happen in front of a crew of trained professionals who can put you through a concussion protocol, whisk you to immediate medical

THE DIRTY DOZEN OF HEAD-BANGING SPORTS

Number of sport-related concussion cases seen in E.R.s in the U.S. in 2009, according to the American Association of Neurological Surgeons

1. **CYCLING** 85,389
2. **FOOTBALL** 46,948
3. **BASEBALL AND SOFTBALL** 38,394
4. **BASKETBALL** 34,692
5. **WATER SPORTS** (including tubing!) 28,716
6. **POWERED RECREATIONAL VEHICLES** 26,606
7. **SOCCER** 24,184
8. **SKATEBOARDS/SCOOTERS** 23,114
9. **FITNESS/EXERCISE/HEALTH CLUB** 18,012
10. **WINTER SPORTS** (skiing, sledding, snowboarding, snowmobiling) 16,948
11. **HORSEBACK RIDING** 14,466
12. **GYMNASTICS/DANCE/CHEERLEADING** 10,223

"If I had a concussion, how long should I wait to go back in the game? I would say 50 years, because we don't know."

attention as needed, and enforce a Sidney Crosby-type vacation until you're healed. "You have to take on that responsibility yourself," says Dr. Gilchrist. "That means the education and actions we're proposing for the school sports fields and in pro sports are even more important for the general population."

But will we actually pay attention?

The first thing Mastrantuono said after his buddies had walked him off the playing field was, "I don't think I have a concussion." Luckily, somebody fetched a trainer, who told him otherwise. The trainer did not insist that Mastrantuono stay sidelined but warned him that it's the second jolt that can kill a person or permanently scar the brain. That was enough to convince Mastrantuono he was done for the day. That night, when he called the nurse on his health plan, she advised him to go to an E.R. So he did what many guys in his situation would do. He conducted a brief self-diagnosis and went home. The next morning, when he could not fully open his drooping eyelids, his girlfriend insisted that he see a doctor.

Mastrantuono did see a doctor, but it was only after a couple of weeks had passed that the real symptoms began to reveal themselves. The slightest movement would give him spasms of nausea; he suffered from vertigo and severe headaches. "There were days when I was walking to or from work that I would have to steady myself on a building," he says.

This was Mastrantuono's first diagnosed concussion. (He suspects he might have had a couple in his teens but says he never sought medical attention for them.) Which brings us to the most sobering finding from recent medical science: One concussion—just one—might permanently change your brain. "To call it a mild TBI is really an oxymoron because it's a serious injury," says Dr. Smith.

Your brain is a 3-pound mass, about the consistency of tofu, floating freely but snugly inside your skull. The familiar gray folds are connected by networks of white matter—nerve cells with long, spindly tendrils called axons that relay signals from cell to cell in milliseconds. The connections among axons account for every function of your brain, including memory, concentration, movement, emotion, and even maintaining consciousness—as long as a jarring hit doesn't deprive you of it.

When your brain is suddenly shocked—the average injury occurs in less than a second—it can't absorb the acceleration, so it's briefly distorted. (Picture what happens if you shake a Jell-O mold.) This sudden stretching of axons can break the internal train tracks that nerve cells use to transport signal-carrying proteins along their length. There's a limit to the elasticity of these transportation lines. Dr. Smith compares it to pulling Silly Putty. Yank it too fast, and it stiffens and breaks.

After impact, proteins that are nor-

Improve Your Game **MH**

mally ferried along the length of the axons are suddenly dumped, piling up like derailed boxcars in places they're not supposed to be. In the frantic rush to repair themselves, nerve cells can summon protection mechanisms that actually make the damage worse. The axons swell. Brain function is interrupted. All this can start instantly and go on for months.

"People ask me, 'If I were playing football and had a concussion, how long should I wait to go back in the game?' I would say 50 years, because we don't know," says Dr. Smith. "We don't know when it's safe again, or if it's ever safe."

Another mystery is why some victims recover quickly while others never do. Research suggests that perhaps 10 percent of people have life-changing symptoms after a single concussion. In another study, this one published in the journal *Brain Pathology* in 2011, Penn researchers reported that victims of a single TBI were more likely than their uninjured peers to show the kind of abnormal hallmarks in brain architecture that occur in Alzheimer's disease.

None of these brain specialists is suggesting that we all cower at home on the sofa. But they all do caution that you should protect your head as if your life depends on it. Because it does. And a brain recovering from a concussion is even more vulnerable to damage from a second blow.

"There seems to be a period of time when doing less activity, both mental and physical, helps your concussion heal," says Stephen Leffler, M.D., chief of emergency medicine at the University of Vermont. Unfortunately, he says, a lot of men don't want to go to a doctor and be given a list of things they shouldn't do. And there's really nothing a doctor can do, or tell a patient to do, that will accelerate healing.

Concussions are serious injuries for which no specific treatment exists. A physician can rule out more severe possibilities, such as bleeding into the brain. He or she can also manage and treat your symptoms and supervise a safe return to your old life. But the brain heals on its own, with rest; medicine doesn't really have much more to offer.

A Surprising Treatment

This is partly because researchers paid little attention to concussions until recently, says Jack Jallo, M.D., Ph.D., director of neurotrauma and critical care at Thomas Jefferson University in Philadelphia. "Patients with mild head injuries were historically ignored," he says. That's changing as researchers look for treatments that can repair the damage. And a female hormone might be one of the saviors emerging from research.

A clinical trial now under way at 17 major U.S. medical centers aims to determine if the female hormone progesterone, which plays an important biological role in maintaining pregnancy, might protect against neurological damage when it's administered within the first few hours following impact. After animal studies suggested that progesterone might protect brain cells, scientists at Emory University conducted a randomized trial of 100 victims of moderate to severe concussions, each of whom received an infusion of either progesterone or a placebo within

11 hours after the injury. This study, published in 2007, was primarily a test of safety, and it revealed no serious side effects. But the study participants who had received progesterone were about half as likely to die, and if their concussions were moderate, they were significantly less disabled.

Those results were promising enough that Emory received a $14.5 million National Institutes of Health grant to oversee the clinical trial, which will test progesterone in more than 1,100 TBI patients. Athletes would not be the only beneficiaries; the military also has a stake in the outcome. If the pregnancy hormone proves to be an effective aid in healing brain cells, it would be the first new treatment for severe brain injuries in three decades.

Almost a year after his concussion, Mastrantuono says most of his symptoms have subsided, but that he still suffers from headaches—sometimes blistering ones.

"It's something I'm going to have to live with from here on out," he says. He's back on the field, but now he wears what he calls "goofy headgear" that might soften another hit. Other players rib him about it sometimes, but he doesn't care. He knows that they probably aren't taking the possibility of a concussion any more seriously than he did. "For a normal guy," he says, "it's not something you really think about until it comes your way."

And when it does, your head ought to be covered. But don't think that guarantees that your guava won't end up pureed.

"Goofy headgear" is usually subjected to a battery of safety tests that can include dropping helmets onto anvils. (As if that can tell you anything about how your own noggin will fare against a competitor's elbow.) The only test that mattered for Shannon Day of Houston was the one that took place one Saturday in September as he was racing motocross. The track curved, but the 46-year-old father of three went straight. The bike and rider catapulted into the air, flipped, and crash-landed upside down.

Though his neck brace probably kept him from being paralyzed, his helmet . . . well, it's harder to say what that did. Day suffered a concussion, even though he'd always thought the headgear would prevent one. "I always made sure to buy the best, safest helmets out there," he says.

But the truth is a little more complicated. No helmet is concussion-proof, despite marketing that has become so commonly overblown that in 2011 the Senate Committee on Commerce, Science, and Transportation held hearings to address safety claims.

"The simple truth is that no current helmet, mouth guard, headband, or other piece of equipment can significantly prevent concussions from occurring," testified Jeffrey Kutcher, M.D., the American Academy of Neurology's chairman of sports neurology. "They occur as the result of the nature of sports. Concussion prevention is much more about teaching proper technique, playing by the rules, and limiting the overall dose of impacts."

Helmets are designed to protect against high-impact collisions that could crack the skull, but they don't have the design or technology to prevent the delicate, enfolded gray matter within from shifting. That may explain a recent finding from Cleveland Clinic researchers that the old leatherhead gear might protect against concussions just as effectively as the modern football helmets. In other words, helmets cannot solve the concussion problem. Experts also share some concern that men (and it is largely men in this case) might take risks while wearing a helmet that they would not take with an exposed head, though research on this is sparse.

"Even with a helmet, you are still at extreme risk of having a traumatic brain injury in any type of sport," says Dr. Smith. After all, the number of sports-related TBIs has not decreased, even though helmet use is now more prevalent than ever.

The bottom line for him? "Wear a helmet, and be careful."

TIMELINE OF A CONCUSSION

Brain injuries happen in a flash, but symptoms can last days or weeks. Here's what to look for, and when.

Pro athletes have doctors standing by for brain assessment. All you have are your buddies, who just want you to man up and play. If you black out or have a seizure or suffer any of the symptoms below, see a doctor or have a teammate dial 911.

HEADACHE:
Ninety-five percent of concussed athletes experience headaches, according to the *American Journal of Sports Medicine.*
When you notice it:
Within 30 minutes (severe pain that day; mild ache after that)

SENSITIVITY:
A concussion can disrupt visual system brain circuits; bright lights and noises may seem especially intense.
When you notice it:
Immediately after the injury or up to a few days afterward

NAUSEA:
Unrelenting or intense nausea or vomiting after a blow to the head may indicate a more severe concussion. Have someone take you to the emergency room, pronto.
When you notice it:
Within the first few hours

DIZZINESS:
Concussion can cause bruising or trauma of the inner ear; you feel dizzy or off balance. You might feel as if you've been whirling around or have vertigo.
When you notice it:
Usually within minutes

MEMORY LOSS:
You might forget the hit that landed you on the ground—or the ambulance ride. This could indicate a particularly severe concussion even if your memory returns in minutes.
When you notice it:
Right after the injury

MENTAL FATIGUE:
If you're tired, you're still recovering. You might be able to work, but you may feel like your daily routine is exhausting.
When you notice it:
The second or third day after the injury

IRRITABILITY:
Lashing out, mood swings, and short tempers all fall into this category. And a Snickers bar won't cure this one.
When you notice it:
A few days later, often after your physical symptoms subside

SOURCES: Mark Lovell, Ph.D., developer of the ImPACT concussion test; Paul Gubanich, M.D., an assistant clinical professor of internal medicine at Ohio State University; and Brian Rieger, Ph.D., director of the concussion management program at SUNY Upstate University Hospital in Syracuse

How to Do Everything Better

With a few simple adjustments, you can up your game, in everything.

Create an Underwater Kingdom

Give our googly-eyed pals the best—a healthy aquarium that can help them live longer and swim happier. (Bonus: You'll spend less time cleaning the tank!) Here are three simple steps from Jonathan Wolf, aquarium design consultant at Chicago's Blue Planet Aquarium Services.

Start fresh. A saltwater tank can support exotic species, but it requires more supplies and is more expensive to maintain. Freshwater fish cost less than saltwater swimmers, so they'll be cheaper to replace if they go belly-up. Try a wedge-shaped corner aquarium with a bowed outer surface. This won't hog space, and it makes your corner a terrific wall of light and color.

Add ambience. Adorn your pals' watery world with rocks, freshwater lily pads, and fake coral. (Real ocean coral and shells will mess with the water's chemistry.) Decorations offer shelter and a sense of security for your fish. Toss in a few submersible LED lights, and add driftwood, sports trophies, action figures ... anything you think would look cool at the bottom of your tank.

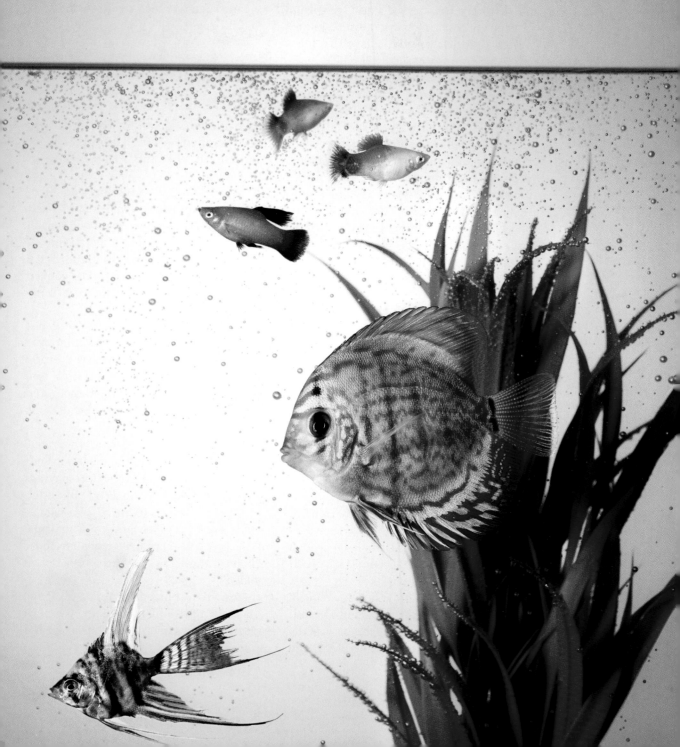

Go fish. Buy hearty fish varieties such as tetra, barb, or danio. They're more likely to survive your learning curve. Once things are going swimmingly, impress your friends with a teacup stingray or snowflake eel. These look just like their larger oceanic counterparts but are perfect for a freshwater tank. But beware: They're predators. Pair rays or eels only with larger species, such as the black ghost knife fish. Otherwise you'll just spawn an underwater battleground. Feed your crew bloodworms, plankton, or other flash-frozen foods instead of dried flakes. These more nutritious options will improve the health of your fish and bring out their most vibrant colors.

Mix the Ultimate Bloody Mary

Use these tips from drink specialist Jeffrey Tascarella of the new NoMad Hotel in New York City.

Make your base. Fresh vegetable juice makes your Bloodys bolder. Blend three celery stalks (with leaves), a large shallot, 1 teaspoon grated horseradish, and 1 tablespoon capers with brine.

Add some spice. To balance rich flavor and spiciness, add $1/4$ cup Worcestershire sauce, the juice of a lemon, 1 teaspoon black pepper, and 1 tablespoon each of celery salt and red-pepper flakes.

Flesh it out. Add about $3^{1}/_{2}$ cups of tomato juice (we like Sacramento brand) and refrigerate the mix overnight. Run the chilled mixture through a strainer, and

then pour it into six glasses. Add about $1^{1}/_{2}$ ounces vodka to each glass, along with a cleaned and trimmed celery stick.

Construct a Philly-Caliber Cheesesteak

Ditch the boring sub for this healthier super-sandwich with these tips from Troy Guard, chef and owner of TAG in Denver.

Start with lean beef. Buy a pound of beef tenderloin, a lower-calorie cut. Coat it with 2 tablespoons of olive oil and season it with salt, pepper, and a few dashes of red-pepper flakes. Grill or broil the meat 6 to 7 minutes, and then freeze the cooked beef for 5 minutes so you can slice it thinly with ease.

Adjust your vegetable ratio. Heat 1 tablespoon of canola oil in a skillet over medium heat. Add $1/2$ small red onion (thinly sliced), cook for 3 minutes, and then add a medium poblano pepper and one red pepper, both thinly sliced. Cook for 1 minute.

Melt the cheese perfectly. Arrange the sliced meat on a baking sheet, top with the vegetables, and add a few thin shavings of Gruyère cheese on top. Broil 1 minute.

Fix the foundation. Slice a wholewheat roll lengthwise and scoop out some of the bread to cut calories and allow more room for the steak. Toast the bread until golden.

Top off. Consider adding a fried egg (its yolk will add moisture), peppery greens such as arugula or frisee, or hot sauce.

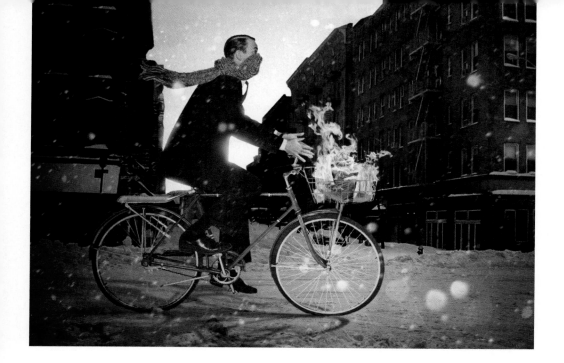

De-Ice Your Driveway

Put down the pickax. There's an easier (and safer) way to thaw a sidewalk or driveway.

Add water. For smaller areas, shovel off any snow and pour warm water on the exposed ice. When you eventually throw on rock salt, you'll create a brine, which should melt the ice faster.

Harness the sun. Coat the ice with a dark-colored abrasive material, such as coal ash or dark sand. The dark color can then absorb heat from the sun and help melt the ice, as well as provide traction for walking and driving.

Shake on the salt. Rock salt lowers the freezing point of water, so when it's added to ice it speeds the melting process. Be wary: Salt can damage concrete and plants if you let it collect, so when the ice is gone, sweep it up and toss it.

Survive a Wintry Ride to Work

A hat and scarf won't cut it on subzero days. Use these tactics from John Hughes, cycling coach and author of *Distance Cycling*; Josh Tack, writer and avid cyclist for Adventure Cycling Association; and Ryan Venis, M.D., co–vice director of emergency services at St. Vincent Hospital Indianapolis, to pedal to the office without freezing your butt off.

Lighten your load. Added weight, such as a gym bag or briefcase, will make the bike more of a slog to pedal, and in winter, a sweaty cyclist is a cold cyclist. Avoid hauling your laptop on days you bike, and stash your work clothes at the office. Store small items in a seat bag such as Jandd's Mountain Wedge Expandable ($30, jandd.com).

Layer up. Start with wind-proof briefs,

such as the breathable Zepher Wind Boxer Brief ($60, ibex.com), to keep your boys comfortable.

For aerodynamics and warmth, add form-fitting athletic tights and a long-sleeved shirt made of synthetic fibers or wool; these help wick moisture away from your body. Protect your knees, which are sensitive to cold, with knee warmers over your pants. Try the ones from SmartWool ($30, smartwool.com).

Cover your head and face with a balaclava, your hands with gloves, and your shoes with waterproof booties. The balaclava can also help counteract chills from your vented helmet. (You are wearing a helmet, right?)

Finish with a waterproof, windproof outer layer. Wet clothes freeze you because your body tries to transfer energy to warm up a cold, wet shirt. Windproof gear protects your body from bone-chilling headwinds. We like Sugoi's lightweight Zap Jacket ($100, sugoi.com).

Go easy on the hills. Overexerting yourself, either while huffing up hills or hurrying because you're late, can also lead to chills—especially if you don't layer up as we recommend. Be sure to leave on time, and spin the pedals at an even cadence regardless of the terrain. Doing this instead of pushing down heavily on every rotation helps you maintain momentum without taxing yourself too hard. (And it's key if you don't have a shower at your office.)

Set Up the Perfect Home Gym

Convert your workout dungeon into a space you'll actually want to spend time in, according to Gabe Valencia, C.S.C.S., co-owner of Focus Integrated Fitness in New York City, and Trip Haenisch, a designer based in Los Angeles.

Fortify your floor. Carpet fibers can trap sweat odors. Opt for roll-out rubber flooring; this can protect your floor from dropped weights and make body-weight exercises, like pushups or planks, more comfortable.

Add some color. Use warm tones like red, yellow, or orange on the walls. In a 2011 study in the journal *Perceptual and Motor Skills*, these colors were seen as stimulating, while cool hues were associated with restfulness.

NO ROOM FOR THIS?	USE THIS INSTEAD
Cable weight station	JC Predator Bands ($50, ihpfit.com) hook to a door or fixed object. You can add resistance by doubling or tripling them up.
Full set of dumbbells	Lift with the Powerblock Sport 5.0 Adjustable Dumbbell set ($300, powerblock.com). They quickly adjust between 5 and 50 pounds.
Bench	Curls, presses—all are more challenging on a Swiss ball ($35 to $55, theragear.com) because your core stabilizes your body.

Motivate! A wall mirror opens up the space and helps you check your form. For inspiration, hang a print of a historic sports moment from artletics.com, or order a canvas photo of your own at canvaspop.com.

Stop gym funk. Place a Smelleze Gym Deodorizer Pouch ($25, noodor.com) in a corner to stanch the stench. Improve the room's airflow with an oscillating fan. (A ceiling fan could interfere with jumping exercises.)

Bonus: See the table on page 350 for fitness gear for a small room.

Type Texts Faster

Tense band muscles slow you down. Rest your forearms on a table instead, says Marco Santello, Ph.D., professor of biomedical engineering at Arizona State University.

Rent a Car without Being Taken for a Ride

Here's the cheaper, faster way to book the wheels you want for an upgraded vacation, according to Paula Lyons, founder of Best-Car-Rental-Tips.com; Denise Meiler, Hurley Travel Experts; and Marybeth Bond, gutsytraveler.com.

Time your call. Rates tend to be lower 3 to 4 weeks in advance; if you call then, you may save $100 to $175 on a weekend rental. If you're planning a 3- or 4-day getaway, try to include a Saturday night, which might qualify you for a weekend rate and can amount to an additional daily savings of $15.

Expand your car pool. Don't limit your search to major companies. You might find cooler cars and better deals (up to 30 percent off) through off-airport rental companies. Check out local tourist sites, which often list these local outfits. Or visit rentawreck.com for great deals on pickups and fun-to-drive classic cars.

Make allies, not adversaries. Rental-car agents might have flexibility to negotiate. Establish a personal connection with the rep and then deliver a line like, "Look, this is my first vacation in 2 years and I've always wanted to drive a convertible. They're expensive, though. Any chance for a discount?" The worst they can say is no.

Shoot a Time-Lapse Movie

Send slow-moving scenes into overdrive—and rake in the YouTube views—with this advice from Doug Urquhart, creative director at the UpThink Lab.

Choose your subject. Try scenes that unfold gradually and show clear progression, such as building a Lego kit or watching an arena fill.

Gear up. Your easiest option is to use an iPhone with the iTimeLapse Pro app ($2, iTunes) or an Android device with TimeLapse! (free, market.android.com). You can also use a digital SLR, which has the manual controls you need for pro results. If your camera has no interval-shooting option, buy an intervalometer.

Try Aputure's Digital Timer Remote ($28, aliexpress.com).

Set up. Optimal playback time is between 8 and 10 seconds with 240 photos. Try to predict how shadows and people will move throughout the shoot so you're not left with dark or empty scenes. For fast-moving subjects, adjust the interval to 1 second between shots. For slower ones, try 6 seconds. Manually lock the focus on the scene and let 'er rip.

Make your movie. The smartphone apps can create the movies for you, or import your sequences into QuickTime 7 Pro, which offers the easiest time-lapse function. For smooth motion, use 30 frames per second; then use video-editing software to add music and effects.

Be a Foosball Wizard

Raw power doesn't bring victory-speed, control and shot setup do. Let Ryan Moore, ranked sixth in the world, help you dominate.

Learn ball control. Position your index finger and thumb in the indents of the handle. A closed-fist grip limits your range of motion and slows you down.

Serve—to yourself. When you serve, place your index finger on the right side of the ball in the serving hole and gently flick it as you release. This adds spin. The ball will exit at an angle—straight toward your players.

Perfect the stop. If you stand firm, the ball will bounce back to your opponent. Instead, turn the handle toward the ball so your little dude's foot traps it underneath.

Develop surefire attacks. Pass shot: Opponents expect direct shots, so pass between players on the same rod before shooting.

Side sweep: Center kicks are easily blocked. Move the ball to the edge of the table and have the player brush the side of the ball for an angled shot.

Organize Your Fridge

A cluttered, sloppy refrigerator is more than just a bacteria buffet: It's inefficient. Michael Ferraro, chef at Delicatessen in New York City, helps you streamline.

Thermometer: To reduce your risk of illness, keep the temperature at 40°F or lower. Buy a fridge thermometer from a hardware or restaurant-supply store and stick it on the fridge's ceiling—the best spot for an accurate reading. We like the easy-to-read Taylor 5 Commercial Digital Freezer/Refrigerator Thermometer ($10, amazon.com).

Top shelf: The back corners of the top shelf are the coldest spots in the refrigerator; this is where manufacturers often locate cooling vents. Store dairy items here to best protect them from temperature fluctuations. And don't stand there all day with the door open!

Leftovers: Place a sticky note on each container to identify the contents and prep date. Most food is safe for 3 to 4 days after it's cooked, the USDA says.

Middle shelf: Stash the items you use most here. Arrange them in rows from front to back, smallest to tallest. That way you're less likely to forget about smaller items, such as caviar. Keep an arm's-width

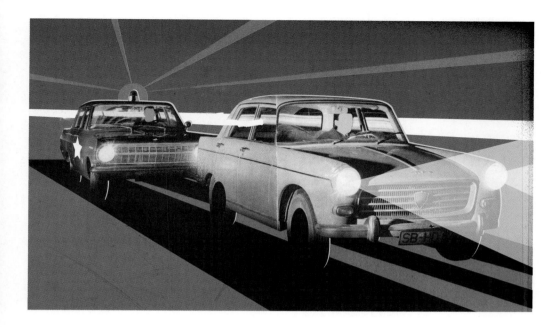

lane between each row so you can reach items easily.

Bottom shelf: Reserve this area for foods such as raw chicken or beef, which could drip onto other items. Keep meats tightly wrapped and as far back as possible to stay as cold as they can.

Drawers: Stash produce in the bins—especially foods you snack on, such as apples and celery. Produce is especially susceptible to cross-contamination if it's next to raw or cooked poultry. Bins are also great for cheese, which can breathe without drying out like it would elsewhere in the fridge.

Dodge a Speeding Ticket

Flashing lights in the rearview? Squeak by without logging any points with these pointers from Steve Pomper, author of *Is* *There a Problem, Officer? A Cop's Inside Scoop on Avoiding Traffic Tickets*, and Seth I. Katz, Esq., a traffic law and vehicle criminal defense attorney in Manhattan.

Start off right. Pull over as soon as you see the officer's lights. Turn on your interior light if it's dark out, and have your license and insurance card ready. This will put him in a good mood.

Don't hem and haw. Officers are lied to so often that it's refreshing when someone just fesses up. Acknowledge where you erred and promise you'll be safer. Throw in an apology as well.

Cop a plea. Now that you've proved your sincerity, ask for a break: "I earned that citation, but would you mind issuing me a warning instead? It won't happen again." Being direct may work.

Win in court. If you do get a ticket, consider lawyering up. A good attorney can turn a 6-point "30 mph over" ticket

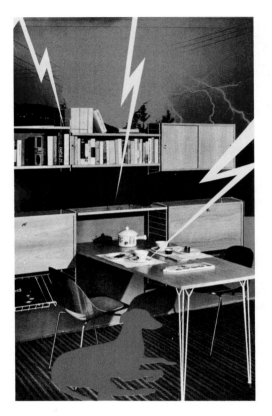

or side of your foot rubs during the hike, stop to relace, skipping the grommet closest to the hot spot. That'll help relieve the pressure.

Calibrate your stride. Rookies tend to stomp over rough terrain. Instead, walk as if you were on the street—naturally. Over time, any unnatural motion in your stride can fatigue and stress your joints. To ensure you're walking without added pressure, use a pair of trekking poles. Leki Teton poles ($140, leki.com) are durable and can take weight off your feet and knees while helping you stay stable.

Don't waste breaks. Damp feet slip more, so keeping your feet dry will prevent blisters. Take off your shoes and socks each time you stop, and cover friction hot spots with duct tape—but with the sticky side facing away from the skin. Hold it down by covering it with another, larger piece of tape facing inward. This will stop the shoe and sock from rubbing against bare skin.

into a 4-point "unsafe lane change" ticket, and you won't have to go to court.

Conquer the Trails

Keep your feet happy with tips from long-distance hiker Justin Lichter and Georganna Morton of Mountain Crossings Outfitter.

Outfit your feet. Go with trail shoes. They lack the stiffness of boots and don't need to be broken in. On a long hike, your feet can swell half a shoe size. When sizing, you should be able to fit a finger between your heel and the shoe. If the top

Pacify Your Pooch

Thunderstorm rolling in? Big vet visit coming up? Train Boozer to keep his cool, with these ideas from Julie Albright, D.V.M., a board-certified veterinary behaviorist at the University of Tennessee college of veterinary medicine.

Recognize stress signs. When a dog encounters an unfamiliar dog, it shows fear by licking its lips, yawning, lowering its head, or rapidly shifting its eyes. It does the same in other threatening situations. You want to recognize these behaviors and shift your dog's attention to you instead of the source of anxiety. If the situation is really stressful, you'll find it almost impossible to distract your dog, so start a desensitization program.

Ace a vet trip. Make a habit of swinging by the vet to score some treats. That way Boozer won't always associate the doc with a scary experience. During the visit, place a towel or bath mat on the exam table (bring your own, or ask the vet). Good footing keeps a canine calmer. Use treats and praise so your pooch's attention stays on you. You're familiar; the doctor isn't.

Weather a storm. To prevent Boozer from skittering under your bed when nature unleashes its fury, train him to associate thunder with a nonthreatening activity. First, find a thunderstorm video on YouTube, or download an ambient-noise app that includes thunderstorms, like White Noise by TMSOFT ($2, Android, iOS). Once or twice a week, play the storm sounds through your stereo while you're playing with the dog. Gradually increase the volume to help Boozer adjust to thunder as the background of something pleasurable. But take a break if your dog shows signs of stress or can't stay focused. Start again with a lower volume, and repeat.

Pop a Perfect Bowl of Popcorn

Use the stove top, not a microwave, for fresher-tasting, more thoroughly popped kernels, says Aida Mollenkamp, host of *FoodCrafters* on the Cooking Channel.

Prep your pot. In a large pot, heat 2 tablespoons canola oil and a few popcorn kernels on medium high. When the kernels begin to pop, the oil is hot enough. Remove the pot from the heat and add ¼ cup popcorn kernels and ½ teaspoon kosher salt. Put on the lid and count to 20, allowing the popcorn and oil to reach the same temperature; otherwise some of the kernels will burn.

Steam and shimmy. With one hand, gently move the pan back and forth over the burner; with your other hand, hold the lid like a shield over the pot, leaving it slightly ajar. The idea is to let the steam escape without letting the popcorn kernels leap out. Heat the popcorn until you notice a delay of several seconds between pops, about 3 minutes total.

Coat the kernels. In a small pot, melt 2 tablespoons unsalted butter and, if you want, add additional flavors. Once the butter is melted, pour it over the popcorn, cover the bowl with a dinner plate, and give it a few shakes of seasoning to coat evenly. Serve immediately. Makes 5 to 6 cups of popcorn.

Amputate a Limb

Remove problem branches the right way, with these tips from Manfred Mielke, Forest Health Specialist, USDA Forest Service.

Time your cut. Prune during the dormant season, when the tree isn't leafy or flowering; for most trees, that's winter or very early spring. That way you limit the tree's exposure to sap-hungry, disease-carrying insects. If you have to cut in

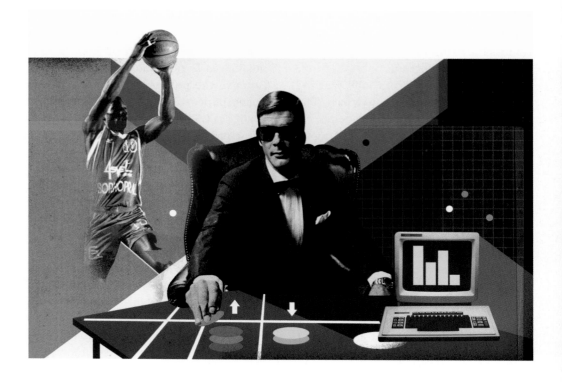

warmer months, avoid pruning in times of rainy weather or high humidity, when fungi and spores thrive.

Find your entry point. Look to remove branches that intersect in a V (as opposed to a U); these intersections are more likely to fail in snowy or windy conditions. Cut the branch half an inch from where it connects to the trunk or another branch. (A flush cut or a longer nub will need more healing time.)

Lop in stages. A sturdy handsaw, such as the Fiskars 15-inch D-handle pruning saw ($21, homedepot.com) is your best bet for limb cutting. Saw the branch off in sections to keep it from tearing away at the joint, unnecessarily exposing more of the tree's flesh.

Let it bleed. Unless the tree is an oak or elm that's wounded during a critical time of year, don't do anything to the exposed wound. Applying synthetic paint, a common wound dressing, could interfere with the healing process.

Pick NCAA Bracket Busters

Most March Madness fans assess the seeds, select an upset or two, and throw down their picks. There's a more informed way to increase your odds, says Howie Schwab, former host of *Stump the Schwab* on ESPN.

Look to last year. Bracket builders tend to focus on the current tournament and forget the teams' past performance. Look for last year's sleeper teams that played hard and lost in tough games but retained the same coach and many players. Bonus points for teams now stocked with seniors.

Scan the score lists. Head to ncaa. org to check out scores for the current season. Blowout games can help you pick winners, but pay more attention to close games from underrated teams. Those are your upset-bound picks.

Analyze the stats. Come tournament time, check out usatoday.com for its in-depth look at detailed stats behind the points. Notice a team that's ranked 60th in three-pointer defense playing a team in the top three for sinking the trey? Lock down the bracket.

Check the odds. Even if you're not a betting man, see what Vegas has to say about the spread. Vegas plays it safe, and if it's saying the opposite of what most sportscasters are predicting, consider siding with the house.

Build a Stand-Up Desk

Improve your health and posture by staying on your feet, courtesy of Jack Dennerlein, Ph.D., ergonomics professor at Harvard school of public health, and Jonathan Scott, cohost of HGTV's *Property Brothers*.

Elevate your screen. Choose an adjustable monitor stand, like the 3M Adjustable Monitor Arm ($100, officede pot.com). Position the screen so it's 18 to 24 inches from your face.

Make your perch. Your shelf should be big enough for the keyboard and mouse. Before attaching legs to it, measure from the floor to your elbows—that's your keyboard height. From that number, subtract the thickness of the shelf and the height of the desk. This leaves you with the length of legs you need. Cut legs to fit, and place antislip adhesive pads below each leg. Predrill the bottom of your shelf and screw in the legs. (Be sure the screws in the legs you buy aren't longer than the shelf is thick.)

Switch things up. Alternate sitting and standing throughout your day—and use a wireless keyboard and mouse.

WEAR THIS, GO FAST

You don't need a yellow wristband to cycle strong. Wearing a large-knit jersey might help you perform better in hot weather, say French scientists. After completing time trials in hot, humid conditions, cyclists reported feeling less hot when they biked in large-knit polyester jerseys than when they wore small- or medium-knit tops. The wider the gap between fibers, the more airflow the fabric allows and the faster your sweat evaporates, says study author Benoit Gonzales, Ph.D. "Thermal comfort is a psychological factor that can help athletes perform at a higher level." Slip into Nalini's light-weight, large-knit Acrab jersey. ($120, carbonconnection.com)

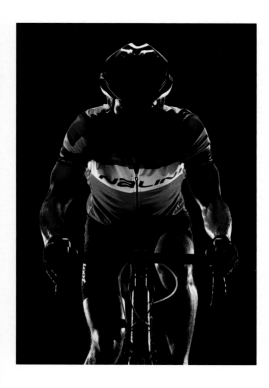

RAISE THE BAR

Why buy specialty snacks? Raisins are effective fuel for endurance events, a new Louisiana State University study found. When cyclists ate raisins, their finish time, power, and perceived exertion were not significantly different from when they ate Jelly Belly Sport Beans. Eat a 90-calorie box of raisins every 20 minutes during long events.

PACE YOURSELF

Running alongside someone might make the time go by faster, but it won't make you any faster, new research from the United Kingdom and South Africa reveals. Although the runners in the study thought their performance improved in the presence of another athlete, their speed, pacing, and heart rate didn't significantly change. "Your pacing strategy is so hardwired that it's not easily altered by something external, like a running partner," says study author Alan St Clair Gibson, M.D., Ph.D. A running buddy could, however, provide you with a psychological edge: He or she may make your workout, whether during training or a race, seem less mentally taxing, he says.

CHECK YOUR RIDE

Your cycling gear might be lulling you into a false sense of invincibility. Here's what the science says.

Helmet: Newer soft-shell helmets

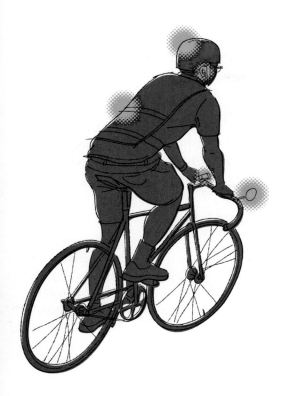

they can distract you, report Rutgers researchers.

PEEL FOR POWER

Bananas pump up more than your potassium. Appalachian State University scientists found that cyclists who ate the fruit experienced the same energizing boost in blood glucose as cyclists who drank liquid carbohydrates.

DRINK UP

Save salty sports drinks for after your workout. Low-carb, low-sodium sports drinks are absorbed the fastest, say New Zealand scientists. Cyclists who downed a drink with lower carb and sodium concentrations than those in an average man's body—thus triggering rapid diffusion into the gut—exercised longer and harder than those who had Gatorade or Powerade. The drink from the study isn't sold here, so try Gatorade G2 instead.

offer significantly less protection than classic hard-shell styles, according to a 2011 review from Norway.

Reflective vest: Wear a vest and ankle and knee reflectors. Illuminating moving parts boosts your visibility, say Australian scientists.

Ear buds: Music can motivate you, but it might also affect your ability to hear traffic. Stay safe by using a single earbud, Dutch scientists recommend.

Bicycle light: Use a beam to light your path; however, Australian researchers warn that it won't help a driver spot you any sooner.

Mirrors: Bike mirrors don't provide a broad enough view to increase safety, and

FOCUS BETTER

Hey, all-world: It's not all about you. Focusing on your team's strengths instead of your own can improve your performance, reveals a new study in the *Journal of Sports Sciences*. The researchers found that players who thought about their team's strengths felt more confident and performed better than those who focused on personal strengths. Emphasizing the group might ease your performance anxiety so you can relax and focus.

GO AIRBORNE

Step lively: Reducing the amount of time your feet touch the turf is the key to acceleration, say Australian scientists. In a study of field sport athletes, the researchers found that players' acceleration was primarily determined by ground contact time—as opposed to the length, rate, or force of their strides. Less time on the ground means more-explosive movement, says study author Robert Lockie, Ph.D. To improve your acceleration, focus on short sprints and plyometrics during training.

SERVE IT UP

Serving in volleyball can be nerve-racking. Stop worrying: Smashing a volleyball

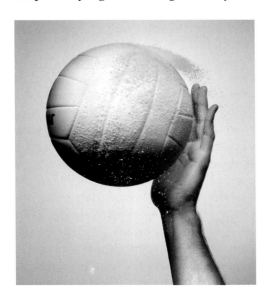

won't help you score, but neither will babying it, new Spanish research reveals. A slow serve makes it easy for your opponent to react, while a fast one is too risky. Moderate velocity is the most effective. The perfect rec-league move? The "jump float" serve, says lead author Bernat Busca, Ph.D. As you run forward, toss the ball up in front of your hitting shoulder, jump, and high-five the ball with a stiff wrist.

STREAKIN'

Hot streaks are real and not just luck, German researchers recently concluded. In their study of volleyball players, nearly half of the athletes experienced streaks that couldn't be explained by mathematical randomness. "Success breeds success due to increased confidence," says study author Markus Raab, Ph.D. However, in sports such as basketball, where defenders can thwart your success (and there's no net separating teams), you're less likely to experience a streak, notes Raab.

FAST FORWARD

Slow start? Just press "play." Listening to music for the first mile of a 5-K can help you finish faster, a study from Brazil reveals. When racers slipped their earbuds in early, they shaved seconds off their times, but cranking music during the final leg had no impact. If you tune in before you feel tired, it's easier to shift your focus from the burn to the beat, which can motivate you, says study author Adriano Lima-Silva, Ph.D.

WEAR TIGHTS

Don't stash those running tights just because winter is over. A new study from Australia reports that wearing compression tights can speed your recovery. Men who wore tights during interval training and recovery had lower heart rates and lactate levels than guys who wore shorts. One explanation: Compression garments boost blood-flow to your heart, says study author Chris McLellan, Ph.D.

TREAD CAUTIOUSLY

Running barefoot or in minimalist shoes is still gaining converts, but you should tread cautiously. "Since most of us wear shoes all the time, the muscles in our feet are essentially dormant," says Carey Rothschild, P.T., C.S.C.S., a physical therapist and instructor at the University of Central Florida. That means you need to gradually make the switch to unshod exercise. Ease the transition with these basic drills and strengthening moves.

Feel

1. Walk barefoot indoors and out.
2. Run barefoot indoors and on grass.

Benefit: "This type of activity helps the sensory receptors in your feet gradually adapt to the increased stimulation of being barefoot, says Rothschild.

Form

1. Land on your forefoot, not your heel
2. Pick up your pace.

3. Shorten your stride.

Benefit: The "quicker, shorter skipping" of minimalist running will feel natural as you focus on form, Rothschild says.

Flexibility

1. Calf stretches on the edge of a step

Benefit: You'll loosen up your lower body. "The barefoot running technique requires increased calf muscle activity and range of motion in your ankle," says Rothschild.

Power

1. Single-leg hops
2. Squat jumps
3. Depth jumps

Benefit: If you strengthen your leg muscles, you'll be more equipped to handle the impact of landing, reducing your risk of injury.

Strength

1. Towel curls
2. Pick up marbles with your toes.
3. Bring the ball of your foot toward your heel without flexing your toes.

Benefit: Stronger feet help maintain arch height and prevent excessive pronation.

Proprioception

1. Stand on a wobble board or Bosu ball.

Benefit: Balance exercises improve your neuromuscular control. This helps prevent injury when you aren't wearing cushioned shoes to absorb the shock of impact.

Q I bet on almost every football game I watch. Do I have a gambling problem?

A: Probably, if you bet on the Browns. (Joking!) Clinically speaking, it depends on how you answer two questions: First, do you ever lie about how often you bet? Second, do you have to increase your bets to get the same thrill?

"If your answer to either question is yes, then you may have a problem," says Timothy Fong, M.D., a psychiatrist and the director of UCLA's gambling studies program.

Here's a bonus question: Do you spend more than 2 percent of your income on wagers? While not as diagnostically definitive as a yes to either of the first two questions, an affirmative here is a bad sign, Dr. Fong's research finds.

If you're still not sure, try this test. Write down the amount of time and money you're willing to spend each week on gambling. Or take out your total budget for the season in cash, stuff it into an envelope, and once it's gone, stop betting. If you can stick to either strategy, you probably have control over your gambling, says Dr. Fong. Otherwise, seek help from a specialist who's certified by the American Society of Addiction Medicine (asam.org).

Q Is coconut water really that great for hydration?

A: This quirky quaff is overhyped, but it has some benefits. The truth is, the perfect beverage for replenishing your body's H_2O and electrolytes—the minerals that help regulate hydration and muscle function—is different for everyone, says Michael F. Bergeron, Ph.D., FACSM, executive director of the National Institute for Athletic Health and Performance.

"The duration and intensity of your activity, combined with the saltiness of your sweat and the rate you sweat, determines what's right."

In general, longer sessions call for more carbs and electrolytes, but check our situation-specific guide. And remember: To gauge how much to guzzle, weigh in before and after exercising. For every pound you lose, slowly drink 16 to 20 ounces.

Best for a day at the beach or working in the yard: Electrolyte drink: These drop-and-dissolve tablets deliver a strong dose of electrolytes, and they're so low in calories that you can sip all day. NUUN Active Hydration (1 tablet) 3 calories, 1 gram (g) carbohydrates, 180 milligrams (mg) sodium, 50 mg potassium

Best for a typical workout (60 minutes or less): Low-calorie sports drink or coconut water? Go with a very low-cal sports drink (such as Gatorade G2 Natural) or Zico coconut water. Both have a good balance of electrolytes, plus a light load of carbs to provide some energy. ConsumerLab.com found that Zico contained exactly what it listed on its label, whereas other coconut water brands fell short. GATORADE G2 NATURAL (16 oz) 40 calories, 10 g carbohydrates, 220 mg sodium, 60 mg potassium; or ZICO NATURAL (14 oz)

Improve Your Game **MH**

60 calories, 13 g carbohydrates, 160 mg sodium, 569 mg potassium
   Best for a long workout (90 minutes or more) sports drink:
   Grab a beverage that has up to 500 mg sodium per 16 oz, and around 6 percent carbs (less than 28 g per 16 oz). Any more and your body will pull water from your blood to your gut for digestion. Keep extra fuel on hand—think dried fruit and salted pretzels.
   SKRATCH LABS "SECRET DRINK MIX" (16.9 oz) 80 calories, 20 g carbohydrates, 310 mg sodium, 40 mg potassium

Q If I'm out running and hit a red light, should I stop or jog on the spot?

A: Neither. If you stand there, you risk cooling down, and if you jog in place, you just look silly, says Rachel Cosgrove, C.S.C.S., co-owner of Results Fitness in Santa Clarita, California. "A smarter strategy is to do a dynamic stretch. This keeps your glutes firing and your ankles and hips mobile, both of which help prevent muscle strains."

Cosgrove recommends this stretch: Stand in a staggered stance, left foot forward, hands on your hips. Bend your left knee and push your hips forward to stretch your hip flexors while engaging your glutes, and press your right heel into the ground. Reach up with your right arm and hold for 5 seconds. Then step back with your left foot and switch sides. Keep at it until the light turns green and you're ready to hit the gas again.

Q Is "performance underwear" for exercise a gimmick?

A: They aren't superhero skivvies, but for slip-on strength? They're great. A recent study published in the *Journal of Strength and Conditioning Research* found that power-lifters who trained for 10 weeks while wearing compression garments added nearly 40 pounds to their squat, while lifters who didn't wear them as they trained added only 6 pounds.

The scientists suggest that the compression design of these garments reduces bloodflow to the muscles in a way that may stimulate hormonal and neural pathways involved in building strength.

Are you more of a cardio guy? In a New Zealand study, fit men who wore compression underwear for 24 hours following aerobic exercise ran faster and felt less fatigued during their next workout than those who didn't don the tights. They also experienced less muscle soreness. "The extra pressure may affect muscle sensory receptors and change their feedback to your brain in a way that alters performance," says study author Michael Hamlin, Ph.D., an exercise scientist at Lincoln University in New Zealand. Try the 2XU Compression Shorts ($80) or Compression Tights ($100), available at 2xu.com.

How can I build the rock-solid, ripped upper body of a UFC fighter?
A: Try this workout by Nick Tumminello, CPT, of Performance University. Set a timer for 3 minutes. Do 2 chinups, 4 shoulder presses per arm, and 6 gorilla cleans per arm. Repeat until time's up. Do 3 rounds. Rest for 2 minutes between each.

Chinup

Grab a chinup bar using a shoulder-width, underhand grip. Hang at arm's length. Bend your elbows and pull your chest to the bar. Pause and lower your body. Repeat.

Dumbbell Alternating Shoulder Press

Stand with dumbbells outside your shoulders, palms in. Press your right hand up until your arm is straight. Lower. Repeat on the left.

Kettlebell Gorilla Clean

Let two kettlebells hang between your legs with your feet slightly beyond shoulder width. Bring the kettlebell in your right hand to the "rack" position—your elbow bent in front of your ribs and the weight resting against your outer wrist. Squat down so your thighs are nearly parallel to the floor. This is the starting position. Simultaneously stand (but not so much that you straighten your legs) and switch the positions of the kettlebells, lowering the right one and racking the left. Squat back down. Repeat the move, racking the right one again. Continue alternating sides.

I'm thinking about trying creatine. What do I need to know?
A: Think of creatine as muscle medicine—the extra-strength formula. When you supplement your diet with this amino acid, you spur the production of proteins your body uses to weave muscle fibers, says Douglas Kalman, Ph.D., R.D., a sports nutritionist at Florida International University.

"Using creatine while weight training typically enhances strength gains by 5 to 15 percent in the first month, with no side effects," he says.

In fact, a landmark study from Belgium confirmed that daily use of creatine by healthy adults for as long as 5 years does not affect the kidneys. That said, people with diabetes or a kidney disorder should steer clear, since their already overworked organs may have trouble processing the extra fuel. As for which type to buy, Kalman recommends sticking with classic creatine monohydrate. It's as effective as newer formulas but less expensive. For the first month, take 5 grams a day, mixed into your postworkout recovery shake. On rest days, consume your 5 grams at any time. After the first month, drink 5 grams after training.

We like BodyTech's 100% Pure Creatine Monohydrate ($20, vitaminshoppe.com) because it has no added sugar and is approved by ConsumerLab.com.

Can nitric oxide supplements really help me pack on muscle?

A: Only if you attach jumbo canisters to each end of a barbell.

"The problem with nitric oxide supplements is the way they're formulated," says nutritionist Mike Roussell, Ph.D., author of *The 6 Pillars of Nutrition*. "Their main ingredient, arginine, can't be absorbed efficiently in this form." Instead, Roussell recommends citrulline, an amino acid that speeds into your system, after which it is converted into arginine. As your arginine levels rise, your body produces more nitric oxide, which in turn dilates your blood vessels to help speed muscle growth and recovery time.

What's the fastest way to stop sweating after my lunchtime workout?

A: Fastest? Find a walk-in freezer. Fastest and most practical? Cold water, inside and out.

"You continue to sweat after a workout because your core temperature is still above normal," explains David Nielson, M.D., a San Antonio physician who specializes in treating excessive sweating. "Lower your core temperature and you'll shut off sweat."

Try Dr. Nielson's "16-15" strategy: After your workout, slowly drink 16 ounces of ice-cold water (avoid "brain freeze" from drinking it too fast). Next, take a 15-minute shower that's as cold as you can stand. If you're still sweating, down another 16 ounces of ice water.

Photo Credits

Cover (left to right): ©Howard Schatz, ©Misha Gravenor, ©Weston Wells, ©Levi Brown.

Interior Images:

©Michael Reh/Fuse/Jupiter: page ix.

©Howard Schatz: pages 3–6, 12, 35, 37.

©Joshua Scott: pages 9, 105, 194 (far left), 196–197, 315, 339.

©Travis Rathbone: pages 15, 48, 69, 70, 106, 162 (right), 208, 219, 259, 292.

©Arne Bellstorf: page 19.

©Arthur Mount: pages 21–23, 359.

©Ian Allen: pages 27, 225, 227.

©Graham Samuels: page 31.

©+ISM: page 33.

©Beth Bischoff: pages 38–39, 50–51, 114–119, 123–127, 130–136, 140–142, 148–152, 162 (left), 166–171.

©Levi Brown: pages 41–44, 58–62, 65, 67 (top), 101, 163, 293, 294, 347, 360.

©Thomas MacDonald/Rodale Images: page 53.

©Chris Brennan: page 57.

©Mitch Mandel/Rodale Images: pages 63, 96–99, 102, 120–121, 172–173, 194 (5), 202–205 (products), 213.

©Jeff Harris: page 67 (bottom).

©Misha Gravenor: pages 75–86, 107.

©Harry Bates: page 87 (5).

©Photodisc: page 89 (top).

©Simon Walker: page 89 (bottom).

©Yunhee Kim: page 90.

©Plamen Petkov: pages 95, 100 (right), 250.

©Lisa Shin: page 100 (left/photo).

©Mike Campau: page 100 (left/illus).

©James Dawe: page 113.

©Scott McDermott: page 129 (photo).

©Bryan Christie: page 129 (illus).

©Oliver Eltinger/Corbis: page 137.

©Randi Berez: pages 139, 143.

©Matt Klitscher, Spartacus: Vengeance© 2011 Starz Entertainment, LLC. All Rights Reserved: page 144.

©Cody Pickens: pages 146–147.

©Craig Cutler: pages 155, 159, 358.

©Bill Diodato: pages 177, 211, 275.

©Jill Greenberg: page 183.

©Nicky Woo: page 193.

©Brooke Nipar: page 199.

©Greg Broom: page 200.

©Terry Richardson/Art Partner: page 203 (Badgley)

©Courtesy: page 203 (humidifier).

©Getty Images: pages 204 (Reynolds), 205 (Cooper), 316 (Prefontaine), 317 (Bolt), 325.

©Isselee/Masterfile: page 209.

©Michael Hoeweler: page 210.

©Michael Byers: pages 231, 233.

©Andrea Manzati: page 237.

©Jason Munn: page 245.

©Chris Philpot: page 252.

©Claire Benoist: page 265.

©Made by Radio: pages 266–269.

©Bill Owens: page 279.

©Jake Chessum/Trunk Archive: page 282.

©Textbook Example: page 283.

©Michael Lewis/Gallery Stock: page 284.

©Zachary Zavislak: page 287.

©Jameson Simpson: page 290.

©Veer: page 295.

©Michael Muller: pages 305, 306, 309–311, 313.

© John Franklin Phillips: pages 307, 312, 317 (bottom).

©Stacy Kranitz: page 319.

©Gijs Van Der Most: pages 331–335.

©Jesse Lenz: page 349.

©Marek Haiduk: pages 353–356.

Index

Boldface page references indicate indicate photographs. Underscored references indicate boxed text.

Dogs, stress in, 354–55
Dopamine, 16, <u>33</u>, 261–62
Dreams, 301
Drinks
    electrolyte, 362
    energy, 68–73
    relaxation, <u>70</u>
    sports, 359, 362–63
Driving, winter, <u>271</u>
Drug addiction, <u>33</u>, **33**, 278–85
Drying your hands, 269
Dumbbell alternating shoulder
        press, 364
Dumbbell bench press, 169, **169**
Dumbbell bottom-half getup, 133,
        133
Dumbbell box squat, overhead
        press, and calf raise, 141,
        141
Dumbbell fly, 169, **169**
Dumbbell high-low farmer's walk,
        135, **135**
Dumbbell hot potato squat, 131,
        131
Dumbbell lawnmower pull, 132,
        132
Dumbbell lunge, curl, and press,
        140, **140**
Dumbbell mountain climber, **127**,
        <u>127</u>
Dumbbell 11/2 pushup, 131, **131**
Dumbbell overhead shouldering,
        132, **132**
Dumbbell rotational deadlift, 133,
        133
Dumbbell Russian twist, 152, **152**
Dumbbell shoveling, 136, **136**
Dumbbell side lunge and curl, 149,
        149
Dumbbell single-arm alternating
        clean, 150, **150**
Dumbbell single-arm snatch, 327
Dumbbell skier swing, **127**, <u>127</u>,
        130, **130**
Dumbbell squat to alternating
        shoulder press and twist,
        148, **148**
Dumbbell stepover, 150, **150**
Dumbbell straight-leg deadlift
        and row, 152, **152**

Dumbbell threaded lunge, 135,
        135
Dynamic stretch, 363

E

Eating
    avoiding mindless, 17
    emotional, 17
    pattern, 36–37
Eccentric stepups, 327
Eden Foods, 61
Electrolyte drinks, 362
Emergency fund, 222
Endorphins, 262–63
Energy chews, 73
Energy drinks, 68–73
Energy shots, 71–72
Enthusiasm, faking, 187–88
Erectile dysfunction, 292
Excess postexercise oxygen
        consumption (EPOC), 28
Exchange rate, 254
Exercise. *See also* Workouts;
        specific exercises
    benefits of
        antidepressant, 164
        brain health, <u>317</u>
        endorphin release, 263
        fat burning, 12–13
        heart health, 32, 290
        inflammation decrease, 24
        lowering blood pressure, 163
        pain control, 156, 158
        weight loss, 32
    with date, 206
    equipment, 112–19, <u>120</u>, <u>121</u>
    heart attacks and, 272–73
    intensity, 28
    weight loss and, 26–32
    at work, 250
Exfoliating pads, 204
External oblique muscles, 128,
        129
Extroverts, 190–91
Eye cream, 204
Eyes
    cell phones as threat to, 252
    circles under, 209–10

F

Facebook, 254
Faking it, 182–91
Fascia, 128, **129**
Fasting, 11
Fat cells, shrinking, 47
Fats, 16, 58, 251. *See also* Body fat
Fiber, 16, 30, 59, 95
Financial issues. *See* Money
Finishers, **126–27**, <u>126–27</u>
Fish, <u>59</u>, 92, 102, 106
5-5 split squat, **126**, <u>126</u>
Flavonoids, 100–101
Flooring, <u>242</u>
Flossing teeth, 269, 292
Foam roller, <u>153</u>, 165
Focus, to improve performance,
        359–60
Folic acid, 71
Food. *See also* Diet; Eating;
        specific foods
    addiction, 14–17, **33**, <u>33</u>
    Asian dishes, 88–93, <u>89</u>
    buying in-season, 221
    choline content of, 251
    color, 62–63, 66
    cost of unhealthy diet, 295
    cravings, 16, 47
    eating pattern, 36–37
    Nutrition Facts label, <u>58</u>, 58–59
    NuVal scale, 63, 104
    "organic" and "natural" labels,
        104
    refrigerator organization,
        352–53
    shopping by profession, <u>59</u>, <u>60</u>,
        <u>63</u>, <u>64</u>
    substitutions, <u>65</u>
    supermarket survival guide,
        56–67
    takeout, 88
    thermic effect of, <u>31</u>
    UPC bar codes on, 60–61
    upgrades, <u>66</u>
    water-rich, 300
Food allergy, <u>64</u>, <u>276</u>
Foosball, 352
Football players, mixed martial arts
        training by, 330–37, <u>336</u>

M

O

Oats, 65
Oberto's jerky line, 61
Obesity, 45, 46. *See also* Weight
Omega-3 supplements, 298
Organic food, 64, 104
Orgasm, faking, 191
Oxycodone, 278–85

P

Pain
    controlling with strength, 156, 158
    discovering reason for, 157
    playing around, 156–59
    when to call a doctor, 158
Panax ginseng, 71
Parents, finances of, 238
Parkinson's disease, 101
Partners, workout, 146
PBDEs, 301
Peanut butter, **48**, 49
Peanut oil, 89
Perfluorooctanoic acid, 301
Pets, hypoallergenic, 276–77
Pharmacies, 278–85
Philly-Cheesesteak, 348
Phthalates, 301
Pickup strategy, 206
Pilates, 161
Plank, 167, **167**
Plank walkup with dumbbell
    drag, 149, **149**
Plantar fasciitis, 314
Plyometrics, 160–61, 312
Polar FT80, 121
Polybrominated diphenylethers
    (PBDEs), 301
Polyphenols, 100–101
Pomegranate juice, 66
Popcorn, 355
Pork
    Four-Alarm Green Chili with
    Pork, 96, **96**
    Ham-and-Pear-Stuffed Pork
    Loin, 85, **85**
Posture, 184–85, 215
Poultry shears, 82
Preacher curls, 170

Prefontaine, Steve (runner), 316, **316**
Probiotics, 293
Productivity, exercising at work
    and, 250
Progesterone, for concussions, 343
Prosciutto
    La Quercia Prosciutto Green
    Label, 105
    Veal Scaloppini with Prosciutto
    and Sage, 84, **84**
Prostate disease, 292
Protein
    body weight and, 45
    daily amount needed, 30
    hydrolyzed, 61
    including in meals, 37–38
    for muscle growth, 146
    on Nutrition Facts label, 59
    on workout days, 153
Prunes, 291
Pruning trees, 355–56
Psychologist, video chat with, 299
Pullup, 50, **50**
Purslane, 109
Pushup, 10, 136
Pushup-position row and squat
    thrust, 151, **151**

Q

Quercetin, 71

R

Radicchio, 109
Radiofrequency skin tightening,
    290
Raisins, 358
Ralph Lauren, **200**, 201
Range of motion, increasing, 165
Recovery, 7–8, 165
Rectus abdominis muscle, 128, **129**
Refrigerator, organizing, 352–53
Relationships, fakery in, 185,
    187–88, 191
Relaxation drinks, 70
Renting out items, 220
Repetitions, number of, 134
Resistance band, 114

Resistance trainers, 324
Respiratory quotient, 5
Rest
    dynamic, 158–59
    between sets, 172
Restaurant discounts, 223
Reverse lunge and rotation, 307, **307**
Reverse lunge and shoulder press, 10
R.I.C.E. acronym, 156
Risk taking, 262–63
Roast, stuffing, 87
Rotator cuff, strengthening, 163
Runner's knee, 314
Running, 304–17
    barefoot, 361
    boredom busters, 311
    carbohydrate use in, 7
    core strengthening for, 316
    diagnosing injuries, 312–14
        Achilles tendinitis, 312
        iliotibial band syndrome,
        312, 314
        plantar fasciitis, 314
        runner's knee, 314
        shinsplints, 314
    drills for, 311
    dynamic stretching during
        pauses, 363
    form, 309–10
    health benefits of, 290, 317
    inspiration, 316–17
    intervals, 308
    learning from others, 312
    music during, 360
    pacing, 358
    shoes, 314–15
    strengthening your weak areas,
        306–7, **307**
    stride length, 312

S

Salad, adding to meal, 44–45
Salad greens, 109
Salivary glands, cell phones as
    threat to, 252
Salmon
    cancer risk decrease with, 102
    Salmon Teriyaki with
    Asparagus, 92